WITHDRAWN

Perspectives in Exercise Science
and Sports Medicine: Volume 11

Exercise, Nutrition, and Weight Control

Edited by

David R. Lamb
The Ohio State University

Robert Murray
The Gatorade Company

Library of Congress Cataloging in Publication Data:
LAMB, DAVID R., 1939-
PERSPECTIVES IN EXERCISE SCIENCE AND SPORTS MEDICINE
VOLUME 11: EXERCISE, NUTRITION, AND WEIGHT CONTROL

Cover Design: Gary Schmitt

Library of Congress Catalog Card number: 98-70205

ISBN: 1-884125-70-0

Printed in the United States of America by Cooper Publishing Group LLC, P.O. Box 562, Carmel, IN 46032

10 9 8 7 6 5 4 3 2 1

The Publisher and Author disclaim responsibility for any adverse effects or consequences from the misapplication or injudicious use of the information contained within this text.

Contents

**Chapter 3   Body Fat Distribution, Exercise and Nutrition:
            Implications for Prevention of Atherogenic
            Dyslipidemia, Coronary Heart Disease, and
            Non-Insulin Dependent Diabetes Mellitus 107**
Jean-Pierre Despres

Contributors

Luis Aragon-Vargas, Ph.D.
The Gatorade Company - Latin America
San Jose, Costa Rica

Oded Bar-Or, M.D.
Children's Exercise & Nutrition Centre
Chedoke Hospital Division
Evel Bldg., Sanatorium Road
Hamilton, Ontario L8N 3Z5
CANADA

Louise Burke, Ph.D.
Australian Institue of Sport
P.O. Box 176
Canberra, AC 2616
AUSTRALIA

JiDi Chen, M.D.
Institute of Sports Medicine
Beijing Medican University
Beijing 100083
CHINA

Priscilla M. Clarkson, Ph.D.
Department of Exercise Science
University of Massachusetts
Boyden Building
Amherst, MA 01003

Edward F. Coyle, Ph.D
Human Performance Lab
University of Texas
Bellmont Hall, Room 222
Austin,TX 78712

J. Mark Davis, Ph.D.
Department of Exercise Science
1300 Wheat Street, Rm. 1011
University of South Carolina
Columbia, SC 29208

Jean-Pierre Despres, Ph.D.
Lipid Research Center
Laval Univ. Medical Research Center
CHUL 2705 Laurier Blvd
Ste Foy, Quebec H2L 4MI
CANADA

E. Randy Eichner, M.D.
Section of Hematology (EB-271)
P.O Box 26901
University of Oklahoma
Health Sciences Center
Oklahoma City, OK 73190

Maria Fiatarone-Singh, M.D., Chief
Human Physiology Laboratory
Jean Mayer USDA Human Nutrition
Res. Center
Tufts University
711 Washington Street
13th Floor
Boston, MA 02111

Carl V. Gisolfi, Ph.D.
Dept. of Exercise Science
N420 Field House
University of Iowa
Iowa City, IA 52242

Bernard Gutin, Ph.D.
Dept. of Pediatrics
Georgia Prevention Institute
Medical College of Georgia
1499 Walton Way
Augusta,GA 30912-3710

Mark Hargreaves, Ph.D.
School of Human Movement
Deakin University
Burwood 3125
AUSTRALIA

Craig A. Horswill, Ph.D.
Exercise Physiology Laboratory
The Gatorade Company
617 West Main Street
Barrington, IL 60010

Linda Houtkooper, Ph.D.
Department of Nutritional Science
University of Arizona
312A FCR #33
Tucson, AZ 85721

Ricardo Javornik, M.D.
c/o Productors Quaker, C.A.
Centro Plaza, Torre C, Piso 16
Avendida Francisco de Miranda
Los Palos Grandes
Caracas, VENEZUELA

Steve Johnsen, B.S.
Nebraska Coaches Association
4701 VanDorn
Lincoln, NE 68510

W. Larry Kenney, Ph.D.
102 Noll Physiological Research
Center
The Pennsylvania State University
University Park, PA 16802-6900

Tom Koto, ATC
Idaho Sports Medicine Institute
1188 University Dr.
Boise, ID 83706

David R. Lamb, Ph.D.
Sport and Exercise Sciences
School of Physical Activity and
Educational Services
The Ohio State University
129 Larkins Hall
337 West 17th Avenue
Columbus, OH 43210

Timothy G. Lohman, Ph.D.
Department of Physiology
Room 114 INA Gitting Building
University of Arizona
Tucson, AZ 85721

Dennis McKay, Ph.D.
College of Pharmacy
Parks Hall
500 West 12th Avenue
Columbus, OH 43210

Ronald J. Maughan, Ph.D.
University Medical School
Dept. Environmental/
Occupational Medicine
Foresterhill
Aberdeen AB9 2ZD, SCOTLAND

Christopher Melby, Dr. P.H.
226 Gifford
Dept. Food Science and Human
Nutrition
Colorado State University
Fort Collins, CO 80523

Robert Murray, Ph.D.
The Gatorade Company
617 West Main Street
Barrington, IL 60010

Ethan R. Nadel, Ph.D.
John B. Pierce Foundation Laboratory
290 Congress Avenue
New Haven, CT 06519

Dennis Passe, Ph.D.
The Gatorade Company
617 West Main Street
Barrington, IL 60010

William Prentice, ATC
214 Fetzer Gym
University of North Carolina
Chapel Hill, NC 27599-8700

Anita Rivera-Brown,M.S.
Centro de Salud Deportiva and
Ciencias del Ejercico
Salinas, PUERTO RICO 00751

Thomas Rowland, M.D
Department of Pediatric Cardiology
Baystate Medical Center
Children's Hospital
759 Chestnut Street
Springfield, MA 01199

Yvonne Satterwhite, M.D.
Kentucky Sports Medicine Clinic, PSC
Orthopedic Surgery
501 Perimeter Drive, Suite 200
Lexington, KY 40517

Mike Sherman, Ph.D.
School of Physical Activity and
Educational Services
The Ohio State University
216 Pomerene Hall
1760 Neil Avenue
Columbus, OH 43210

Xiaocai Shi, Ph.D.
Exercise Physiology Lab
The Gatorade Company
617 W. Main Street
Barrington, IL 60010

Lawrence Spriet, Ph.D.
University of Guelph
Human Biology & Nutritional
Sciences
John Powell Building
East Ring Road
Guelph, Ontario NIG 2WI
CANADA

Suzanne Nelson-Steen, D.Sc., R.D.
Immaculata College
Graduate Division-Nutrition
P.O. Box 500
Immaculata, PA 19345-0500

Janet Walberg-Rankin, Ph.D.
Human Nutrition & Foods Dept.
Drill Field
215 War Memorial Hall
Virginia Tech
Blacksburg, VA 24061-0351

Clyde Williams, Ph.D.
Dept Physical Education, Sports
Science & Recreation Management
Loughborough University
Loughborough
Leicestershire, LE11 3TU
ENGLAND, UK

Melvin H. Williams, Ph.D
2204 Woodlawn Avenue
Virginia Beach, VA 23455

Acknowledgement

For over a decade, The Gatorade Company has been proud to sponsor the textbook series, *Perspectives in Exercise Science and Sports Medicine*. The publication of this eleventh volume is part of our continuing commitment in support of research and education programs in sports science. As in previous years, this textbook resulted from a meeting of scientific experts in the areas of sports medicine, exercise science, and sports nutrition. The topics that comprise each of the chapters were presented and extensively discussed. The end result is captured in this text on *Exercise, Nutrition, and Weight Control*. The authors, reviewers, and editors worked hard to produce a superior result. We hope you find this to be a valuable addition to your professional library.

Susan D. Wellington
President, Gatorade - U.S.
The Quaker Oats Company
Chicago, IL

Preface

If there is a single contemporary theme for a book in the field of exercise science and sports medicine that is of interest to most scientists and physicians, men and women, athletes and non-athletes, young and old, it surely is the theme of this volume–exercise, nutrition, and weight control. Obesity is a major risk factor for degenerative diseases, and a cultural emphasis on leanness for both health and cosmetic reasons causes us to spend billions of dollars annually in often-misguided attempts to reduce body fat. For some, these attempts at fat reduction develop into bulimia, anorexia, and other eating disorders that can be devastating to the afflicted individuals. For many athletes, especially those who compete in endurance events or in events such as gymnastics or ballet in which most judges place a high priority on leanness, control of body fat is absolutely critical to success. Accordingly, we anticipate that this 11th volume of *Perspectives in Exercise Science and Sports Medicine* will perhaps be the most well-received volume in the series to date.

The authors of these chapters are to be congratulated for having written such concise yet comprehensive and up-to-date manuscripts, and the chapter reviewers likewise did excellent work in helping the authors refine their work. Much of this refinement occurred as an outgrowth of a conference held in Palm Springs, California, in the summer of 1997, and we are grateful to The Gatorade Company, which has sponsored these conferences and the *Perspectives* series annually since 1987. Throughout the history of the series, The Gatorade Company has generously donated all proceeds from the sale of the books to The American College of Sports Medicine.

We express our sincere appreciation to Betty Dye and Sharon Roberts, who so expertly and expeditiously transcribed the conference discussions, and to Paula Darr and her associates at McCord Travel Management for organizing the travel and the conference events; they were superb.

David R. Lamb
Robert Murray

1

Exercise, Macronutrient Balance, and Weight Control

Christopher L. Melby, Dr. P.H.
S. Renee Commerford, Ms.
James O. Hill, Ph.D.

INTRODUCTION

Despite heightened public awareness in the United States of the un-toward health consequences of being overweight, the prevalence of obesity in adults, children, and adolescents is increasing. Based on data from the National Health and Nutrition Examination Surveys, for adults aged 20 and above, an estimated 35% of all women and 31% of all men are overweight (Kuczmarski et al., 1994). The percentage of women who are overweight reaches a maximum of 38.5% in women between 65 and 74 years of age. An estimated 22% of all children and adolescents are overweight (Troiano et al., 1995). The data indicate that rates of obesity are especially high in certain US populations, including African-Americans and Mexican-Americans (Kuczmarski et al., 1994). Women in these populations appear to be at particularly high risk for the development of obesity.

Obesity, particularly that characterized by excessive central body fat deposition, is a risk factor for cardiovascular disease (Rimm et al., 1995; Willett et al., 1995), non-insulin dependent diabetes mellitus (NIDDM) (Colditz et al. 1990, 1995), certain cancers (Lew & Garfinkel, 1979), osteoarthritis (Staff, 1996; Voigt et al., 1994) and peripheral vascular disease (Vogt et al., 1993). Whether or not the associations between obesity and each of these sequelae are causal is not entirely clear. Nevertheless, because excess body fat is a risk factor for several of the leading causes of death in the US adult population, the prevention and treatment of obesity have become priorities among health care providers.

Diet and physical activity are two critical components in any analysis of factors related to obesity. This chapter includes an examination of the impact of physical activity on energy expenditure and intake, macronutrient balance, and regulation of body weight and composition. The purpose of the chapter is to: 1) define body weight regulation in terms of energy and nutrient balance; 2) emphasize the importance of fat balance in body weight regulation; and 3) describe the ways in which physical activity affects energy and nutrient balance.

BODY WEIGHT REGULATION

Prior to examining the effects of exercise on macronutrient balance and weight control, a brief discussion is warranted regarding the factors that influence energy and macronutrient requirements. While there appears to be a systematic increase in body weight across the adult life span, the degree to which body weight is maintained constant suggests that some variable associated with body weight is regulated. This could be body weight, body fatness, body temperature, energy intake, energy expenditure, or energy balance itself (Bray, 1989). Some suggest that body weight is regulated about a *set-point*, i.e., physiological systems act to maintain an established body weight (Keesey et al., 1984). Others prefer the term *settling-point*, which suggests that there is not an optimal weight being defended, but rather that the weight maintained over time is a result of inherent characteristics of the individual combined with the environment in which that individual lives (Hill et al., 1994).

We have previously described a conceptual model for studying factors that contribute to and alter energy and macronutrient requirements in humans (Hill et al., 1995). Figure 1-1 illustrates this concept of body weight control as a settling point regulated over time by the individual's functional phenotype. The latter results from the interaction of both genetic and behavioral factors (e.g., the amount and composition of food intake and the amount of physical activity). According to this model, because of different functional phenotypes, two individuals with similar food intakes and levels of physical activity may defend different settling points. Changes in food intake and/or physical activity can influence the settling point, and the magnitude of this influence depends on the functional phenotype. This model proposes that the components of the system affecting energy and macronutrient utilization are interrelated so that a change in any one component can influence other components.

According to this model, obesity results from the interaction of genetic and environmental (behavioral) factors, with the accumulation and maintenance of excess body fat resulting from the individual's functional phenotype. That is, the body fat level "settles" at a point that allows the individual to reach equilibrium between energy intake and expenditure and between macronutrient intake and oxidation, but at the cost of obesity.

There are numerous central and peripheral factors involved in regulation of energy balance. While a detailed discussion of these regulators is beyond the scope of this chapter, it is important to identify several

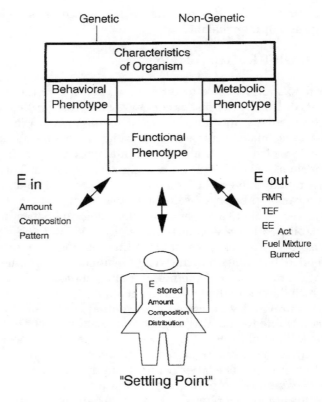

FIGURE 1-1. *The maintenance of a constant body weight and body composition requires achievement of a steady state in which the amount and composition of energy ingested is equal to the amount and composition of fuel burned*. E_{in} = energy intake; E_{out} = energy expenditure; RMR = resting metabolic rate; TEF = thermic effect of food; EE_{ACT} = energy expended in physical activity. Reprinted with permission from Hill et al. (1994), copyright CRC Press, Boca Raton, FL.

peptides that are of current research interest. Recent studies that have examined the impact of acute and chronic exercise on these peptides will be reviewed later in the chapter.

The extent to which brain peptides and monoamines regulate body weight is presently unclear. The recent cloning of leptin, the product of the *ob* gene, has triggered renewed interest in the central regulation of body weight. Leptin is produced by the adipocyte, and serum leptin levels in both rodents and humans correlate closely with percent body fat and body mass index (Considine et al., 1995; Lonnqvist et al., 1995). Leptin appears to be produced in greater quantities by larger fat cells (Hamilton et al., 1995), but the mechanism behind this greater rate of production is unknown. There is some speculation that the degree of stretch of the adipocyte cell membrane may be involved in the regulation of the production of leptin by the adipocyte. Because leptin interacts with receptors in the hypothalamus, a known control center for food intake, some have proposed that leptin is an important factor in communicating peripheral energy status to the hypothalamus (Rohner-Jeanrenaud et al., 1996).

A body of evidence suggests that one of the actions of leptin, at least in rodents, is to serve as a satiety factor. Administration of leptin to obese *ob/ob* mice, a strain of mice unable to produce leptin due to a defect in the *ob* gene, results in decreased food intake and normalization of body weight (Halaas et al., 1995; Pelleymounter et al., 1995). More recent data indicate that leptin might be an acute modulator of food intake in rodents, but not in humans. For instance, prolonged periods of fasting in both rodents (Frederich et al., 1995) and humans (Kolaczynski et al., 1996a) precipitated increases in serum leptin levels, though body fat content was unaltered. Likewise, acute overfeeding in humans without significant alterations in body fat has been associated with declines in serum leptin. (Kolaczynski et al., 1996b). Ironically, serum leptin concentrations are significantly higher in obese compared to lean humans, with concentrations positively correlated with body fat mass. Thus, it is unclear how and to what extent serum leptin levels explain the development of human obesity. Some have hypothesized the defect in leptin action to be in the postreceptor signaling cascade (Considine & Caro, 1996).

Another brain peptide that has received a great deal of attention in recent years is neuropeptide Y (NPY). Intracerebroventricular infusions of NPY into normal-weight rats brought about increased food intake and body weight gain (Vettor et al., 1994). In addition, basal and glucose-induced increases in plasma insulin and basal ACTH and corticosterone levels increased significantly in these animals upon administration of NPY (Rohner-Jeanrenaud et al., 1996; Sainsbury et al., 1996). Finally, lipoprotein lipase activity of white adipose tissue was increased and insulin action at the skeletal muscle was reduced in these rats (Vettor et al., 1994; Zarjevski et al., 1994). Taken together, these data imply that, if its regulation goes unchecked, NPY may be an important factor in the development of both obesity and non-insulin dependent diabetes (NIDDM).

Because recent data indicate that leptin reduces the production of NPY, some have proposed the existence of an NPY-leptin loop (Rohner-Jeanrenaud et al., 1996), with leptin acting as a peripheral signal for negative feedback on the release of NPY and on food intake. Further evidence of the existence of an interaction between NPY and leptin comes from the demonstration that insulin increases the production of leptin by white adipocytes (Cusin et al., 1995). Elevated NPY levels may stimulate food ingestion, resulting in a rise in plasma insulin, which then stimulates leptin production by white adipocytes. Leptin may then interact with receptors in the hypothalamus to act both as a satiety factor and to decrease NPY production. Impairment in any of the steps within this loop could result in an increased risk for the development of obesity, due in part to poor regulation of food intake.

FACTORS CONTRIBUTING TO INCREASED OBESITY RISK

The laws of thermodynamics dictate that an energy surplus is at the root of all obesity; if energy intake (E_{IN}) exceeds energy expenditure (E_{OUT}), then energy storage will occur. While this may seem obvious, it is important to state this at the outset. With all the recent attention devoted to the effect of diet composition on body fat accumulation, one must not forget that diet composition will affect long-term changes in body composition only when there is an imbalance in E_{IN} versus E_{OUT}. The reasoning behind this statement will become clear in subsequent sections of this chapter.

Genetic versus Environmental Contributors to Obesity

Specific risk factors associated with increased weight gain in adults have been identified in some populations, such as Caucasians and Pima Indians (Ravussin & Swinburn, 1993; Swinburn et al., 1991; Zurlo et al., 1990). These include: 1) a low rate of resting energy expenditure relative to the predicted rate for body size; 2) a high whole-body insulin sensitivity; 3) a high 24-h respiratory quotient, indicative of higher carbohydrate oxidation and lower fat oxidation; and 4) a low level of spontaneous physical activity. Insufficient data are available at this time to determine if these four risk factors for weight gain are characteristic of other population groups. Also, these risk factors are not entirely supported by animal data, as prospective data in rats show a negative relationship between insulin sensitivity and weight gain. Also, the relative contribution of genetic versus environmental factors to each of the above four metabolic parameters is presently unclear.

There has been substantial research interest in recent years regarding the role of genetic factors in the etiology of obesity. As previously discussed, the identification and sequencing of the ob gene and the leptin peptide that it encodes, and the discovery that a defect in this gene appears to be the single cause of obesity in the ob/ob mouse (Zhang et al., 1994), have generated considerable interest in the genetics of obesity. Even more recently, the discovery of two new uncoupling proteins (UCP-2 and UCP-3) and their genes has heightened the interest in genetic causes of obesity (Boss et al., 1997; Fleury et al., 1997). The UCP-2 gene appears to be expressed in a wide variety of adult human tissues, including white adipose tissue, and produces a protein that uncouples mitochondrial fuel oxidation from the synthesis of adenosine triphosphate (ATP). Because it is ubiquitous and may be inducible by feeding a high-fat diet, it appears that the UCP-2 may be very important. It is possible that the individual who is obesity-resistant, compared to the obesity-prone, expresses more UCP-2 and more readily "wastes" excess energy in response to overfeeding. The UCP-3 appears to expressed primarily in skeletal muscle and may be a particularly important protein involved in regulation of skeletal muscle respiration and nonshivering thermogenesis (Boss et al., 1997).

However, even if an individual were genetically susceptible to obesity, the genotype does not necessarily dictate an obese phenotype, if the individual matches a low rate of energy expenditure with a low rate of energy intake. It is noteworthy that the prevalence of overweight and obesity in the United States has increased substantially even within the last 20 y, a duration of time in which the gene pool has not changed. This phenomenon argues strongly for the importance of dietary and physical activity patterns interacting with genetic polymorphism to explain the accumulation of excess body fat in a large portion of the American population.

Physical Inactivity and Obesity

Intuitively, one would expect that individuals who are sedentary would exhibit greater risk for excess body fat accumulation compared to their physically active counterparts. Inverse relationships between measures of physical activity (usually self-reports) and indices of obesity (usually body mass index, BMI) are seen in many data sets obtained from the general US population (Eck et al., 1992; Obarzanek et al., 1994; Slattery et al., 1992; Williamsen et al., 1993). In a study of energy balance and body fat in weight-stable runners with differing amounts of training, Maughan and Aulin (1997) reported that percent body fat was inversely related to total training distance covered per week ($r = 0.68$, $P < 0.001$) and to energy intake. Among African-Americans, adults who exercised two or more times per week had, on average, a lower body mass index (weight/height^2) and a smaller waist circumference than did adults who exercised once per week or less (Melby et al., 1991). At least two studies using doubly-labeled water to measure the energy expended in physical activity have shown a significant inverse relationship between physical activity and indices of fatness (Davies et al., 1995; Schulz & Schoeller, 1994). In a recent report of a cohort of over 5000 men and women in Finland followed for 10-y, a decreased level of leisure-time physical activity was associated with large gains in body mass in comparison with those individuals who increased their level of physical activity (Haapanen et al., 1997).

Although there are strong associations between physical activity and obesity, there are insufficient data to conclude that a low level of physical activity is a cause of obesity. It is equally possible that a low level of physical activity is a consequence of obesity. There are a few data sets in which changes in physical activity and changes in BMI have been assessed longitudinally. Williamson (1993) and Williamson et al. (1983) performed follow-up studies on 3515 men and 5810 women in the NHANES I study. Records of BMI and level of physical activity were obtained 10 y later in subjects who participated in NHANES I (1971–75). Although a significant relationship was identified between BMI and level of physical activity at baseline and follow-up, physical activity at baseline was not significantly correlated with change in BMI after 10 y. However, level of physical activity at follow-up was negatively correlated with major weight gain (>13 kg). The authors hypothesized that a low level of physical activity may be both a cause and consequence of weight gain. A few other studies in adults and children have found that a low level of physical activity is associated with weight gain over time (Klesges et al., 1992; Owens et al., 1992).

Macronutrient Balance and Obesity

Within the same individual, there is considerable day-to-day variability in physical activity and in intakes of energy and macronutrients. These variations will cause fluctuations in daily macronutrient storage and oxidation. However, in the obesity-resistant individual, body weight and body composition remain stable over the course of many years. Maintenance of a constant body weight and body composition indicates that the individual must be in a steady state, in which the total energy ingested is equal to the total energy expended. In addition, over some period of time, the composition of the energy ingested must equal the composition of substrate oxidized (Hill et al., 1994). Any disruption of energy and macronutrient balance elicits compensatory responses to restore these balances. The relative stability of body weight over time suggests that compensatory adaptations occur in energy expenditure and intake and in macronutrient oxidation and intake; these compensatory adaptations enable the weight stable-individual to remain in long-term balance.

Any change in body weight must be a result of an imbalance in one or more macronutrients and in total energy. However, changes in body weight and body composition will occur only until homeostasis is reestablished. Reestablishing the steady states of energy and macronutrient balances can occur at the same or at different levels of body weight and body fat mass, depending on the individual's functional phenotype.

Measurement of Energy Expenditure and Macronutrient Oxidation. To clarify how macronutrient balance is determined over time, a brief discussion of calorimetry is warranted. Energy expenditure can be measured either directly or indirectly. Direct measurement of heat production in a given time can be made, but this direct calorimetry provides no information regarding substrate utilization. Measurement of energy expenditure by direct calorimetry in humans is difficult, and few laboratories throughout the world use this procedure. Indirect calorimetry, on the other hand, is less difficult, requires less-costly equipment, and allows calculation of both whole-body energy expenditure and rates of substrate oxidation. Isotopic tracers are also used to measure rates of substrate mobilization, clearance, and oxidation, but a discussion of tracer technology with its specific uses and limitations is beyond the scope of this chapter; Wolfe (1992) can be consulted for a comprehensive explanation of the use of tracers. The principles that guide the use of indirect calorimetry based on pulmonary gas exchange to measure substrate oxidation rates will be covered in some detail in order to help the reader better understand some of the issues related to macronutrient balance that are presented in subsequent sections of the chapter.

Indirect calorimetry is based on the analysis of expired air, from which determinations are made of the respiratory exchange ratio (RER), calculated as the amount of carbon dioxide produced (VCO_2) relative to the amount of oxygen consumed (VO_2) in cellular respiration. Urinary nitrogen excretion is measured as an index of protein (amino acid) oxidation. Because the amount of CO_2 produced in relation to oxygen consumed varies according to the substrate metabolized, the RER along with the VO_2 can be used to determine the amounts of fat and carbohydrate oxidized using stoichiometric equations (Ferrannini, 1988; Jequier et al., 1987). In humans under steady-state conditions, whole-body RER determined from pulmonary gas exchange should accurately reflect the rates of O_2 consumption and CO_2 production at the cellular level (i.e., the respiratory quotient (RQ). However, as discussed below, under certain conditions, the RER does not accurately reflect the true cellular RQ, which limits the use of gas exchange measurements in determining macronutrient oxidation rates.

The nonprotein respiratory exchange ratio (NPRER) is used to determine the relative amounts of oxygen used for carbohydrate and fat oxidation in a given time period, after accounting for the amount of oxygen used in protein oxidation, which is calculated from estimates of urinary nitrogen excretion.

The NPRQ for carbohydrate (glucose) is 1.0, i.e.:

$$C_6H_{12}O_6 + 6\ O_2 \rightarrow 6\ CO_2 + 6\ H_2O; NPRQ = 6\ CO_2/6\ O_2 = 1.0$$

Because fatty acids, in comparison to carbohydrates, contain proportionately more carbon and hydrogen atoms relative to oxygen atoms, the NPRQ for fat is approximately 0.7. Thus, relatively more oxygen is needed to metabolize fatty acids to CO_2 and H_2O than is needed for carbohydrates. When the NPRQ = 0.7, the entire nonprotein VO_2 is used for fat oxidation. This can be seen in the following equation demonstrating the oxidation of palmitic acid.

$$C_{16}H_{32}O_2 + 23\ O_2 \rightarrow 16\ CO2 + 16\ H_2O;\ NPRQ = 16\ CO_2/23\ O_2 = 0.696 \simeq 0.7$$

The RQ for protein is about 0.82, although it varies somewhat depending on the amino-acid composition of the protein. Determination of the contribution of protein to energy expenditure is based on the amount of urinary nitrogen produced (deamination of amino acids occurs prior to their oxidation). Because protein metabolism is only a minor contributor to energy needs, and thus has a fairly small influence on whole-body RQ, indirect calorimetry is often used without measuring the amount of protein oxidized. This is especially true when conducting measurements over a brief time interval, when urinary nitrogen values may not accurately reflect protein oxidation rates. For example, urinary nitrogen values obtained during exercise cannot typically be used to estimate protein oxidation because exercise alters renal perfusion and thus urinary nitrogen output. However, it is important to obtain urinary nitrogen excretion values when examining substrate oxidation rates over an extended period, such as occurs with 24 h indirect calorimetry measurements in a respiratory chamber.

The energy equivalent per liter of oxygen consumed varies among the three macronutrients. By measuring the total amount of oxygen consumed and carbon dioxide produced during a given time period, the energy expended, the relative contributions of carbohydrate and fat to energy expenditure, and the grams of carbohydrate and fat oxidized can be readily calculated.

One difficulty encountered in using indirect calorimetry to estimate substrate utilization is that the RER can be influenced by bicarbonate-ion kinetics. During periods of depletion and repletion of bicarbonate ions, the RER will not accurately represent the true cellular RQ and, thus, cannot be reliably used for determination of substrate oxidation rate at any given time. Because pools of bicarbonate ions can undergo substantial perturbations during and after exercise, such shifts must be considered when estimating fuel oxidation rates. During high-intensity exercise, respiratory VCO_2 values are often higher than cellular CO_2 production, which will elevate the RER above the true cellular respiratory quotient (RQ) (e.g., during measurement of $\dot{V}O_2$max, the RER value should be well above 1.0 because the additional amount of CO_2 that is expired is in excess of that produced in cellular respiration). Conversely, for a period of time following high-intensity exercise, the RER may be much lower than the true cellular RQ, owing to replenishment of the body's bicarbonate ion concentrations. For example, during the first hour following an intense bout of weight lifting, the RER will often drop to a value as low as 0.60 (Melby et al., 1992). Obviously this value is outside the usual range, but it is not due to measurement error. The VCO_2 is reduced as some of the metabolically produced CO_2 is not expired, but rather is used to re-equilibrate the bicarbonate pool.

At any time when the RER does not accurately reflect cellular RQ, estimates of fuel utilization will be in error. However, if the period of indirect calorimetry encompasses these transient periods of depletion and repletion of bicarbonate ions, the average RER during the entire period can be used to estimate fuel utilization. Room calorimeters are especially useful in measuring substrate utilization over an extended period because the respiratory exchange measurements will encompass any transient changes in ventilation.

The hepatic ketogenesis that accompanies uncontrolled diabetes, starvation, and hypoenergetic, low-carbohydrate diets interferes with accurate indirect calorimetry. The production of ketone bodies (acetoacetic acid, β-hydroxybutyric acid, and acetone) consumes oxygen, yet there is no attendant liberation of carbon dioxide unless the ketones undergo subsequent oxidation. Thus, if production of ketones exceeds the rate of their oxidation and ketone bodies are excreted via respiration or urine, the measured RER can be less than 0.7.

Another source of error in using gas-exchange measurements to quantify energy expenditure and substrate oxidation during ketogenesis involves changes in the bicarbonate pool. The formation of acetoacetic acid and β-hydroxybutyric acid releases hydrogen ions; this disturbs the bicarbonate pool and increases VCO_2 to values greater than can be accounted for by CO_2 production via oxidative metabolism. Measuring urinary and breath ketone excretion allows for use of correction factors (Ferrannini, 1988) to more accurately estimate the true RQ.

Measured RER values outside the range of 0.7–1.0 should not always be attributed to ventilatory shifts or to errors in measurement. One such situation occurs with de novo lipogenesis from carbohydrate. Because of the greater number of oxygen atoms in carbohydrate molecules relative to fatty acids, the synthesis of fat from glucose will liberate O_2 that can be used for macronutrient oxidation. Less atmospheric O_2 is then used, even though the normal amount of CO_2 is released during metabolism. In response to carbohydrate overfeeding, RER values greater than 1.0 are indicative of net lipid synthesis. It should be noted that de novo lipogenesis can occur during periods when the RER value is less than 1.0, but because of simultaneous lipid oxidation, the RER is below 1.0, and there is no **net** lipid synthesis (i.e., the rate of de novo lipogenesis remains lower than the rate of whole-body lipid oxidation).

On the intake side, the food quotient (FQ) can be calculated as the ratio of carbon dioxide produced to oxygen consumed during the oxidation of foods in the diet. When balance is achieved between energy intake and expenditure and between macronutrient intake and oxidation, the FQ and the RQ will be equivalent (i.e., RQ/FQ = 1.0). Overfeeding a mixed diet will initially lead to RQ/FQ > 1.0, which is indicative of a higher rate of fat intake relative to oxidation. An energy deficit situation will yield an average RQ lower than the FQ (RQ/FQ < 1.0), which will result in negative fat balance and weight loss.

Effect of Diet on Macronutrient Oxidation. The ability of the human body to adjust energy expenditure and macronutrient oxidation to energy and macronutrient intake is essential for maintenance of stable body weight and body composition. Underfeeding is associated with reductions in resting metabolic rate and in the thermic effect of feeding, as well as a decrease in the RER (reflecting increased fat oxidation and decreased carbohydrate oxidation). Overfeeding produces increases in these components of energy expenditure as well as increases in RER. However, despite these diet-induced alterations, if an energy imbalance is sustained for a sufficient period of time, changes in body energy storage will occur. These changes in body composition will in turn influence macronutrient utilization. Although the focus of this chapter is on exercise and macronutrient oxidation rather than on diet, it is important within the context of weight regulation to briefly examine the impact of energy intake and diet composition on macronutrient oxidation.

Carbohydrate Intake and Oxidation. Carbohydrate oxidation is strongly influenced by carbohydrate intake, such that increased carbohydrate consumption leads to marked increases in postprandial carbohydrate oxidation (Acheson et al., 1988; Flatt et al., 1985). Acheson et al. (1982) found that in young men, the RER values remained close to 1.0 during an 8-h postprandial period following ingestion of 500 g of carbohydrate in a single meal. The increased plasma insulin concentration in response to a carbohydrate-rich meal stimulates both carbohydrate oxidation and storage, and suppresses lipolysis.

Protein Intake and Oxidation. Changes in the body's protein content are typically measured by the nitrogen balance method, wherein nitrogen intake in the form of protein is compared to nitrogen losses (fecal and urinary). Because there is no large pool of stored amino acids in the human body, an increase in protein intake will cause greater amino acid storage (or even greater protein synthesis unless an anabolic situation such as growth exists). Instead, an elevation in protein intake results in increased amino acid oxidation rather than storage. The small increases and decreases in body protein content result in corrective responses by way of increases and decreases in amino acid oxidation. Thus, the body maintains protein balance by closely matching protein oxidation to intake, in a manner similar to that for carbohydrate intake and oxidation.

Fat Intake and Oxidation. Dietary fat is transported by plasma chylomicrons following meal ingestion, with the fatty acids found in the triacylglycerols cleared primarily by adipose tissue, where the majority of lipoprotein lipase enzyme protein is located. Several studies have shown that the addition of fat to a mixed meal does not significantly increase the rate of fat oxidation during the postprandial period (Bennett et al., 1992; Flatt et al., 1985; Schutz et al., 1989). Flatt et al. (1985) found no differences in the RER values during 9 h following a low-fat breakfast (73 g carbohydrate, 30 g protein, 6 g fat) compared to a high-fat breakfast (73 g carbohydrate, 30 g protein, 40 g fat). When 80 g of fat was added to a similar low-fat breakfast, the RER values were lower during a 6 h postprandial period compared to the low-fat meal (Griffiths et al., 1994). However, rarely would an individual consume this much fat in a single meal. Thus, it appears that under conditions in which up to 40–50 g of fat are included in a mixed meal, the partitioning of dietary fat is toward storage rather than immediate oxidation. In fact, consumption of a mixed meal containing both fat and carbohydrate will result in a decrease in fat oxidation relative to the preprandial condition. As previously discussed, the elevation of postprandial plasma insulin levels serves to increase glucose oxidation and storage while enhancing fat storage (insulin induces lipoprotein lipase activity) and suppressing lipolysis.

In several studies, the carbohydrate and fat contents of the diet have been varied over periods ranging from a single meal to 2 wk of meals (Acheson et al., 1988; Astrup, 1993; Horton et al., 1995; Stubbs et al., 1995a, 1995b; Thomas et al., 1992). A consistent finding has been that alterations in carbohydrate intake produce rapid and substantial changes in carbohydrate oxidation that serve to maintain carbohydrate balance. Acute lipid balance, however, is not well regulated. Alterations in fat intake produce little if any immediate changes in fat oxidation, so that there is little effort to maintain fat balance acutely. Thus, weight changes are due primarily to disruptions in fat balance, which account for most of the imbalance produced in total energy. Because carbohydrate and protein balances are maintained over a short period of time, any surplus of dietary energy must necessarily be accommodated by expansion of the fat stores. Even if body carbohydrate stores were doubled, body mass would not increase by more than 1–2 kg.

It is important to recognize that this fat storage in humans eating mixed diets is usually not the result of *net* de novo lipogenesis. Indeed, overfeeding studies have shown that the average daily RER remains below 1.0 (Horton et al., 1995). Rather, the positive fat balance that occurs with overfeeding appears to result from greater storage of dietary fat relative to whole-body fat oxidation. It is possible, of course, for an individual to become obese even on a low-fat diet if energy intake exceeds expenditure— not because of lipogenesis from carbohydrate, but because much of the dietary fat is stored as the body rapidly adjusts to oxidizing carbohydrates and protein to meet its energy needs, at the expense of fat oxidation.

Alcohol Intake and Oxidation. Although beverage alcohol (ethanol) is not typically viewed as a nutrient, it is a potential source of energy. Ethanol has an energy density (29.3 kJ/g) that is closer to that of fat (38.1 kJ/g) than to that of carbohydrate and protein (16.7 kJ/g). Because of its relatively high energy density, alcohol is viewed by many as a possible cause of obesity. However, this is a controversial issue. A well-controlled, prospective cohort study (Liu et al., 1995) and two comprehensive reviews of the epidemiological data (Hellerstedt et al. 1990; MacDonald, 1993) show either no association or an inverse association between alcohol consumption and body weight gain. This is in contrast to what would be expected based on its acute metabolic effects. Ethanol is rapidly oxidized as an energy source, which in turn decreases the oxidation rate of fat. This effect was best identified by Suter et al. (1992) in a short-term energy balance study involving eight men of normal weight. They showed that ethanol consumption produced substantial reductions in 24 h lipid oxidation and concluded that regular, moderate alcohol consumption, because of its suppressive effect on lipid oxidation, would favor fat storage and the subsequent development of obesity. Tremblay et al. (1995) found that ethanol consumption was not associated with a compensatory reduction in lipid and non-alcohol energy intake. In other words, alcohol added to daily energy intake rather than substituted for other macronutrients. These short-term effects of dietary ethanol are difficult to reconcile with the findings from prospective epidemiologic data, and more research is needed to clearly identify the effect of consuming alcoholic beverages on long-term energy balance and weight regulation.

Body Fat Mass and Fat Balance

Although the majority of evidence suggests that fat balance is not well regulated acutely, it must be regulated over the long term because the body-weight regulation system must eventually reachieve energy and nutrient balance. Changes in body composition can alter fat oxidation to bring it into balance with fat intake and stabilize body weight. While carbohydrate balance can be achieved with little alteration of endogenous carbohydrate stores, changes in the body fat mass can contribute substantially to achieving fat balance. Individual differences in achieving fat balance may play a primary role in determining the body weight and level of body fatness that results. Fat intake, fat oxidation, and the size of the body fat mass all may play a role in determining how fat balance is achieved.

Flatt (1987, 1995) and Schutz (1995) have suggested that obesity is fundamentally a problem caused by a lower rate of fat oxidation relative to fat ingestion, leading to expansion of the adipose mass. They suggest that the increased adiposity, which may or may not be coupled with adipocyte insulin resistance, increases the release of free fatty acids into the blood plasma, and the greater concentration of circulating fatty acids thus enhances cellular lipid oxidation. When the fat mass has increased sufficiently, fat balance will be reestablished, and the fat mass will stabilize as shown in Figure 1-2. These changes allow the body to reach a new equilibrium, a point at which the rates of fat oxidation and intake are equal, albeit at a cost of obesity. Similarly, when fat intake is less than fat oxidation, the body fat mass will decline to bring about a reduction in fat oxidation.

Body fat mass is maintained at widely different levels in different people. This suggests that some individuals are able to achieve fat balance with a small body fat mass while others require a larger fat mass. Theoretically, any factor that reduces fat intake or that increases fat oxidation (such as exercise) should contribute to differences in the level of body fat mass at which fat balance can be achieved.

Integration of Macronutrient Intake and Oxidation

Because the human body acutely adjusts carbohydrate, protein, and ethanol oxidation rates to match their intakes, the amount of fat oxidized in a given time period will be the difference between total energy expenditure and energy expenditure due to protein and carbohydrate oxidation. When energy balance and stable body composition prevail, the fuel mix oxidized (RER) equals the macronutrient composition of the diet (FQ). During days of energy surplus on a regular mixed diet, the fuel mix oxidized will be higher in carbohydrate, and fat oxidation will decrease (RER > FQ), with the surfeit of energy largely stored as fat. When food intake is inadequate to meet the body's energy demands, the average RER is lower than the FQ, which reflects the increased oxidation of both dietary and endogenous fat. To lose body fat the average RER/FQ must be less than 1.0. Although this can be accomplished by dietary restriction, it should be apparent that increasing energy expenditure and fat oxidation via regular exercise could also yield an RER/FQ < 1.0. The role of exercise in weight loss and maintenance of fat balance at a low percentage of body fat will be discussed in subsequent sections of this chapter.

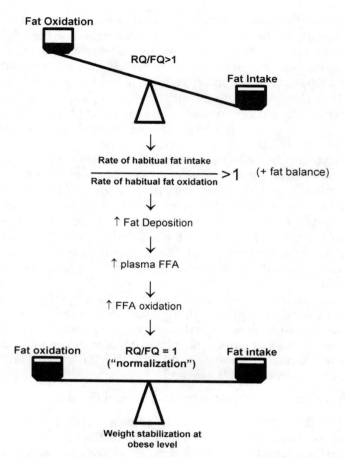

FIGURE 1-2. *Obesity appears to be fundamentally a problem caused by a positive fat balance leading to expansion of the adipose tissue mass.* The increased adiposity leads to elevated plasma free fatty acids, which enhances cellular lipid oxidation. When the fat mass has increased sufficiently, fat balance will be reestablished, and the fat mass will stabilize when the rates of fat oxidation and intake are equal, albeit at a cost of obesity.

In exploring diet composition and food intake, Flatt (1995) has suggested that carbohydrate balance regulates eating behavior and macronutrient selection. This theory is based on observations of mice exposed to negative carbohydrate balance on one day, followed by increased carbohydrate intake on the following day, presumably to restore hepatic glycogen levels to some regulated level. Accordingly, weight stability was achieved over time based on modulation of food intake (i.e., RQ/FQ =1.0). If this were true of humans, in those individuals with a high daily rate of carbohydrate oxidation and a low daily rate of fat oxidation, the drive to adjust carbohydrate intake to match carbohydrate oxidation over the course of several days would necessarily result in overfeeding when the meals were of high fat content. In other words, carbohydrate balance is achieved by regulating carbohydrate intake, at the expense of positive fat balance when the diet is high in fat. Some studies in humans, in which dietary carbohydrate has been displaced by fat, have offered support for this hypothesis (Kendall et al., 1991; Lissner et al., 1987; Thomas et al., 1992; Tremblay et al., 1989), whereas others have not (Shetty et al., 1994; Stubbs et al., 1993). In the latter two studies, dietary manipulation of glycogen stores had little impact on subsequent ad-libitum food intake. However, energy and fat balance were profoundly positive when men were given ad-libitum access to high-energy, high-fat diets for 7 d, whereas energy balance was slightly negative for these same men fed low-fat, high-carbohydrate diets (Stubbs et al., 1993). They have suggested that carbohydrate balance is maintained, not by modulation of carbohydrate intake, but rather by adjustments of RQ to FQ. In a study of overfeeding and underfeeding assessed for 12 consecutive days in a room calorimeter, this same research group (Jebb et al., 1996) concluded that metabolic fuel selection is dominated by the need to maintain carbohydrate balance, which results in inappropriate counterregulatory alterations in fat oxidation during a surplus of energy. An important finding from these studies and others (Tremblay et al., 1989) that must not be overlooked is that humans are much more likely to overeat and to exhibit positive fat balance when the diet is high in fat.

Fat Oxidation and Obesity Risk

Regardless of how closely carbohydrate balance regulates carbohydrate intake, it is clear that overfeeding occurs much more readily on a high-fat diet. Such a diet would clearly increase risk for obesity, especially among individuals who also exhibit a relatively low daily rate of fat oxidation. An excess of calories and fat in the diet does not acutely increase fat oxidation, so a positive fat balance (RQ/FQ > 1.0) leads to fat storage. It follows that a lower rate of fat oxidation could be a predisposing factor to body fat accumulation if dietary fat were widely available, whereas a higher rate of fat oxidation could impart some protection against obesity.

Astrup (1993) and colleagues (1994) in Denmark have suggested that the formerly obese individual (one who has lost substantial weight and has achieved weight stability at a normal body weight) may be a useful model to identify characteristics of those who are obesity prone. That is, the individual who was once obese likely has characteristics similar to those in persons who are likely to become obese; these characteristics presumably increased the susceptibility of the formerly obese to excessive fat accumulation in the first place. These researchers have shown that post-obese women, in comparison to never-obese women, have impaired ability to increase fat oxidation when fed a high-fat diet (50% of energy), with greater partitioning of dietary fat toward storage (Astrup et al., 1994). Larson et al. (1995) have shown that in comparison to normal-weight control subjects, post-obese subjects had a significantly lower 24 h rate of fat oxidation, even when fed diets containing only 30% energy as fat.

An obvious limitation of the post-obese model is that abnormalities identified in the post-obese state may be irreversible defects subsequent to obesity, rather than primary defects causing obesity. Additionally, not all studies of post-obese individuals have found the increased susceptibility to weight gain to be associated with low rates of fat oxidation. For example, Weinsier et al. (1995) compared 24 post-obese women who had lost an average of 12.9 kg to a control group of 24 never-obese women matched for age and body composition. All metabolic variables (resting energy expenditure, thermic effect of food, and fasting and postprandial substrate oxidation) were similar between the post-obese and never-obese women. Four years later, the post-obese women had gained a mean of 10.9 kg, compared to only 1.7 kg for the never-obese controls. However, the substantially greater weight gain of the post-obese women could not be explained by rates of resting and postprandial substrate oxidation. Rather, a low level of physical activity explained much of the 4 y weight gain in the post-obese women. The authors concluded that weight gain in obesity-prone women resulted more from physical inactivity than from a reduced resting energy requirement and a low rate of fat oxidation. The discrepant findings regarding fat oxidation in post-obese subjects indicate the complexity of the etiologies of obesity and, probably, individual differences in functional phenotypes.

Possible Role of Skeletal Muscle. Possible reasons for reduced fat oxidation in obesity-prone individuals are presently unclear but may include enhanced insulin sensitivity in peripheral tissues that favors carbohydrate utilization and reduced lipolysis in adipocytes (Swinburn et al., 1991) and/or reduced plasma epinephrine concentrations with a resultant reduction in rates of lipolysis (Anderson et al., 1994). As mentioned earlier, lower expression of UCP-2 in response to overfeeding (Fleury et al., 1997) could play a role in the reduced fat oxidation of the obesity prone. Also, a reduction in the capacity of skeletal muscle to utilize fatty acids (Abou Mrad et al., 1992; Wade et al., 1990) could be a factor. This latter possibility is discussed in some detail below because of the obvious link between exercise and skeletal muscle function. Note again that a genotypic susceptibility to low rates of fat oxidation will not necessarily result in the phenotypic expression of obesity, unless there is an excess of fat and energy in the diet.

Skeletal muscle morphology and metabolism have been associated with body weight regulation by way of macronutrient oxidation rates. Skeletal muscle fibers exhibit substantial diversity and have been popularly (if somewhat inappropriately) dichotomized into two broad categories based on myosin ATPase activity levels, which also correlate with the fiber's mechanical properties. Type I fibers have been labeled slow-twitch fibers because of their lower rates of force development relative to type II fibers (fast-twitch fibers) that are specialized for rapid force development. Owing to their greater mitochondrial density and higher concentrations of oxidative enzymes, Type I fibers are especially suited for fatty acid oxidation. Type II fibers have been subclassified according to their metabolic characteristics. The so-called type IIa fibers exhibit rapid contraction speed coupled with a relatively high capacity for both aerobic and anaerobic ATP production, while the type IIb fibers exhibit the highest glycolytic and anaerobic capacities. Approximately 25% of the energy expended by lean body tissue occurs in skeletal muscle, with substantial fat oxidation occurring in type I skeletal muscle under conditions of rest and submaximal exercise.

Some evidence suggests that skeletal muscle with a greater glycolytic capacity and lower capacity for oxidation of fat may be related to obesity risk in both experimental animals (Abou Mrad et al., 1992) and humans (Wade et al., 1990). In a study of relatively sedentary men, Wade et al. (1990) found that the proportion of Type I muscle fibers was inversely related to percentage body fat, with approximately 42% of the variance in fatness explained by the proportion of slow- versus fast-twitch fibers. They also found that the rate of fatty acid oxidation at a fixed work intensity of 100 W was inversely related to body fatness. This study has been criticized because the authors failed to control the subjects' diets, and their subjects exhibited a wide range of fitness levels. In an attempt to replicate these findings, Geerling et al. (1994) did not observe an association of body fatness with substrate oxidation during exercise. These discrepant findings are not entirely unexpected, given that the excessive accumulation of body fat is likely to "normalize" the rates of fat oxidation in some obese individuals, thus diluting any differences in substrate utilization in lean versus obese subjects. Despite this caveat, there is other evidence that skeletal muscle characteristics are related to whole-body substrate oxidation and risk of obesity.

Zurlo et al.(1994) found a striking inverse correlation (r = −0.75) between β-hydroxyacyl CoA dehydrogenase activity (involved in beta oxidation of fatty acids) in skeletal muscle and 24-h RQ in 14 Caucasians.

Also, Kriketos et al. (1995) reported that in 62 adult Pima Indians, percent body fat was positively related to percent type IIB fibers, and Simoneau et al. (1995) observed that skeletal muscle of obese, insulin-resistant individuals exhibited reduced oxidative capacity and increased storage of fat. Furthermore, Kelley and Simoneau (1994) found that obese subjects with noninsulin-dependent diabetes mellitus (NIDDM) exhibited reduced postabsorptive and postprandial utilization of free fatty acids in skeletal muscle. These studies indicate that skeletal muscle characteristics are related to macronutrient utilization, NIDDM, and obesity.

EXERCISE AND ENERGY EXPENDITURE

The three components of daily energy expenditure are resting metabolic rate (RMR), the thermic effect of feeding (TEF), and the thermic effect of physical activity (TEPA). The total energy expended in physical activity will vary with the exercise (i.e., frequency, intensity, and duration) and with the subject (body weight, aerobic capacity, etc.).

Energy expenditure does not return to baseline levels immediately following physical activity. The magnitude and duration of this postexercise energy expenditure is controversial (Poehlman et al., 1991). Exercise intensity affects the magnitude of the postexercise elevation of metabolic rate more than does exercise duration (Bahr & Sejersted, 1991; Sedlock et al., 1989). Exercise of the intensity and duration that can be sustained by most nonathletes (40–70% of $\dot{V}O_2$max for 15–40 min) typically results in energy expenditure returning to baseline within 5–40 min following exercise; this accounts for only 21–125 additional kJ expended beyond the exercise bout itself (Freedman-Akabas et al., 1985). In individuals capable of performing high-intensity, long-duration exercise, the postexercise energy expenditure may be higher and might be a significant contributor to total daily energy requirements (Bahr & Sejersted, 1991). Less is known about the effects on energy expenditure following resistance exercise, but high-intensity weightlifting exercise may elevate energy expenditure above baseline levels for several hours (Melby et al., 1993). However, it appears doubtful that individuals untrained in such resistive exercise would be capable of sustaining the exercise intensity necessary to produce a prolonged elevation of postexercise energy expenditure.

Changes in chronic physical activity may influence the other components of energy expenditure, specifically the TEF and RMR. The thermic effect of food is generally considered to account for about 10% of daily energy expenditure. The elevation in energy expenditure above resting values that occurs with food consumption results from both obligatory and facultative components. The former involves the digestion, absorption, and assimilation of macronutrients, whereas the latter involves the elevation of energy expenditure above that attributed to the obligatory component. Presumably, facultative postprandial thermogenesis is caused by increased sympathetic nervous system activity stimulated by high concentrations of plasma insulin. In some studies (Segal et al., 1992a, 1992b) obese individuals exhibited a blunted TEF, which may or may not have implications for weight gain and obesity. It is unclear whether or not the lower TEF in obese individuals is a contributor to or a consequence of excess adiposity. Ravussin et al. (1985) concluded that the blunted TEF characteristic of obesity results from a reduced rate of cellular macronutrient storage due to insulin resistance. When the reduced rate of glucose transport was overcome by hyperinsulinemia, the TEF was similar between obese individuals and lean individuals. Segal and colleagues (1992a, 1992b) found that acute exercise enhanced TEF in obese and diabetic men, possibly by improving insulin sensitivity.

There is no consistent picture of how a change in physical activity affects TEF. Some investigators reported an increase in TEF with increased physical fitness level (Hill et al., 1984), others reported the opposite (Gilbert et al., 1991; Leblanc et al., 1984; Poehlman et al., 1989), and some found no effect (Owen et al., 1986). Witt et al. (1993) proposed that the magnitude of TEF is influenced by the length of time between the last exercise bout and the TEF measurement. Studies in which TEF was measured 12-16 h following strenuous exercise (LeBlanc et al., 1984; Poehlman et al., 1989) often found a lower TEF in trained individuals in comparison to studies in which TEF was measured 36 h or more following exercise (Davis et al., 1983; Hill et al., 1984). With enhanced insulin sensitivity during the 12-16 h following exercise, the lower insulin concentrations may lead to lower sympathetic nervous system activity and reduced facultative thermogenesis.

Other studies have focused on the combined effect of exercise and food intake on thermogenesis. Segal and Gutin (1983) suggested that acute exercise potentiates the thermic effect of feeding such that the combined effects of exercise and food intake on thermogenesis are more than additive. However, Gilbert and Misner (1993) found that meal consumption 30 min prior to exercise did not increase TEM during exercise in either trained or untrained subjects. With all the conflicting data, it is difficult to arrive at a single conclusion regarding exercise and TEF. However, it is likely that the effect of exercise on TEF is fairly small, with the benefits of exercise on weight control resulting more from the increased energy expenditure during exercise, rather than from its impact on this specific component of 24 h energy expenditure.

It is unclear whether changes in physical activity alter RMR independently of changes in fat-free mass because conflicting data have been reported. In several cross-sectional investigations, an elevated RMR was seen in endurance-trained individuals compared to sedentary, untrained subjects, independent of differences in body composition (Burke et al., 1993; Poehlman, 1989; Poehlman et al., 1990). Arciero et al. (1993) compiled data on more than 500 healthy men and women and reported that peak VO_2 was a significant predictor of RMR, independent of body weight and body composition. However, other studies have found that highly-fit, trained subjects have RMR values that are similar to those for sedentary controls (Broeder et al., 1992a, 1992b; Lundholm et al., 1986). As one example, Sharp et al. (1992) used a whole-room calorimeter to perform a cross-sectional study of the relationships among RMR, body composition, and physical fitness in subjects 24 h or more after their last bouts of exercise. They reported that physical fitness (assessed as maximum oxygen consumption) was unrelated to RMR, TEF, energy expenditure of physical activity (EE_{ACT}), or total daily energy expenditure independent of body composition. The reasons for the discrepant findings are unknown but may be related to differences between studies in the time interval between the last bout of exercise and measurement of RMR and to the level of energy intake during the days immediately preceding RMR measurement. Further, it is impossible to determine cause-and-effect relationships from cross-sectional analyses.

Several of the studies that first identified higher RMR values in trained athletes allowed 24 h between the last exercise bout and RMR measurement. Because subjects abstained from exercise for this relatively long period (compared to the usual 10–12 h fast), an acute effect of exercise on RMR was largely discounted, and investigators suggested the increased RMR values in athletes might be due to adaptations to chronic exercise (Poehlman et al., 1989). Several well-conducted studies that used a longer interval (48–56 h) between previous exercise and RMR measurement failed to find elevations of RMR in trained subjects (Herring et al., 1992; Schulz et al., 1991). Taken together, these studies suggest that any elevation of RMR in trained athletes may reflect the acute perturbations of strenuous exercise, rather than an adaptation to training.

Because acute changes in energy intake and energy balance can influence RMR, it is important to separate the effects of exercise from the effects of alterations in energy intake. Contrary to several of the aforementioned studies, Ballor et al. (1992) observed an elevation of RMR in trained women who had abstained from exercise for at least 36 h. Energy consumption was not controlled during the period of exercise abstention, and if the subjects failed to lower their usual energy intakes during this period, they would have been acutely overfed. Overfeeding carbohydrate or mixed diets containing largely carbohydrate is associated with a rapid increase in energy expenditure (Acheson et al., 1988; Horton et al., 1995). In another study (Bingham et al., 1989), RMR was not increased in subjects who underwent an exercise training program for 9 wk, but the subjects were found to be underfed according to energy expenditure determinations using doubly-labeled water. Melby et al. (1990) have previously observed that RMR decreases in exercising athletes when they move to an energy-deficit state. From earlier studies, it was suggested that the combination of high energy expenditure and energy intake (high energy flux or turnover) could elevate RMR in endurance-trained athletes, even when they are in energy balance (Poehlman et al., 1989). A report from our laboratory supports this hypothesis (Bullough et al., 1995). Resting metabolic rate in exercise-trained individuals was influenced by the total flux of energy through the body (total energy expenditure at steady state). Also, in trained versus untrained subjects, RMR was elevated under acute conditions of high exercise-induced energy expenditure and high energy intake, but this elevation was attenuated as the time interval increased from the last exercise bout to the measurement of RMR. These data suggest that RMR may be chronically elevated in individuals who engage in daily, high-intensity, prolonged exercise, due to an effect of acute exercise rather than an adaptation to chronic exercise. It should be noted that the amount of exercise performed by nonathletes for the purpose of weight control is typically of much lower intensity and duration and would likely have little, if any, impact on RMR.

In summary, TEPA changes directly with changes in physical activity. Whether or not other components of energy expenditure are affected by changes in physical activity is controversial. It appears that the major impact of physical activity on energy expenditure occurs during the activity itself.

EXERCISE AND CARBOHYDRATE BALANCE

Carbohydrate Utilization During Exercise

The two sources of carbohydrate used during exercise are skeletal muscle glycogen and plasma glucose. The rate of utilization of the glucose derived from glycogenolysis and from plasma glucose is dependent on the intensity and duration of exercise. Muscle glycogen and plasma glucose both play minor roles in meeting the increased energy demand associated with low-intensity exercise (e.g., 25% of VO_2max); plasma free fatty acids are the predominant fuel (Romijn et al., 1993b). With prolonged moderate-intensity exercise (60–75% VO_2max), muscle glycogen provides most of the carbohydrate energy, but as the exercise progresses in duration, there is greater reliance on plasma glucose

(Coyle et al., 1986, Romijn et al., 1993b). With high-intensity exercise (>75% $\dot{V}O_2$max), muscle glycogen is the major fuel.

Although there is not yet a clear picture of all of the biochemical events involved in coupling glycogenolysis with the contractile activity of the muscle cell, one scenario is as follows. At the onset of exercise, calcium released from the sarcoplasmic reticulum into the cytosol becomes bound to troponin C and calmodulin. Both of these two calcium-binding proteins can activate phosphorylase kinase b to the more active phosphorylase kinase a, resulting in glycogen phosphorylase activation and glycogen degradation. In this manner, the release of Ca^{++} in skeletal muscle when stimulated by nerve impulses is linked to both muscle contraction and glycogen degradation. The increased carbohydrate utilization with increasing exercise intensity also results from increased sympathetic nervous system activity and the accompanying increase in plasma epinephrine that elevates cyclic AMP, leading to the phosphorylation (and thus activation) of glycogen phosphorylase. Carbohydrate utilization also increases due to enhanced contraction-mediated glucose transport from plasma to muscle and from increased muscle fiber recruitment, especially of the glycolytic type II fibers.

The amount of carbohydrate utilized during exercise depends not only on the intensity of the exercise bout but also on the training status of the individual performing the exercise. It is widely recognized that training produces several adaptations within skeletal muscle that enhance the utilization of fat and decrease carbohydrate oxidation at a given absolute submaximal exercise intensity (Gollnick, 1985). These adaptations include increased mitochondrial reticular mass (Davies et al., 1981; Kirkwood et al., 1987) and associated enzymes (Oscai et al., 1982) and decreased concentrations of circulating catecholamines at a given absolute submaximal workload (Deuster et al., 1989). Exercise training may also increase skeletal muscle fatty-acid binding proteins and carnitine acyl transferase activity (needed for transport of long-chain fatty acids into the mitochondrial matrix) (Kiens, 1997). Other exercise-induced training adaptations that appear to enhance skeletal muscle fatty acid oxidation include an increase in the activity of β-hydroxy-acyl CoA dehydrogenase, a key enzyme needed in β-oxidation of fatty acids, and an increase in skeletal muscle capillarization that increases the surface area exposed to blood flow, thus promoting the uptake of free fatty acids (Saltin & Gollnick, 1983). Because of these adaptations, exercise training enhances fat uptake and oxidation during low- and moderate-intensity exercise. The greater rates of fat oxidation that occur with training result in less severe increases in P_i, AMP, and ADP during a given submaximal power output, resulting in less stimulation of glycogenolysis and glycolysis. This increased reliance on fat during exercise apparently contributes to the glycogen sparing effect demonstrated with increased levels of fitness (Baldwin et al., 1977; Gollnick, 1985; Karlsson & Saltin, 1971).

Other training-induced cellular adaptations enhance carbohydrate utilization. These adaptations include increased concentrations of glucose transporter protein 4 (GLUT 4) and increased insulin sensitivity in skeletal muscles (Houmard et al., 1991). However, even with these adaptations, in humans who undergo endurance training there is a decrease in skeletal muscle glucose uptake at the same absolute submaximal exercise intensity, and possibly also during exercise performed at the same relative intensity (Coggan, 1997; Coggan et al., 1995). These observations help explain how exercise training improves an individual's resistance to exercise-induced hypoglycemia, which likely contributes to enhanced exercise performance. On the other hand, in rats, training-induced resistance to hypoglycemia seems to be primarily due to improved hepatic gluconeogenesis (Donovan & Sumida, 1997).

Thus, exercise training increases the ability to use both fat and carbohydrate, with fat oxidation predominant at low- and moderate-exercise intensities and carbohydrate the dominant fuel for high-intensity exercise. Brooks and Mercier (1994) have reviewed exercise macronutrient utilization based on the interaction between intensity-induced responses and training-induced adaptations. They described the "crossover point" as the power output at which energy derived from carbohydrate predominates over energy derived from lipid, with further increases in exercise intensity producing incremental increases in carbohydrate utilization and concomitant decreases in fat oxidation. Exercise training produces a rightward shift in the crossover point, so that at low and moderate exercise intensities the training adaptations enable the individual to oxidize more lipids than does the untrained individual. During high-intensity exercise, the carbohydrate-related adaptations in the trained individual allow the utilization of large amounts of glucose needed for high power output.

Impact of Exercise and Carbohydrate Intake on Carbohydrate Balance

Carbohydrate intake promotes its own oxidation (Acheson et al., 1982, 1988), and while it appears that exercise of sufficient duration and intensity may well deplete glycogen stores in the body, these stores are typically replenished within 24 h, depending upon the quantity and type of carbohydrate consumed (Coyle, 1995). Thus, the intake and oxidation, as well as the restoration of carbohydrate stores within the body, appear to be carefully regulated. As previously discussed, there is some suggestion that food intake may be driven by the body's need to maintain carbohydrate stores at a certain level (Flatt, 1987, 1995). In addition, there is evidence that exercise requiring greater utilization of carbohydrate is associated with postexercise macronutrient selection that favors carbohydrate (King et al., 1994; Verger et al., 1992). Thus, it appears that carbohydrate balance is carefully regulated, primarily by adjusting carbohydrate oxidation to intake. There remains the possibility that spontaneous increases in carbohydrate intake following carbohydrate depletion also serve to maintain carbohydrate balance.

Obviously, the energy expended with exercise has implications for weight regulation. However, the depletion of glycogen stores that accompanies regular exercise may also be of importance in body weight regulation. Flatt (1995) has argued that regular depletion of glycogen stores and maintenance of hepatic glycogen levels far below saturation will lead to a decrement in carbohydrate oxidation that will be offset by an increment in daily fat oxidation. A high-fat, low-carbohydrate diet can deplete glycogen stores and over time lead to enhanced adipocyte lipolysis and greater fat oxidation (Carroll & Klein, 1995). However, given that high-fat diets tend to produce positive energy and fat balance in both humans and laboratory animals (Salmon & Flatt, 1985), the most viable means of regularly depleting glycogen stores and stimulating daily fat oxidation would seem to be habitual exercise rather than a high-fat, low-carbohydrate diet.

Several recent studies provide evidence that acute glycogen-depleting exercise enhances fat oxidation during recovery. Schrauwen et al. (1997) tested the effect of glycogen-lowering exercise on fat oxidation during a 36 h postexercise period measured in a respiratory chamber. They found that glycogen-depleting exercise followed by a high-fat diet (60% fat energy, 25% carbohydrate energy, and 15% protein energy) consumed during the ensuing 36 h period caused greater fat oxidation (156 g fat oxidized per 36 h) compared to a control condition (124 g fat oxidized per 36 h) in which subjects did not exercise but were fed the same diet composition. For both the exercise and no-exercise conditions, subjects were fed to achieve energy balance during the 36 h period in the chamber. However, subjects were able to achieve fat balance on the high-fat diet only when they followed the exercise treatment. On the high-fat diet without exercise, fat balance was substantially positive (+ 24 g). The authors concluded that among lean subjects, fat oxidation increases to match fat intake after glycogen-lowering exercise. Tuominen et al. (1997) determined the rate of lipid oxidation in 14 males under basal conditions and during a euglycemic, hyperinsulinemic clamp 44 h following a bout of glycogen-depleting exercise compared to a control condition of no exercise. Following exercise, there was a two-fold higher rate of fat oxidation in the basal state and almost a three-fold increase during hyperinsulinemia. Data from these studies demonstrate that glycogen-lowering exercise enhances fat oxidation for up to 44 h after exercise, a finding that has important implications for fat balance.

EXERCISE AND PROTEIN BALANCE

Protein Utilization During Exercise

Endurance exercise, whether acute or chronic, could potentially impact protein metabolism in one of two ways. First, the increased need for ATP could require increased protein oxidation to meet these demands. Second, higher rates of protein turnover might result if muscle damage were to occur with endurance exercise.

A single bout of endurance activity increases protein oxidation, as estimated by leucine oxidation (Evans et al., 1983; Lemon et al., 1982, 1985; Rennie et al., 1980; White & Brooks, 1981) in an intensity-dependent manner (Rennie et al., 1981); this is likely associated with alterations in the activity of the enzyme branched-chain keto-acid dehydrogenase (Kasperek & Snider, 1987; Odessey et al., 1974). It is unclear whether or not the source of this protein oxidized during exercise is from skeletal muscle. Some evidence indicates such to be the case (Dohm et al., 1982), whereas other information suggests that tissues other than skeletal muscle are the source of the proteins being catabolized (Decombaz et al., 1979; Radhu & Bessman, 1983). Regardless of the tissue source, it appears that a single bout of endurance exercise may increase the rate of whole-body protein oxidation. However, the contribution of protein oxidation to total energy expenditure remains fairly small compared to carbohydrate and fat utilization. Over 24 h or more, protein oxidation roughly equals intake, i.e., about 12–15% of energy intake for most people. During prolonged exercise, the proportion of protein oxidized relative to energy demand decreases to 5–6% or less, primarily due to increases in the oxidation of other substrates.

Endurance Training and Protein Balance

Two studies suggest that there may be some adaptation in protein metabolism that ultimately offsets the initial increase in protein loss seen at the onset of a training program (Gontzea et al., 1974, 1975). Sedentary men who began an endurance training program of moderate intensity (8-10 kcal(min^{-1}) demonstrated negative nitrogen balance, even when protein intake was increased from 1.0 g·kg^{-1}·day^{-1} to 1.5 g·kg^{-1}·day^{-1} (Gontzea et al., 1974). Only after 12 d of training did nitrogen balance begin to approach zero (Gontzea et al., 1975), suggesting that with endurance training, protein metabolism may become more efficient, thereby negating any need for increased protein intake. Conversely, the return to zero nitrogen balance could also be explained by a decline in the relative intensity of the exercise bouts, since the subjects were becoming better trained. There is some evidence to suggest that lower-intensity endurance exercise does not increase protein oxidation or protein requirements (Butterfield & Calloway, 1984; Todd et al., 1984; Wolfe et al., 1982). Thus, it is unclear whether or not endurance training of moderate intensity results in more efficient protein metabolism. However, a number of investigations provide evidence of increased protein needs in individuals who participate in high-intensity endurance exercise (Brouns et al., 1989; Friedman & Lemon, 1989; Meredith et al., 1989; Tarnopolsky et al., 1988). It is doubtful, however, that a sedentary person who begins an exercise program will need to increase protein intake to maintain nitrogen balance because the exercise bouts will not, at least initially, be strenuous or prolonged.

Resistance Exercise and Training: Protein Balance

To date, there has been little investigation of the impact of a single bout of resistance training on protein turnover. The available data suggest either increased protein catabolism (Dohm et al., 1982) or no effect on protein catabolism following a single bout of strength training (Hickson et al., 1986). Protein oxidation appears to be unaffected by a single session of strength training (Tarnopolsky et al., 1991), but further investigation is necessary. The equivocal responses could be at least partly explained by different intensities of the exercise bouts and different levels of training status of the participants among the investigations. For instance, participants in a study that demonstrated increased levels of urinary 3-methylhistidine (an indicator of skeletal muscle catabolism) in response to a single strength-training session were well trained, and the exercise session was fairly intense (Dohm et al., 1982) compared to the study that failed to demonstrate any effects on protein metabolism (Hickson et al., 1986).

Most investigations of the impact of regular participation in strength training have been designed to evaluate whether or not there is a need for increased protein intake as a consequence of training. The results from several of these investigations permit some generalizations to be made. First, because those who consumed the higher protein intake (above the RDA of 0.8 $g \cdot kg^{-1} \cdot d^{-1}$) consistently demonstrated either positive nitrogen balance (Lemon et al., 1992; Walberg et al., 1988), greater whole-body protein synthesis (Fern et al., 1991; Tarnopolsky et al., 1992), or greater gains in body mass (Fern et al., 1991) or size (Frontera et al., 1988), protein intake above the recommended RDA should be considered by those who participate in strength training on a regular basis. Second, there appears to be a threshold of protein intake above which no significant benefits result, at least in terms of protein oxidation relative to protein synthesis. For instance, in subjects who consumed 2.4 $g \cdot kg^{-1} \cdot d^{-1}$, the rate of oxidation of amino acids (estimated by leucine oxidation) was greater than in persons consuming only 1.4 $g \cdot kg^{-1} \cdot d^{-1}$. However, protein synthesis between these two groups was similar, suggesting the optimal quantity of protein intake had been exceeded, somewhere in the range of 1.4 and 2.4 $g \cdot kg^{-1} \cdot d^{-1}$ (Tarnopolsky et al., 1992). Other investigations have reported similar results (Fern et al., 1991). Finally, some evidence suggests that increasing protein intake above the RDA for protein when first beginning a strength training regimen may be beneficial in terms of gains in both body mass and size (Frontera et al., 1988) as well as in avoiding negative nitrogen balance (Lemon et al., 1992).

Impact of Exercise and Protein Intake on Protein Balance

As with carbohydrate, protein intake and its subsequent oxidation are closely linked, so that an increase in protein intake causes higher rates of protein oxidation (Flatt et al., 1985; Flatt, 1987). Thus, protein balance appears to be tightly regulated. Because of this close association between protein intake and its subsequent oxidation, there is no reason to believe that increased protein intake should lead to alterations in body composition due to increased lean body mass, unless the appropriate stimuli are present for muscle hypertrophy (i.e., progressive overload resistance exercise). High protein intakes are generally not viewed as contributing to positive energy balance. However, it is possible that a high protein intake coupled with a dietary energy surplus could contribute to fat accumulation—most likely not the result of enhanced lipogenesis from amino acid carbons but because amino-acid oxidation would replace a portion of the fat normally oxidized.

EXERCISE AND FAT BALANCE

As discussed earlier, it is possible that a low rate of fat oxidation, for whatever reason, could predispose an individual to obesity when faced with a highly palatable mixed diet. Conversely, an increased rate of 24 h fat oxidation can provide some protection against excessive body fat accumulation. We have already seen that unlike carbohydrate and protein intakes, which increase their respective oxidation rates when ingested, increasing fat intake does little to acutely increase fat oxidation. How then can fat oxidation be increased?

Fat oxidation is enhanced by a deficit of energy intake relative to energy expenditure. Obviously, the greater the energy deficit, the greater the reliance on stored fat as a fuel to meet energy demands in the face of the energy deficit. Energy restriction leads to lower insulin levels and less suppression of lipolysis. Although dieting can clearly enhance fat oxidation and produce weight loss, long-term weight loss is often not achieved by changes in diet alone. Several components of daily energy expenditure (RMR and TEF) are reduced with dieting. Additionally, weight stability at the lower body weight will be accompanied by decreased fat oxidation compared to fat oxidation at the higher body weight (Schutz et al., 1992). These reductions in energy expenditure and fat oxidation would facilitate weight regain if the individual returns to the usual diet.

As previously explained, another factor that can increase fat oxidation is an increase in body fat mass. Obese individuals often have higher circulating concentrations of plasma free fatty acids (Schutz et al., 1992), especially as insulin resistance develops. The increase in fat utilization that accompanies obesity helps re-establish a new equilibrium between fat intake and fat oxidation that stabilizes the higher body weight. Obviously, this is not an effective means of increasing fat oxidation to prevent obesity.

A low-carbohydrate, moderate-to-high-fat diet is another means to increase fat oxidation. This type of diet has received considerable recent interest in lay periodicals and books, and is advocated by some to promote both body fat loss and improved endurance exercise performance. Advocates of this type of diet suggest that a high-fat diet will enhance fat utilization by inducing the oxidative enzymatic machinery of skeletal muscle, and that such a diet will lower plasma insulin concentrations, result in less suppression of lipolysis, and lead to enhanced fat oxidation.

While it is true that a high-fat, low-carbohydrate diet will lead to greater fat oxidation, there is a significant lag time between the increase in fat oxidation in response to increased fat intake (Horton et al., 1995). Also, the purported benefits of a low-carbohydrate, high-fat diet are mostly anecdotal, with the few experimental studies performed plagued by weaknesses that limit conclusions regarding the beneficial effects of such a diet for enhancing weight loss or exercise performance.

The final means of increasing fat oxidation, and arguably the most viable approach for those attempting to decrease body fat stores, is an increase in physical activity. An increase in fat oxidation is seen in virtually all forms of exercise. As discussed below, the amount of fat oxidized *during* exercise depends on the characteristics of the exercise and of the individual engaged in the exercise.

Fat Utilization During Exercise

There are two different sources of fat for oxidation during exercise: plasma free fatty acids mobilized from adipose tissue and fatty acids stored in intramuscular triacylglycerols. Adipose tissue contains an abundance of triacylglycerols, easily enough to fuel an 800-km walk in a lean person. Obviously, for use during exercise, adipocyte triacylglycerols must undergo lipolysis and transport to skeletal muscle mitochondria where oxidation occurs. During exercise, the increase in plasma epinephrine concentrations stimulates β-receptors in the adipocyte membrane that signal cAMP formation, which in turn activates cAMP-dependent protein kinase. This latter enzyme covalently modifies hormone-sensitive lipase by phosphorylation, leading to its activation. Hormone-sensitive lipase then hydrolyzes (de-esterifies) the fatty acids from the glycerol backbone of the triacylglycerol. Under basal or resting conditions, many of the free fatty acids formed in lipolysis will undergo re-esterification within the same adipocyte. However, during low-intensity exercise, the majority of free fatty acids formed in the adipocyte by lipolysis will enter the plasma. Because of their hydrophobic nature, the fatty acids must be bound to plasma albumin for transport. These free fatty acids are then taken up by skeletal muscle in a poorly understood process and transported by intramuscular proteins to the mitochondria where they undergo β-oxidation.

Exercise Intensity and Fat Oxidation

Much of our understanding of fat mobilization and oxidation during exercise at various intensities comes from research using isotopic tracers combined with indirect calorimetry (Klein et al., 1994, 1995, 1996; Romijn et al., 1993a, 1995; Coyle, 1995). A brief summary of the research findings is discussed in the following paragraphs.

During low-intensity exercise (e.g., walking at 25% $\dot{V}O_2$max), there can be a five-fold increase, compared to resting conditions, in the rate of appearance of free fatty acids (FFA) (R_a FFA) in the plasma (Klein et al., 1994; Romijn et al., 1993c; Wolfe et al., 1990). The oxidation of plasma FFA accounts for most of the energy needed for exercise, with much smaller contributions from blood glucose and intramuscular triacylglycerols.

As the exercise intensity increases from 25% to about 65% of $\dot{V}O_2$max (e.g., a jogging pace that could be sustained for several hours), muscle glycogen contributes substantially to meeting the energy demand. Tracer studies have shown that the rate of FFA appearance into plasma decreases with this increase in exercise intensity, but total fat oxidation as measured by indirect calorimetry (i.e., VO_2 and RER measurements) actually increases (Romijn et al., 1993b). The most logical explanation for this phenomenon is that intramuscular triacylglycerols provide the additional fatty acids to account for this increase in fat oxidation (Hurley et al., 1986; Martin, 1997). Direct measurement of changes in intramuscular triglycerides from muscle biopsies is plagued with difficulties and as yet has yielded little useful information regarding this source of energy during exercise.

As the exercise intensity increases to about 85% $\dot{V}O_2$max, muscle glycogen serves as the primary fuel. Plasma concentrations of FFA actually decrease as the rate of appearance of FFA (R_a FFA) decreases even further (Romijn et al., 1993b). The explanation for the declining R_a FFA is not clear. One might surmise that because the concentration of plasma catecholamines increases dramatically with high-intensity exercise, lipolysis should also occur at a high rate, leading to an increase in the R_a FFA. Tracer studies using labeled glycerol suggest that a substantial rate of lipolysis occurs during high-intensity exercise (Klein et al., 1996), but for unexplained reasons most of the adipocyte FFA fail to enter the plasma (i.e., the R_a of glycerol is high, but the R_a FFA is low). Coyle (1995) suggests that a reduced blood flow to adipose tissue during high-intensity exercise may provide inadequate plasma albumin concentrations needed to mobilize the adipocyte FFA. Regardless of the reason, it is apparent that during high-intensity exercise, both plasma FFA and intramuscular triacylglycerols contribute less to meeting the energy demands than does skeletal muscle glycogen.

It should be noted the studies examining fuel utilization at exercise intensities of 25%, 65%, and 85% of $\dot{V}O_2$max have used highly trained endurance athletes. Presumably, at each of the same exercise intensities, untrained subjects would exhibit greater reliance on carbohydrate and less reliance on fat, compared to the trained subjects.

It is well recognized, then, that for exercise of high- compared to low-intensity, a greater portion of the oxygen consumed is used for carbohydrate and less for fat oxidation during the exercise bout. This has led some fitness practitioners to suggest that low-intensity exercise is better than high-intensity exercise for regulating body weight and body composition because the former produces greater fat oxidation. However, such advice fails to consider the higher energy expenditure with exercise of greater intensity as well as the impact of high-intensity activity on postexercise resting substrate utilization.

Several studies (Bahr & Sejersted, 1991; Bielinski et al., 1985) have reported that the postexercise RER is depressed during recovery from exercise that provokes greater fat oxidation. For example, Bielinski et al. (1985) found that among trained male subjects there was a significantly higher contribution of fat to total fuel utilization during a 5 h postexercise period compared to a similar time period on a control day of no exercise. Broeder et al. (1991) reported lower RER values in males during a 3 h period following exercise at 60% $\dot{V}O_2$max compared to the same period following exercise at 30% $\dot{V}O_2$max. Phelain et al. (1997) examined the effects of low- and high-intensity exercise, of similar energy output, on exercise and postexercise energy expenditure and substrate oxidation in eight active, eumenorrheic females. Continuous indirect calorimetry was performed during cycle ergometry exercise and for 3 h following each of three protocols administered in random order: 1) low-intensity exercise (LIE: 500 kcal @ 50% $\dot{V}O_2$max), 2) high-intensity exercise (HIE: 500 kcal @ 75% $\dot{V}O_2$max), and 3) control condition (C) of quiet sitting for 1 h. They found that, as expected, carbohydrate oxidation was significantly greater for the high-intensity protocol than for the low-intensity. Total fat oxidation (exercise plus 3 h recovery) was greater during the low-intensity exercise treatment. However, at the end of the 3 h recovery period (whole blood bicarbonate levels had returned to preexercise values within the first hour after exercise) the calculated rate of fat oxidation was 23.8 percent higher following high-intensity compared to low-intensity exercise. These data indicate that the recovery period must also be considered when determining the impact of different exercise intensities on total energy expenditure and fat and carbohydrate utilization.

Endurance Training and Fat Oxidation

With endurance-exercise training, the same amount of submaximal work can be performed at a lower RER value (indicating greater fat oxidation) than before training (Gollnick, 1985). One might suggest that the posttraining RER is lower because adaptations lead to less lactic acid formation at the same absolute exercise intensity. Thus, less bicarbonate buffer would be needed and less CO_2 would be expired, resulting in the lower RER. However, training-induced decreases in submaximal exercise RER are apparent even under steady-state conditions, when any disturbances in the bicarbonate pool would be minimal (Gollnick, 1985), which suggests the lower RER does, in fact, reflect greater fat oxidation. This is partly due to the lower relative intensity of the exercise. Even so, fat oxidation may be increased at the same relative work intensity in trained versus untrained individuals (Bergstrom & Hultman, 1967; Turcotte et al., 1992). Increased fat oxidation in trained subjects is greatly facilitated by morphological and enzymatic adaptations in skeletal muscle following training (Holloszy & Coyle, 1984; Hoppeler, 1986) combined with increased availability of lipid substrate (Romijn et al., 1993c).

There is some indication that high levels of fitness or training may affect the way that dietary fat is partitioned between oxidation and storage. Simsolo et al. (1993) studied regulation of lipoprotein lipase, a key enzyme in the uptake of triglyceride-derived free fatty acids, in adipose tissue and skeletal muscle before and after detraining in runners. After detraining, lipoprotein lipase activity was increased in adipose tissue and decreased in skeletal muscle. This suggests that detraining may have influenced fat partitioning by shunting it away from muscle (presumably for oxidation) toward adipose tissue (presumably for storage). Thus, a high level of physical activity may favor dietary fat being transported to muscle for oxidation rather than to adipose tissue for storage.

Resistance Exercise and Training: Fat Oxidation

Few studies have focused on the impact on fat oxidation during acute resistance exercise for improving strength. It is well recognized that during strength-training exercise, phosphocreatine and muscle glycogen are the major sources of fuel for ATP synthesis. However, it is possible that during rest periods between sets of exercise and during the postexercise recovery period, fat may contribute to energy needs. In apparent support of this contention is the fact that RER values are low during the hours following strenuous strength-training exercise (Gillette et al., 1994; Melby et al., 1993). However, a major contributor to the low postexercise RER is the replenishment of the bicarbonate pool (metabolically produced CO_2 is conserved, resulting in a lower VCO_2 and RER); thus, it is unclear how much fat is actually oxidized. However, in one of our studies (Melby et al., 1993), we found the RER to be lower 15 h following a strenuous bout of strength training, a finding that likely reflects greater fat oxidation. Thus, it appears that fat oxidation may be enhanced during recovery from strength training, as well as from other high-intensity exercise, serving to spare available carbohydrate for glycogen resynthesis.

Little is known about the effect of strength training on daily fat oxidation. Treuth et al. (1995) examined the effect of a 16-week strength-training program in healthy older women on 24 h substrate utilization as measured in an indirect room calorimeter. At the end of the training program, they found daily fat oxidation to be almost double compared to the pretraining values. Findings from this study await confirmation. Future research should address the impact of both acute and chronic strength-training exercise on 24 h macronutrient oxidation.

The fat oxidation associated with exercise (both during exercise and recovery) has significant implications for body weight regulation. Flatt (1995) suggests that exercise is a substitute for expansion of the adipose tissue mass, allowing the physically active individual to achieve fat balance at a lower body fat mass. In other words, exercise increases daily fat oxidation to become commensurate with fat intake, obviating the need to expand the body fat mass. He also suggests that the reverse is true: obesity is a substitute for exercise in bringing about positive fat balance and body weight maintenance at a higher body weight. This is an oversimplification of a complex issue, as there are obviously individuals who do not exercise and yet maintain a low body fat mass, and some obese individuals are regular exercisers. However, it does suggest the importance of exercise in elevating daily energy expenditure and fat oxidation, so that in the face of a highly palatable diet, there would be less likelihood of positive fat balance leading to excessive body fat storage.

EXERCISE AND ENERGY COMPENSATION

In a review of weight-loss studies, Stefanick (1993) highlighted the substantial variability in the amount of body fat losses by study participants in response to similar weight-loss interventions. Reasons for this marked variability in fat mass loss include differences in the amount of energy expended during or after the exercise sessions and/or differences among the participants in the extent to which they compensated for the exercise bout by increasing their energy intakes. Exercise contributes to weight loss only if it creates negative energy balance. Negative energy balance will not occur if energy intake increases to meet the energy demands brought on by exercise and/or if spontaneous physical activity declines. Factors that influence the degree of energy compensation seen in response to exercise are not well understood but clearly have an important impact on energy balance.

Although the effects of physical activity on energy expenditure and substrate oxidation have been studied extensively, much less in known about the effect of physical activity on food intake. Because active people generally have higher levels of energy expenditure, energy intake also should be higher. This is generally found in cross-sectional studies (Maughan & Aulin, 1997; Montoye et al., 1976; Stefanick, 1993). However, investigations that attempt to characterize the impact of exercise on subsequent energy and macronutrient intake are often limited by the inability to accurately assess food intake in humans. Because of this limitation, some investigators have employed laboratory animals to study the impact of exercise on food intake. However, although food intake is more accurately assessed in laboratory animals, forced exercise, such as weighted swimming or treadmill running using shock grids, may affect food intake independent of exercise. That is, eating behavior after exercise may be confounded by the stress that accompanies these forced exercise bouts. Given this phenomenon, as well as obvious differences between rats and humans, data from laboratory animal studies of exercise and food intake may not accurately characterize the human condition. There is yet much to learn regarding the effects of acute and chronic exercise on food intake.

One of the first human studies to address the effect of physical activity on energy intake was conducted by Mayer et al. (1956). They proposed that some minimal level of physical activity was necessary for energy expenditure to effectively regulate energy intake. More recently, because it appears that acute fat intake and its subsequent oxidation are not as tightly linked as carbohydrate and protein intake and oxidation (Flatt, 1987; Tremblay et al., 1991), research has focused on the impact of exercise on subsequent macronutrient selection and energy balance (King & Blundell, 1995; Tremblay et al., 1994).

Effect of Acute Exercise on Immediate Postexercise Appetite and Energy Intake

Several investigations have examined the impact of exercise on appetite and subsequent food intake following exercise in humans (King & Blundell, 1995; King et al., 1994; Oscai, 1973; Saris, 1991; Wilmore, 1983). In humans, there appears to be an acute decrease in appetite during the period immediately following exercise (King & Bludell, 1995; King et al., 1994), with appetite returning by 15 min following exercise cessation. Evidence suggests that exercise of greater intensity may be more likely to bring about a postexercise suppression of appetite than does exercise of lower intensity (Katch et al., 1979; King et al.,1994; Kissilef et al., 1990; Reger et al., 1984; Thompson et al., 1988). Finally, there is some indication that the duration of exercise may be associated with the degree to which appetite is suppressed following exercise, independent of exercise intensity (King et al., 1994). However, while appetite is an interesting outcome variable, the key question is how exercise affects actual food intake.

The phenomenon of exercise-induced anorexia observed following an exercise bout has been documented in a number of investigations in both humans (Staten, 1991; Thompson et al., 1988) and rats (Kissilef et al., 1990; Larue-Achagiotis et al., 1992, 1993, 1994; Richard et al., 1986; Satabin et al., 1991). Other investigations have failed to demonstrate any impact on energy consumption immediately following exercise (Applegate et al., 1984; Garthwaite et al., 1986; Jen et al., 1992; Oscai et al., 1974). Why discrepancies exist among investigations concerning the impact of exercise on food intake during the postexercise period might be partially explained by differences in gender, exercise intensity, exercise mode, whether or not the exercise bout was forced or voluntary (animal investigations), and macronutrient composition of the diet provided following exercise. For instance, some studies indicated that food intake is reduced following exercise in male rats but not female rats (Applegate et al., 1982), whereas other studies reported no alteration in food intake following exercise in either gender (Applegate et al., 1984). Larue-Achagiotis and associates (1992) concluded that there appears to be an increase in food intake in response to exercise in female rats, while food intake declines following exercise in male rats (Larue-Achigiotis et al.,

1992, 1993, 1994). Titchenal (1988) summarized the findings from 33 different studies, all of which had examined the impact of exercise on food intake in rats. In response to forced low-intensity, long-duration exercise, food intake was lower in male compared to female rats. However, when exercise was voluntary, gender differences were not apparent. This review suggests that in laboratory rats, there is an interaction between gender and exercise intensity that affects postexercise food intake. Whether or not such an interaction is characteristic of humans is unclear.

Effect of Acute Exercise on 24 h Postexercise Energy Intake

Although numerous investigations in humans and rats have demonstrated a decline in appetite and food intake during the early postexercise period, whether or not a negative energy balance results over prolonged periods becomes clear only when the energy cost of the exercise is considered relative to energy intake. In a study comparing food intake following both low- and high-intensity cycling bouts that demanded similar energy expenditure, there were no differences in either 24 h energy intake or macronutrient intake following the cycling bouts when compared to a sedentary control day (King et al., 1994). Thus, whereas exercise intensity may impact food intake during the period immediately following exercise, long-term energy balance may be unrelated to exercise intensity. In this same study, when two high-intensity cycling bouts of different durations were compared, the longer-duration bout resulted in energy intake that was no different from that seen following a high-intensity, short-duration cycling bout. However, when the energy expended during the exercise bout was taken into consideration, energy balance following the high-intensity, long-duration bout was negative for the subsequent 24 h (King et al., 1994). Thus, at least in terms of energy balance, a "relative energy intake," in which the energy expended during the exercise bout is considered along with the subsequent food intake, is likely the more appropriate means by which to describe the relationship between exercise and food intake.

Whether or not any relationship between relative energy intake and energy balance exists for exercise of lower intensities is unknown. Research in this area is warranted, given the fact that low-intensity exercise does not suppress appetite immediately after exercise (King et al., 1994). Lower- intensity exercise could conceivably be associated with increased energy intake over the subsequent 24 h, especially if an individual takes exercise as a license to eat more with no regard to energy balance. In addition, those populations that exercise at lower intensities, such as the elderly or obese, are also those who may not accurately regulate energy intake. For instance, Woo and colleagues (Woo & Pi-Sunyer,

1985; Woo et al., 1982a, 1982b) have shown that obese women fail to increase energy intake in the face of increased activity levels, whereas lean women increased energy intake to match increased energy expenditure. It should be noted that in these studies there was substantial variability in the responses of both the obese and lean subjects, indicating that body composition alone explains only a small part of the variability in energy intake in response to exercise.

Exercise and Macronutrient Selection

The notion that exercise might impact subsequent macronutrient selection is not new. In 1954, Andik and colleagues demonstrated that rats undergoing low-intensity, long-duration training ingested more lipid throughout the investigation compared to sedentary conditions, and because of this increased fat consumption, a positive energy balance resulted (Andik et al., 1954). Conversely, rats that underwent high-intensity, short-duration exercise consumed more carbohydrate, and energy intake and energy balance were similar to those for sedentary rats (Parízková et al., 1964). More recently, Larue-Achagiotis et al. (1994) compared food intake and macronutrient selection over a period of 20 d in exercised rats (2 h of treadmill running each day) to rats that remained sedentary during this time. During the 2 h in which the trained rats exercised, the sedentary rats were deprived of food. On average for the 20 d, the exercise-trained rats consumed less total energy, less fat, and more carbohydrate than did rats that remained sedentary. For the first 6 h following treadmill running, fat intake decreased with no change in carbohydrate or protein intake in the exercise-trained rats; there was an overall negative energy balance in these rats. Conversely, fat intake of the sedentary rats increased throughout the study. Perhaps more interesting was the pattern of food intake prior to either the 2 h exercise session or 2 h fast; exercise-trained rats increased daytime intake of both carbohydrate and protein during the investigation. Conversely, sedentary rats did not increase daytime food intake significantly, but in the few hours prior to commencement of the 2 h fast, fat intake increased significantly in the sedentary rats throughout the 20 d study. These data suggest that the substrates utilized, both during exercise and during periods of fasting, may potentially drive patterns of macronutrient intake in rats.

The association between fuel utilization during exercise and subsequent macronutrient selection in humans has been investigated, and a positive correlation was found between RQ during exercise and postexercise macronutrient selection (King et al., 1994). Thus, exercise that demands more carbohydrate as fuel may also drive greater carbohydrate consumption following exercise. In support of this hypothesis, exercise of greater intensity and duration was associated with a greater proportion of the energy intake coming from carbohydrate during the postexercise period than was exercise of lower intensity (Verger et al., 1992); however, the same investigators failed to reproduce these results in a subsequent study (Verger et al., 1994).

Impact of Postexercise Meal Composition on Energy Intake

The emphasis of most research regarding exercise and dietary compensation has been on the impact that exercise has on energy intake, macronutrient selection, and energy balance. However, recent work in several laboratories has focused on the impact of postexercise macronutrient selection on energy balance. The findings thus far are consistent: after exercise, people provided with foods containing large amounts of fat consume more total energy than when the foods provided are high in carbohydrate (King & Blundell, 1995; Tremblay et al., 1994). Tremblay et al. (1994) demonstrated that exposure to a high-fat diet over a 2 d period offset the negative energy balance brought on by exercise. In a subsequent investigation, energy intake in a meal provided immediately after exercise was significantly greater if the meal was high in fat compared to one high in carbohydrate (King & Blundell, 1995). Taken together, these investigations demonstrate that any impact exercise might have on body weight by promoting negative energy balance can be completely offset if available food is high in fat. Again, this reinforces the concept that it is *fat balance* that is important, not just fat intake or fat oxidation.

There appears to be an effect of the time interval between cessation of exercise and food availability on postexercise food intake, at least in humans. In one study (Verger et al., 1992), the greater the delay in food accessibility following exercise, the greater was the total energy intake. The increased energy intake was explained solely by increased carbohydrate intake; fat and protein intake remain unchanged regardless of how long food access was denied (Verger et al., 1992). In rats, whether access to food was denied 0, 30, or 90 min following 2 h of forced treadmill running, total energy intake was significantly less over the subsequent 24 h, relative to energy intake in sedentary rats deprived of food for 2 h. However, although food intake decreased similarly regardless of how long access to food was delayed, carbohydrate intake decreased and protein intake increased with longer periods of denial (Larue-Achagiotis et al., 1993).

Because plasma levels of leptin and NPY affect food intake, might exercise influence energy intake by way of its impact on these regulatory peptides? Only recently have studies been undertaken to examine the effects of exercise on serum leptin concentrations and leptin mRNA. In rodents, an acute bout of exercise significantly reduced *ob* mRNA levels both immediately following exercise and 3 h after exercise. Four weeks of exercise training reduced serum leptin by 48% from pretraining levels (Zheng et al., 1996). Conversely, Hickey et al. (1997) failed to show any change in serum leptin levels in lean, endurance-trained, male distance runners following an acute exhaustive exercise bout (20 mi run at 70% $\dot{V}O_2$max). Thus, the acute effect of exercise on serum leptin levels may differ between rodents and humans. Other data also suggest that serum leptin levels in humans and rodents may respond differently to exercise. For instance, a recent study in rats compared the effect of 7 wk of voluntary wheel running on the expression of leptin mRNA. Rats were either sensitive or resistant to the development of dietary-induced obesity. Exercise training in both groups of rats was associated with lower leptin mRNA in epididymal adipose tissue, lower serum leptin levels, and increased food intake, suggesting that the impact of exercise on the expression of leptin can occur independent of obesity susceptibility (Zachwieja et al., 1997). However, in women aged 60–72 y, a 9 mo training program failed to produce any changes in serum leptin levels that were independent of changes in body fat content, even though serum leptin levels declined 23% (Kohrt et al., 1996). Clearly, further work is needed to better describe the impact of exercise on leptin action in humans. It may be that serum leptin concentration is a poor indicator of leptin action.

The impact of exercise on NPY and subsequent energy balance has also been investigated. In rats, chronic exercise increases immunoreactive NPY levels in several areas of the brain (Lewis et al., 1993). The mechanism by which this occurs is unknown, but there is no evidence that exercise alone increases NPY levels. Some have speculated that insulin may be involved (Richard, 1995); lower insulin levels in the brain are associated with elevated concentrations of NPY (Schwartz et al., 1994), and exercise is known to reduce serum insulin levels (LeBlanc et al., 1979; Lohmann et al., 1978). It is equally conceivable that exercise may act through leptin to bring about the elevation in NPY levels. Exercise that promotes negative energy balance requires that energy demands be met by deriving energy from adipocytes, thus reducing adipose tissue stores and cell size. Because leptin is produced in proportion to body fat content and adipocyte cell size (Hamilton et al., 1995; Lonnqvist et al., 1995), any reduction in these variables should also bring about a reduction in serum leptin concentrations. Given the impact of leptin on NPY production (Cusin et al., 1996; Schwartz et al., 1996), the elevation in NPY in response to chronic exercise may be explained by the reduction in adipocyte size and body fat content and the subsequent reduction in serum leptin levels. There is yet much to learn regarding the influence of acute and chronic exercise on energy intake and on the roles of these regulatory peptides.

Exercise and Physical Activity Compensation

Surprisingly little is known about the impact of acute exercise on 24 h spontaneous physical activity. It seems reasonable that a vigorous bout of exercise might induce a degree of fatigue that could limit the amount of physical activity performed during the remaining hours of the day. Goran and Poehlman (1992) reported that despite initiating an exercise program, elderly individuals failed to increase total daily energy expenditure as measured by doubly-labeled water. Presumably their subjects were more sedentary than usual during nonexercise times. Their data suggested total compensation for the exercise energy expenditure, i.e., the reduction in the subjects' 24 h spontaneous activity levels matched the increase in their daily exercise energy expenditures. In this study, the subjects were exercising at 85% of $\dot{V}O_2$max, which is much more intense than exercise regimens practiced by most individuals who exercise for health-related purposes. Had this study been continued for a longer period to allow the subjects greater opportunity to adapt to the high-intensity exercise program, the apparent decline in spontaneous activity may have been different.

Studies of exercising lean and obese women (Meyer et al., 1991; Van Dale et al., 1989) did not find reductions in spontaneous physical activity outside of the exercise training hours. Furthermore, in lean males and obese boys, exercise training appeared to actually stimulate physical activity during the nonexercising part of the day (Blaak et al., 1992; Meyer et al., 1991). Possibly, compensation for exercise by decreases in normal daily physical activities occurs more readily in older adults than in young people. On the other hand, older subjects with physical limitations in strength, flexibility, agility, and stamina may benefit from strength-training exercise; such training may increase spontaneous activity by improving the strength and agility needed to carry out routine daily tasks. Currently, it is unclear what is the optimal mode and intensity of exercise that both maximizes exercise energy expenditure and minimizes compensatory decreases in spontaneous activity. Future research should address this important question.

EXERCISE VERSUS DIETING FOR WEIGHT LOSS

Many studies have addressed, either alone or in combination, the contributions of diet and exercise to weight loss. It has become clear that dieting alone produces greater weight loss than does exercise alone (Saris, 1995) and that exercise in combination with dieting often adds little to the weight loss achieved by dieting alone. These findings have led some investigators to discount the importance of exercise (Garrow,

1995). However, it is unrealistic to expect that a sedentary person who initiates an exercise program can achieve the same magnitude of energy deficit that can be achieved by a low energy diet. Thus, a greater and more rapid weight loss should occur with dieting compared to exercise. However, this does not suggest that exercise would have only a marginal impact on weight loss over an extended period of time. As an individual becomes exercise trained, there is an increased capacity to exercise at higher intensities for longer durations. The trained individual also has a greater capacity for fat oxidation. These training adaptations may enable a physically active individual to gradually lose fat mass and to successfully maintain the weight loss that was initially achieved by dieting.

PRACTICAL IMPLICATIONS

Table 1-1 illustrates the theoretical impact on energy balance produced by a chronic increase in physical activity. For the purposes of this example, assume that a moderately overweight, sedentary woman initiates an exercise program in which she expends 1425 kJ/h (340 kcal/h) in low-intensity physical activity. Because the energy necessary for internal work (i.e., RMR) would have been approximately 251 kJ (60 kcal) during that same hour had she not been active, the net increase is 1174 kJ (280 kcal). If she engaged in exercise for a total of 5 h/wk, this would in-

TABLE 1-1. *Theoretical impact on energy balance of adding 5 h/wk of low-intensity exercise to an individual's normal daily activities.* See text for details.

No Energy Compensation		
Length of Program	Energy Deficit	Body Weight Loss
12 weeks	70.32 MJ (16,800 kcal)	1.9–2.2 kg
20 weeks	117.20 MJ (28,000 kcal)	3.1–3.7 kg
52 weeks	304.71 MJ (72,800 kcal)	8.1–9.7 kg
25% Energy Compensation		
Length of Program	Energy Deficit	Body Weight Loss
12 weeks	52.74 MJ (12,600 kcal)	1.4–1.7 kg
20 weeks	87.90 MJ (21,000 kcal)	2.3–2.8 kg
52 weeks	228.53 MJ (54,600 kcal)	6.1–7.3 kg
50% Energy Compensation		
Length of Program	Energy Deficit	Body Weight Loss
12 weeks	35.16 MJ (8,400 kcal)	1.4–1.7 kg
20 weeks	58.60 MJ (14,000 kcal)	2.3–2.8 kg
52 weeks	152.36 MJ (36,400 kcal)	6.1–7.3 kg

crease TEPA by 5870 kJ/wk (1400 kcal/wk) or an average increase in energy expenditure of 840 kJ/d (200 kcal/d).

This increase in chronic physical activity represents a perturbation to the steady state of energy and macronutrient balance. To maintain the steady state, the system must completely compensate for the effects of the increased physical activity. This can occur if total energy intake increases to match the increased energy expenditure due to activity and if the composition of fuel consumed is changed to match the composition of fuel oxidized. Most available data suggest this is not the case and that energy compensation for alterations in physical activity is incomplete. If there were no energy compensation for the exercise, the subject would be in a negative energy balance of 840 kJ/d (200 kcal/d). At 25% compensation, the negative energy balance would be 630 kJ/d (150 kcal/d), and at 50% compensation, it would be 420 kJ/d (100 kcal/d). Unless energy compensation is complete, the energy deficit will eventually affect body weight and body composition. Note in Table 1-1 that the projected weight loss due to participation in exercise programs of 12-, 20-, or 52-wk duration, with varying degrees of energy compensation, is only estimated. In actuality, weight loss is accompanied by decreases in RMR and in the energy cost of physical activity, which can attenuate the magnitude of the energy deficit over time. Also, the amount of body weight lost over time will depend on the amount of fat versus lean tissue lost. Because this energy imbalance cannot be maintained indefinitely, the final effect of the activity on energy requirements cannot be determined until the system reaches a new steady-state.

If energy compensation is not complete, some loss of body mass will occur. The degree of energy imbalance will determine the amount of body mass lost, and the nature of the macronutrient imbalance will affect the composition of the body mass lost. Body weight will stabilize when enough body mass is lost so that energy expenditure is reduced to match energy intake. Body composition will stabilize when the composition of fuel oxidized matches the composition of ingested energy. For example, the weight loss that occurs with increased aerobic exercise appears to come largely from body fat stores. This is illustrated in a study by Bouchard et al. (1994), who produced negative energy balance over 93 d by exercise alone (with a constant energy intake) in identical twins. The subjects averaged 5 kg of weight loss, all from body fat. Because fat oxidation is proportional to fat mass, a reduction in body fat stores will eventually result in a decline in fat oxidation. Body fat mass will continue to decline until fat oxidation is aligned with fat intake.

Figure 1-3 illustrates two ways in which the steady state of energy and macronutrient balance might be disrupted and reestablished in an overweight subject who increases chronic physical activity with a net

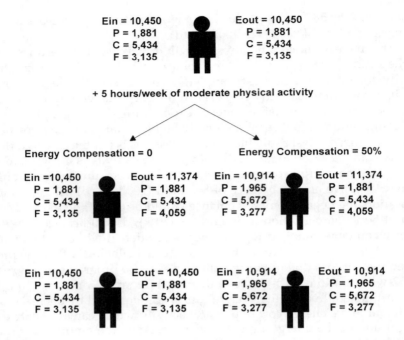

FIGURE 1-3. *The extent to which a chronic change in physical activity alters body weight and body composition depends both on the composition of fuel oxidized for physical activity and the composition of energy compensation.* All values are kJ/day. E_{in}, energy intake, E_{out}, energy expenditure; P, protein; C, carbohydrate; F, fat. See the text for details. Adapted from Hill et al. (1995).

energy cost of 924 kJ/d (220 kcal/d). In one case, we assume there is no energy compensation and that the exercise creates an imbalance only in fat. This would reduce fat mass until fat oxidation is equated with fat intake and the subject would reestablish the steady state of energy and macronutrient balance(but at a lower body weight and body fat content. In this case total energy intake and expenditure would still be 10.45 MJ/d (2,500 kcal/d). In the second example, we assume that the subject compensated for 50% of the energy expended in exercise and that the composition was the same as the usual diet. A new steady state of energy and macronutrient balance will be reached at 10.914 MJ/d (2,610 kcal), and body weight and body composition will be altered. In this case, there may be a slight increase in FFM because a state of positive protein balance is created by the exercise. In both cases, the net result will be a change in the settling point and a new functional phenotype. The latter will reflect the change in behavior (i.e., altered energy intake) and the change in the adaptive metabolic state.

DIRECTIONS FOR FUTURE RESEARCH

To begin to quantify the change in the settling point, it is important to consider the effects of physical activity on long-term macronutrient intake and oxidation. More research is needed to understand how a change in physical activity affects macronutrient balance. There is still uncertainty regarding the net effects of physical activity on daily oxidation rates of protein, carbohydrate, and fat. Little information is available about the effects of different modes, intensities, and durations of exercise on 24 h (or longer) substrate oxidation rates in human subjects. For example, whereas carbohydrate oxidation may predominate during an activity such as weight lifting, fat oxidation may increase following this activity, as the available carbohydrate may be used more for restoration of glycogen stores than for oxidation. Carefully controlled studies are needed to determine the net 24 h effects of different types of exercise on nutrient oxidation.

The largest source of differences in energy requirements among individuals is differences in the amount of physical activity performed. In light of this, it is somewhat surprising that so much attention has been focused on understanding the reasons for individual differences in RMR and TEF and so little on understanding the reasons for differences in the energy expended in physical activity. Future research should focus on elucidating the reasons for individual differences in amounts of physical activity. Such reasons may include genetic factors, environmental factors, and their interactions.

We know very little about the extent to which energy compensation occurs following exercise. It is likely that characteristics of both the exercise and of the subject contribute to this compensation. Finally, the net effects of a chronic change in physical activity depend on how the steady state of energy and macronutrient balance is reestablished. We need to understand how and over what period of time this occurs and to identify the factors that influence this process. Individual differences in how this steady state is reestablished would be expected to contribute to individual differences in the extent to which a change in physical activity would alter energy requirements and change the settling point.

In summary, future research is needed to address the following specific questions:

1) What exercise mode and intensity maximizes energy expenditure? What exercise regimen minimizes the energy compensation that can occur via diet and physical activity? The answers to these questions may well vary among male, female, lean, and obese subjects.

2) What are the impacts of different exercise modes and intensities on 24 h macronutrient oxidation and balance?

3) How does exercise training affect 24-h macronutrient oxidation in response to acute exercise?

4) Do acute and chronic exercise affect the rate at which macronutrient oxidation adjusts to changes in macronutrient intake?

5) What is the role of skeletal muscle morphology and metabolism in macronutrient oxidation and obesity risk? Do the training adaptations that occur in skeletal muscle with chronic exercise contribute to maintenance of fat balance at a lower body fat mass?

SUMMARY

The ability of the human body to adjust energy expenditure and macronutrient oxidation to energy and macronutrient intakes is essential for maintenance of homeostasis and stable body weight and body composition. Although a single bout of exercise presents a challenge to the maintenance of homeostasis owing to the increased energy expenditure and macronutrient oxidation necessary to fuel the activity, its impact is short-lived and has little if any impact of body weight and composition. However, chronic changes in physical activity may be the factor most capable of producing chronic changes in energy requirements, leading to changes in the levels at which body weight and body composition are maintained over time.

The overall impact of a change in physical activity on energy and macronutrient requirements is not simple to predict because a change in one component of energy-nutrient balance can affect other components. For example, a change in physical activity that increases energy expenditure can also affect the amount and composition of subsequent energy intake. If a change in physical activity produces energy imbalance, that imbalance cannot be maintained indefinitely and must lead to further changes in energy intake and/or expenditure. The net effect on energy and macronutrient requirements of a change in physical activity will be influenced by how the individual re-achieves energy and nutrient balance following these changes. This in turn will depend on the characteristics of the subject and of the physical activity.

The accumulation of excess body fat appears to be a problem that results from inadequate fat oxidation relative to intake. An increase in body fat mass increases plasma free fatty acid concentrations, which, in turn, are associated with increased fat oxidation. The increase in fat utilization that accompanies obesity helps re-establish a new equilibrium between fat intake and fat oxidation that serves to stabilize body weight, albeit at the cost of obesity. Because exercise can increase total daily energy expenditure and fat oxidation, chronic exercise may substitute for expansion of the adipose tissue mass, allowing the physically active individual to achieve fat balance at a lower body fat mass.

ACKNOWLEDGEMENTS

Supported by Colorado Agricultural Experiment Station Project 616 (CLM), and NIH grants DK42549 and DK38088 (JOH). Special thanks are extended to Drs. Ron Maughan, Clyde Williams, and Mel Williams for their critiques of this chapter.

BIBLIOGRAPHY

Abou Mrad, J., F. Yakubu, D. Lin, J.C. Peters, J.B. Atkinson, and J.O. Hill (1992). Skeletal muscle composition in dietary obesitysusceptible and dietary obesityresistant rats. *Am. J. Physiol.* 262:R684R688.

Acheson, K.J., J.P.Flatt, and E. Jequier (1982). Glycogen synthesis versus lipogenesis after a 500 g carbohydrate meal in man. *Metabolism* 31:1234–1240.

Acheson, K.J., Y. Schutz, T. Bessard, K. Anantharaman, J.P. Flatt, and E. Jequier (1988). Glycogen storage capacity and de novo lipogenesis during massive carbohydrate overfeeding in man. *Am. J. Clin. Nutr.* 48:240247.

Andik, I., J. Bank, I. Moring, and G. Y. Szegvari (1954). The effects of exercise on the intake and selection of food in the rat. *Acta Physiol. Hung.* 5:457–461.

Applegate, E. A., D. E. Upton, and J. S. Stern (1984). Exercise and detraining: effect on food intake, adiposity and lipogenesis in Osborne-Mendel rats made obese by a high fat diet. *J. Nutr.* 114:447–459.

Applegate, E. A., D. E. Upton, and J. S. Stern (1982). Food intake, body composition and blood lipids following treadmill exercise in male and female rats. *Physiol. Behav.* 28:917–920.

Arciero, P. M.I. Goran, and E.T. Poehlman (1993). Resting metabolic rate is lower in women than in men. *J. Appl. Physiol.* 75:2514–2520.

Astrup, A. (1993). Dietary composition, substrate balances and body fat in subjects with a predisposition to obesity. *Int. J. Obes.* 17(Suppl. 3):S32S36.

Astrup, A., B. Buemann, N.J. Christensen, and S. Toubro (1994). Failure to increase lipid oxidation in response to increasing dietary fat content in formerly obese women. *Am. J. Physiol.* 266:E592–599.

Bahr, R., and S. Maehlum (1986). Excess postexercise oxygen consumption A short review. *Acta Physiol. Scand.*128 (Suppl 556):99104.

Bahr, R., and O.M.Sejersted (1991). Effect of intensity of exercise on excess postexercise oxygen consumption. *Metabolism* 40:836–841.

Baldwin, K.M., P.J. Campbell, and D.A. Cooke. (1977). Glycogen, lactate, and alanine changes in muscle fiber types during graded exercise. *J. Appl. Physiol.* 27:691–695.

Ballor, D.L., and E.T. Poehlman (1992). Resting metabolic rate and coronary heart disease risk factors in aerobically and resistance-trained women. *Am. J. Clin. Nutr.* 56:968–974.

Bennett, C., G.W. Reed, J.C. Peters, N.N. Abumrad, M. Sun, and J.O. Hill (1992) Shortterm effects of dietaryfat ingestion on energy expenditure and nutrient balance. *Am. J. Clin. Nutr.* 55:10711077.

Bergstrom, J., and E. Hultman (1967). A study of the glycogen metabolism during exercise in man. *Scand. J. Clin. Lab. Invest.* 19:218–228.

Bielinski, R., Y. Schutz, and E. Jequier (1985). Energy metabolism during the postexercise recovery in man. *Am. J. Clin. Nutr.* 42:69–82.

Bingham, S.A., G.R. Goldberg, W.A. Coward, A.M. Prentice, and J.H. Cummings (1989). The effect of exercise and improved physical fitness on basal metabolic rate. *Br. J. Nutr.* 61:155–173.

Blaak, E.E., K.R. Westerterp, O. Bar-or, L.J.M. Wouters, and W.H.M. Saris (1992). Total energy expenditure and spontaneous activity in relation to training in obese boys. *Am. J. Clin. Nutr.* 55:777–782.

Boss O, S. Samec, A. Paoloni-Giacobino, C. Rossier, A. Dulloo, J. Seydoux, P. Muzzin, and J.P. Giacobino (1997). Uncoupling protein-3: a new member of the mitochondrial carrier family with tissue specific expression. *Fed. Europ. Biochem. Soc. Let.* 408:39–42.

Bouchard, C., A. Tremblay, J-P Despres, G. Theriault, A. Nadeau, P.J. Lupien, F. Moorjani, D. Prudhomme, and G. Fournier (1994). The response to exercise with constant energy intake in identical twins. *Obes. Res.* 2:400–411.

Bray, G.A. (1989). 1989 McCollum Award Lecture. Genetic and hypothalamic mechanisms for obesity—Finding the needle in the haystack. *Am. J. Clin. Nutr.* 50:891902.

Broeder, C.E., M. Brenner, Z. Hofman, I.J. Paijmans, E.L. Thomas, and J.H. Wilmore (1991). The metabolic consequences of low and moderate intensity exercise with or without feeding in lean and borderline obese males. *Int. J. Obes.* 15:95–104.

Broeder, C.E., K.A. Burrhus, L.S. Svanevik, and J.H. Wilmore (1992a). The effects of aerobic fitness on resting metabolic rate. *Am. J. Clin. Nutr.* 55:795801.

Broeder, C.E., K.A. Burrhus, L.S. Svanevik and J.H. Wilmore (1992b). The effects of either highintensity resistance or endurance training on resting metabolic rate. *Am. J. Clin. Nutr.* 55:802810.

Brooks, G.A., and J. Mercier (1994). Balance of carbohydrate and lipid uilization during exercise: the "crossover" concept. *J. Appl. Physiol.* 76:2253–2261.

Brouns, F., W.H.M. Saris, E. Beckers, H. Adlercreutz, G.J. van der Vusse, H.A. Keizer, H. Kuipers, P. Menherre, A.J. Wangenmakers, and F. Ten Hoor (1989). Metabolic changes induced by sustained exhaustive cycling and diet manipulation. *Int. J. Sports Med.* 10(Suppl. 1):S49–S62.

Bullough, R.C., M.A. Harris, C.G. Gillette, and C.L. Melby (1995). Interaction of acute changes in exercise energy expenditure and energy intake on resting metabolic rate. *Am. J. Clin. Nutr.* 61:473–481.

Burke C.M., R.C.Bullough, and C.L.Melby (1993). Resting metabolic rate and postprandial thermogenesis by level of aerobic fitness in young women. *Eur. J. Clin. Nutr.* 47:575–85.

Butterfield, G.E., and D.H. Calloway (1984). Physical activity improves protein utilization in young men. *Br. J. Nutr.* 51:171–184.

Carroll, R.M., and S. Klein (1995). Effect of energy compared with carbohydrate restriction on the lipolytic response to epinephrine. *Am. J. Clin. Nutr.* 62:757–760.

Coggan, A.R. (1997). Plasma glucose metabolism during exercise: effect of endurance training in humans. *Med. Sci. Sports Exerc.* 29:620–627.

Coggan, A.R., C.A. Gaguso, B.D. Williams, L.S. Sidossis, and A. Gastaldelli (1995). Glucose kinetics during high-intensity exercise in endurance-trained and untrained humans. *J. Appl. Physiol.* 78:1203–1207, 1995.

Colditz, G.A., W.C. Willett, A. Rotnitzky, and J.E. Manson (1995). Weight gain as a risk factor for clinical diabetes in women. *Ann. Internal Med.* 122:481–486.

Colditz, G.A., W.C. Willett, M.J. Stampfer, J.E. Manson, C.H. Hennekens, R.A. Arky, and F.E. Speizer (1990). Weight as a risk factor for clinical diabetes in women. *Am. J. Epidemiol.* 132:501–513.

Considine, R.V., and J. F. Caro (1996). Leptin: genes, concepts and clinical perspective. *Horm. Res.* 46:249–256.

Considine, R.V., E.L. Considine, C.J. Williams, M.R. Nyce, S.A. Magosin, T.L. Bauer, E.L. Rosato, and J. F. Caro (1995). Evidence against either a premature stop codon or the absence of obese gene mRNA in human obesity. *J. Clin. Invest.* 95:2986–2988.

Coyle, E.F. (1995). Substrate utilization during exercise in active people. *Am. J. Clin. Nutr.* 61(suppl):968S-979S.

Coyle, E.F., A.R. Coggan, M.K. Hemmett, and J.L. Ivy (1986). Muscle glycogen utilization during prolonged strenuous exercise when fed carbohydrate. *J. Appl. Physiol.* 61:165–172.

Cusin I., A. Sainsbury, P. Doyle, F. Rohner-Jeanrenaud, and B. Jeanrenaud (1995). The ob gene and insulin. A relationship leading to clues to the understanding of obesity. *Diabetes* 44:1467–1470.

Cusin I., F. Rohner-Jeanrenaud, A. Stricker-Krongrad, and B. Jeanrenaud (1996). Weight-reducing effect of intracerebroventricular bolus injection of leptin in genetically obese fa/fa rats: reduced sensitivity compared with lean animals. *Diabetes* 45:1446–1451.

Davies, K.J, L. Packer, and G.A. Brooks (1981). Biochemical adaptation of mitochondria, muscle, and whole-animal respiration to endurance training. *Arch. Biochem. Biophys.* 209:539–554

Davies, P.S.W., J. Gregory, and A. White (1995). Physical activity and body fatness in pre-school children. *Int. J. Obes.* 19:6–10.

Davis, J.R., A.R. Tagliafero, R. Ketzer, T. Gerardo, J. Nichols, and J. Wheeler (1983). Variations in dietary induced thermogenesis and body fatness with aerobic capacity. *Eur. J Physiol.* 50:319–329.

Decombaz, J., P. Reinhardt, K. Anantharaman, G. Von Glutz, and J.R. Poortmans (1979). Biochemical changes in a 100 km run: free amino acids, urea, and creatinine. *Eur. J. Appl. Physiol.* 41:61–72.

Deuster, P.A., G.P. Chrousos, A. Luger, J.E. DeBolt, L.L. Bernier, U.H. Trostmann, S. B. Kyle, L.C. Montgomery, and D.L. Loriaux (1989). Hormonal and metabolic responses of untrained, moderately trained, and highly trained men to three exercise intensities. *Metabolism* 38:141–148.

Dohm, G.L., R.T. Williams, G.J. Kasperek, and A.M. Van Rij (1982). Increased excretion of urea and N-methylhistidine by rats and humans after a bout of exercise. *J. Appl. Physiol.* 52:27–33.

Donovan, C.M., and K.D. Sumida (1997). Training enhanced hepatic gluconeogenesis: the importance for glucose homeostasis during exercise. *Med. Sci. Sports Exerc.* 29:628–634.

Eck, L.H., C. HackettRenner, and L.M. Klesges (1992). Impact of diabetic status, dietary intake, physical activity, and smoking status on body mass index in NHANES II. *Am. J. Clin. Nutr.* 56:329333.

Evans, W.J., E.C. Fisher, R.A. Hoerr, and V.R. Young (1983). Protein metabolism and endurance exercise. *Phys. Sports Med.* 11:63–72.

Fern, E.B., R.N. Bielinski, and Y. Schutz (1991). Effects of exaggerated amino acid and protein supply in man. *Experientia* 47:168–172.

Ferrannini, E. (1988). The theoretical bases of indirect calorimetry: a review. *Metabolism* 37:287–301.

Flatt, J.P. (1987). Dietary fat, carbohydrate balance, and weight maintenance: effects of exercise. *Am. J. Clin. Nutr.* 45:296–306.

Flatt, J.P. (1995). Use and storage of carbohydrate and fat. *Am. J. Clin. Nutr.* 61(suppl):952S-959S.

Flatt, J.P., E. Ravussin, K.J. Acheson, and E. Jequier (1985). Effects of dietary fat on postprandial substrate oxidation and on carbohydrate and fat balances. *J. Clin. Invest.* 76:10191024.

Fleury, C., M. Neverova, S. Collins, S. Raimbault, O. Champaigny, C. Levi-Meyrueis, F. Bouillard, M.F. Seldin, R.S. Surwit, D. Ricquier, and C.H. Warden (1997). Uncoupling protein-2: a novel gene linked to obesity and hyperinsulinemia. *Nature Genetics* 15:269–272.

Frederich R.C., B. Lollman, A. Hamann, A. Napolitano-Rosen, B.B. Kahn, B.B. Lowell, and J.S. Flier (1995). Expression of ob mRNA and its encoded protein in rodents. *J. Clin. Invest.* 96:1658–1663.

Freedman-Akabas, S., E. Colt, H.R. Kissileff, and F.X. Pi-Sunyer (1985). Lack of a sustained increase in VO_2 following exercise in fit and unfit subjects. *Am. J. Clin. Nutr.* 41:545–549.

Friedman, J.E., and P.W.R. Lemon (1989). Effect of chronic endurance exercise on the retention of dietary protein. *Int. J. Sports Med.* 10:118–123.

Frontera, W.R., C.N. Meredith, K.P. O'Reilly, H.G. Knuttgen, and W.J. Evans (1988). Strength conditioning in older men: skeletal muscle hypertrophy and improved function. *J. Appl. Physiol.* 64:1038–1044.

Garrow, J.S. (1995). Exercise in the treatment of obesity: a marginal contribution. *Int. J. Obes.* 19:S126–S129.

Garthwaite, S. M., H. Cheng, J. E. Bryan, B. W. Craig, and J. O. Holloszy (1986). Aging, exercise and food restriction: effects on body composition. *Mech. Aging Devel.* 36:187–196.

Geerling, B.J., M.S. Alles, P.R. Murgatroyd, G.R. Goldberg, M. Harding, and A.M. Prentice (1994). Fatness in relation to substrate oxidation during exercise. *Int. J. Obes.* 18:453459.

Gilbert, J.A., and J.E. Misner (1993). Failure to find increased TEM at rest and during exercise in aerobically trained and resistance trained subjects. *Int. J. Sports Nutr.* 3:55–66.

Gilbert, J.A., J.E.Misner, R.A. Boileau, L. Ji, and M.H. Slaughter (1991). Lower thermic effect of a meal post-exercise in aerobically trained and resistance-trained subjects. *Med. Sci. Sports. Exerc.* 23:825–830.

Gillette, C.A., R.C. Bullough, and C.L. Melby (1994). Postexercise energy expenditure in response to acute aerobic or resistive exercise. *Int. J. Sport Nutr.* 4:347–360.

Gollnick, P.D. (1985). Metabolism of substrates: energy substrate metabolism during exercise as modified by training. *Fed. Proc.* 44:353–357.

Gontzea, I., R. Sutzescu, and S. Dumitrache (1975). The influence of adaptation of physical effort on nitrogen balance in man. *Nutr. Reports Int.* 11:231–236.

Gontzea, I., P. Sutzescu, and S. Dumitrache (1974). The influence of muscle activity on nitrogen balance and the need of man for proteins. *Nutr. Reports Int.* 10:35–43.

Goran, M.I., and E.T. Poehlman (1992). Endurance training does not enhance total energy expenditure in healthy elderly persons. *Am. J. Physiol.* 263:E950–E957.

Griffiths, A.J., S.M. Humphreys, M.L. Clark, B.A. Fielding, and K.N. Frayn (1994). Immediate metabolic availability of dietary fat in combination with carbohydrate. *Am. J. Clin. Nutr.* 59:53–59.

Haapanen, N., S. Miilunpalo, M. Pasanen, P. Oja, and I Vuori (1997). Association between leisure time physical activity and 10–year body mass change among working-aged men and women. *Int. J. Obes.* 21:288–296.

Halaas, J.L., K.S. Gajiwala, M. Maffei, S.L. Cohen, B.T. Chait, D. Rabinowitz, R.L. Lallone, S.K. Burley, and J.M. Friedman (1995). Weight-reducing effect of the plasma protein encoded by the obese gene. *Science* 269:543–546.

Hamilton B.S., D. Paglia, A.Y.M. Kwan, and M. Deitel (1995). Increase obese mRNA expression in omental fat cells from massively obese humans. *Nature Med.* 1:953–956.

Hellerstedt, W.L., R.W. Jeffrey, and D.M. Murray (1990). The association between alcohol intake and adiposity in the general population. *Am. J. Epidemiol.* 132: 594–611.

Herring, J.L., P.A. Mole, C.N. Meredith, and J.S. Stern (1992). Effect of suspending exercise training on resting metabolic rate in women. *Med. Sci. Sports Exerc.* 24:59–64.

Hickey M.S., R.V. Considine, R.G. Israel, T.L. Mahar, M.R. McCammon, G.L. Tyndall, J.A. Houmard, and J.F. Caro (1997). Leptin is related to body fat content in male distance runners. *Am. J. Physiol.* 271:E938–E940.

Hickson, J.F., I. Wolinsky, G.P. Rodriquez, J.M. Pivarnik, M.C. Kent, and N.W. Shier (1986). Failure of weight training to affect urinary indices of protein metabolism in men. *Med. Sci. Sports Exerc.* 18:563–567.

Hill, J.O., S.B. Heymsfield, C.B. McManus, and M. DiGirolamo (1984). Meal size and thermic response to food in male subjects as a function of maximum aerobic capacity. *Metabolism* 33:743–749.

Hill, J.O., C. Melby, S.L. Johnson, and J.C. Peters (1995). Physical activity and energy requirements. *Am. J. Clin. Nutr.* 62(suppl):1059S-1066S.

Hill, J.O., M.J. Pagliassotti, and J.C. Peters (1994). Nongenetic determinants of obesity and fat topography. In Genetic Determinants of Obesity, C. Bouchard (ed.), Boca Raton:CRC Press Inc., pp. 35–48.

Holloszy, J.O., and E.F. Coyle (1984). Adaptations of skeletal muscle to endurance exercise and their metabolic consequences. *J. Appl. Physiol.* 56:831–838.

Hoppeler, H. (1986). Exercise-induced ultrastructural changes in skeletal muscle. *Int. J. Sports Med.* 7:187–204.

Horton, T.J., H. Drougas, A. Brachey, G.W. Reed, J.C. Peters, and J.O. Hill (1995). Fat and carbohydrate overfeeding in humans: different effects on energy storage. *Am. J. Clin. Nutr.* 62:19–29.

Houmard, J.A., P.C. Egan, P.D. Neufer, J.E. Friedman, W.S. Wheeler, R.G. Israel, and G.L. Dohm (1991). Elevated skeletal muscle glucose transporter levels in exercise-trained middle-aged men. *Am. J. Physiol.* 261:E437–E443.

Hurley, B.F., P.M. Nemeth, W.H. Martin, J.M. Hagberg, G.P. Dalsky, and J.O. Holloszy (1986). Muscle triglyceride utilization during exercise: training effect. *J. Appl. Physiol.* 60:562–567.

Jebb S.A., A.M. Prentice, G. Goldberg, P.R. Murgatroyd, A.E. Black, and W.A. Coward (1996). Changes in macronutrient balance during over- and underfeeding assessed by 12–d continuous whole-body calorimetry. *Am. J. Clin. Nutr.* 64:259–66.

Jen, K.L.C., R. Almario, J.Ilagan, S. Zhong, P. Archer, and P.K. H. Lin (1992). Long-term exercise training and retirement in genetically obese rats: effect on food intake, feeding efficiency and carcass composition. *Int. J. Obes.* 16:519–527.

Jequier, E., K.J. Acheson, and Y. Schutz (1987). Assessment of energy expenditure and fuel utilization in man. *Ann. Rev. Nutr.* 7:187208.

Karlsson, J., and B. Saltin (1971). Muscle glycogen utilization during work of different intensities. In: B. Pernow and B. Saltin (eds.) *Muscle Metabolism During Exercise.* New York: Plenum Press, pp. 289–299.

Kasperek, G.J., and R.D. Snider (1987). Effect of exercise intensity and starvation on the activation of branched-chain keto acid dehydrogenase by exercise. *Am. J. Physiol.* 252:E33–E37.

Katch, V. L., R. Martin, and J. Martin (1979). Effects of exercise intensity on food consumption in the male rat. *Am. J. Clin. Nutr.* 23:1401–1407.

Keesey, R.E., S.W. Corbett, M.D. Hirvonen, and L.N. Kaufman (1984). Heat production and body weight changes following lateral hypothalamic lesions. *Physiol. Behav.* 32:309317.

Kelley D.E., and J.A. Simoneau (1994). Impaired free fatty acid utilization by skeletal muscle in non-insulin dependent diabetes mellitus. *J. Clin. Invest.* 94:2349–56.

Kendall, A., D.A. Levitsky, B.J. Strupp, and L. Lissner (1991). Weight loss on a lowfat diet: consequence of the imprecision of the control of food intake in humans. *Am. J. Clin. Nutr.* 53:11241129.

Kiens, B. (1977). Effect of endurance training on fatty acid metabolism: local adaptations. *Med. Sci. Sports Exerc.* 29:640–645.

King, N. A., and J. E. Blundell (1995). High-fat foods overcome the energy expenditure induced by high-intensity cycling or running. *Eur. J. Clin. Nutr.* 49:114–123.

King, N. A., V. J. Burley, and J. E. Blundell (1994). Exercise-induced suppression of appetite: effects on food intake and implications for energy balance. *Eur. J. Clin. Nut.* 48:715–724.

Kirkwood, S.P., L. Packer, and G.A. Brooks (1987). Effects of endurance training on mitochondrial reticulum in limb skeletal muscle. *Arch. Biochem. Biophys.* 255:80–88.

Kissilef, H. R., F. X. Pi-Sunyer, K. Segal, S. Meltzer, and P. A. Foelsch (1990). Acute effects of exercise on food intake in obese and nonobese women. *Am. J. Clin. Nutr.* 52:240–245.

Klein, S., E.F. Coyle, and R.R. Wolfe (1995). Effect of exercise on lipolytic sensitivity in endurance-trained athletes. *J. Appl. Physiol.* 78:2201–2206.

Klein, S., E.F.Coyle, and R.R. Wolfe (1994). Fat metabolism during low-intensity exercise in endurance trained and untrained men. *Am. J. Physiol.* 267:E934–E940.

Klein, S., J.M. Weber, E.F. Coyle, and R.R. Wolfe (1996). Effect of endurance training on glycerol kinetics during strenuous exercise in humans. *Metabolism* 45:357–361.

Klesges, R.C., L.M. Klesges, C.K. Haddock, and L.H. Eck (1992). A longitudinal analysis of the impact of dietary intake and physical activity on weight change in adults. *Am. J. Clin. Nutr.* 55:818822.

Kohrt W.M, M. Landt, and S.J. Birge (1996). Serum leptin levels are reduced in response to exercise training, but not hormone replacement therapy, in older women. *J. Clin. Endocrin. Metab.* 81:3980–3985.

Kolaczynski J.W., R.V. Considine, J. Ohannesian, C. Marco, I. Opentanova, M.R. Nyce, M. Myint, and J.F. Caro (1996a). Responses of leptin to short-term fasting and refeeding in humans: a link with ketogenesis but not ketones themselves. *Diabetes* 45:1511–1515.

Kolaczynski J.W., J. Ohannesian, R.V. Considine, C. Marco, and J.F. Caro (1996b). Response of leptin to short term and prolonged overfeeding in humans. *J. Clin. Endocr. Metab.* 91:4162–4165.

Kriketos A.D., S.Lillioja, G.J. Cooney, M. Milner, J.R. Sutton JR, D.A. Pan, M.M.L. Wiersma, L.A. Baur, and L.H. Storlien (1995). Relationships between muscle metabolism and obesity. *Int. J. Obes.* 19(Suppl. 4):S133 (Abstract).

Kuczmarski, R.J., K.M. Flegal, S.M. Campbell, and C.L. Johnson (1994). Increasing prevalence of overweight among U.S. adults. The National Health and Nutrition Examination Surveys, 1960 to 1991. *J. Am. Med. Assoc.* 272:205–211.

Larson, D.E., R.T. Ferraro, D.S. Robertson, and E. Ravussin (1995). Energy metabolism in weight-stable postobese individuals. *Am. J. Clin. Nutr.* 62:735–739.

Larue-Achagiotis, C., C. Martin, P. Verger, M. Chabert, and J. Louis-Sylvestre (1993). Effects of acute treadmill exercise and delayed access to food on food selection in rats. *Physiol. Behav.* 53:403–408.

Larue-Achagiotis, C., C. Martin, P. Verger, and J. Louis-Sylvestre (1992). Dietary self-selection or standard complete diet: body weight gain and meal pattern in rats. *Physiol. Behav.* 51:995–999.

Larue-Achagiotis, C., N. Rieth, and J. Louis-Sylvestre (1994). Exercise training modifies nutrient self-selection in rats. *Physiol. Behav.* 56:367–372.

LeBlanc, J., P. Diamond, J. Cote, and A. Labrie (1984). Hormonal factors in reduced postprandial heat production of exercise-trained subjects. *J. Appl. Physiol.* 57:772–776.

LeBlanc J., A. Nadeau, M. Boulay, and S. Rousseau-Migneron (1979). Effects of physical training and adiposity on glucose metabolism and 125–I insulin binding. *J. Appl. Physiol.* 46:235–239.

Lemon, P.W.R., M.J. Benevenga, J.P. Mullin, and F.J. Nagle (1985). Effects of daily exercise and food intake on leucine oxidation. *Biochem. Med.* 33:67–76.

Lemon, P.W.R., F.J. Nagle, J.P. Mullin, and N.J. Benevenga (1982). In vivo leucine oxidation at rest and during two intensities of exercise. *J. Appl. Physiol.* 53:947–954.

Lemon, P.W.R., M.A. Tarnopolsky, J.D. MacDougall, and S.A. Atkinson (1992). Protein requirements and muscle mass/strength changes during intensive training in novice bodybuilders. *J. Appl. Physiol.* 73:767–775.

Lew, E.A., and L. Garfunkel (1979). Variations in mortality by weight among 750,000 men and women. *J. Clin. Epidemiol.* 32:563–576.

Lewis D.E., L. Shellard, D.G. Koeslag, D.E. Boer, D. McCarthy, P.E. McKibbin, J.C. Russell, and G. Williams (1993). Intense exercise and food restriction cause similar hypothalamic neuropeptide Y increases in rats. *Am. J. Physiol.* 264:E279–E284.

Lissner, L., D.A. Levitsky, B.J. Strupp, H.J. Kalkwarf, and D.A. Roe (1987). Dietary fat and the regulation of energy intake in human subjects. *Am. J. Clin. Nutr.* 46:886892.

Liu, S., M.K. Serdula, D.F. Williamson, A.H. Mokdad, and T. Byers (1995). A prospective study of alcohol intake and change in body weight among US adults. *Am. J. Epidemiol.* 140:912–920.

Lohmann, D., F. Liebold, W. Heilmann, H. Senger, and A. Pohl (1978). Diminished insulin response in highly trained athletes. *Metabolism* 27:521–524.

Lonnqvist F., P. Arner, L. Nordfors, and M. Schalling (1995). Overexpression of the obese (ob) gene in adipose tissue of human obese subjects. *Nature Med.* 1:950–953.

Lundholm, K., G. Holm, L. Lindmark, B. Larsson, L. Sjostrom, and P. Bjorntorp (1986). Thermogenic effect of food in physically well-trained elderly men. *Eur. J. Appl. Physiol.* 55:486–492.

MacDonald, I (1993). Alcohol and overweight. In P.M. Verschuren (ed). *Health Issues Related to Alcohol Consumption.* Washington DC:ILSI Press, pp. 263–280.

Martin, W.H. (1997). Effect of endurance training on fatty acid metabolism during whole body exercise. *Med. Sci. Sports Exerc.* 29:635–639.

Maughan, R., and K.P. Aulin (1997). Energy costs of physical activity. *World Rev. Nutr. Diet* 82:18–32.

Mayer, J., P. Roy, and K. Mitra (1956). Relation between caloric intake, body weight, and physical works in an industrial male population in West Bengal. *Am. J. Clin. Nutr.* 4:169–171.

Meredith, C.N., M.J. Zackin, W.R. Frontera, and W.J. Evans (1989). Dietary protein requirements and protein metabolism in endurance-trained men. *J. Appl. Physiol.* 66:2850–2856.

Melby, C.L., D.G. Goldflies, and G.C. Hyner (1991). Blood pressure and anthropometric differences in regularly exercising and nonexercising black adults. *Clin. Exper. Hypert.* 13:1233–48.

Melby, C.L., C. Scholl, G. Edwards, and R. Bullough (1993). Effect of acute resistance exercise on postexercise energy expenditure and resting metabolic rate. *J. Appl. Physiol.* 75:1847–1853.

Melby, C.L., W.D.Schmidt, and D. Corrigan (1990). Resting metabolic rate in weight-cycling collegiate wrestlers compared with physically active, noncycling control subjects. *Am. J. Clin. Nutr.* 52:409–14.

Melby, C.L., T. Ticknell, and W.D. Schmidt (1992). Energy expenditure following a bout of non-steady state resistance exercise. *J. Sports Med. Phys. Fit.* 32:128–135.

Meyer, G.A.L., G.M.E. Janssen, K.R. Westerterp, F. Verhoeven, W.H.M. Saris, and F. Ten Hoor (1991). The effect of a 5 month endurance-training programme on physical activity: evidence for a sex-difference in the metabolic response to exercise. *Eur. J. Appl. Physiol.* 62:11–17.

Montoye, H.J., W.D. Block, H.L. Metzner, and J.B. Keller (1976). Habitual physical activity and serum lipids: males, age 16–64, in a total community. *J. Chron. Disease* 29:697–709.

Obarzanek, E., G.B. Schreiber, P.B. Crawford, S.R. Goldman, P.M. Barrier, M.M. Frederick, and E. Lakatos (1994). Energy intake and physical activity in relation to indexes of body fat: the National Heart, Lung, and Blood Institute Growth and Health Study. *Am. J. Clin. Nutr.* 60:1522.

Odessey, R., E.A. Khairallah, and A.L. Goldberg (1974). Origin and possible significance of alanine production by skeletal muscle. *J. Biol. Chem.* 249:7623–7629.

Oscai, L. B. (1973). The role of exercise in weight control. In: J. H. Wilmore (ed.) *Exercise and Sport Sciences Reviews, Vol.1.* New York: Academic Press, pp. 103–123.

Oscai, L. B., S. P. Babviac, F. B. Dubach, J. A. McGarr, and C. N. Spirakis (1974). Exercise or food restriction: effect on adipose tissue cellularity. *Am. J. Physiol.* 227:901–904.

Oscai, L.B., R.A. Caruso, and A.C. Wergeles (1982). Lipoprotein lipase hydrolyzes endogenous triacylglycerols in muscle of exercised rats. *J. Appl. Physiol.* 52:1059–1063.

Owen, O.E., E. Kavle, and R.S. Owens (1986). A reappraisal of caloric requirements in healthy women. *Am. J. Clin. Nutr.* 44:1–19.

Owens, J.F., K.A. Matthews, R.R. Wing, and L.H. Kuller (1992). Can physical activity mitigate the effects of aging in middleaged women. *Circulation* 85:12651270.

Parízková, J., and L. Standova (1964). Influence of physical activity on a treadmill on the metabolism of adipose tissue in rats. *Br. J. Nutr.* 18:325–332.

Pelleymounter, M.A., M.J. Cullen, M.B. Baker, R. Hecht, D. Winters, T. Boone, and F. Collins (1995). Effects of the obese gene product on body weight regulation in ob/ob mice. *Science* 269:540–543.

Phelain, F.J., E. Reinke, M.A. Harris, and C.L. Melby (1997). Postexercise energy expenditure and substrate oxidation in young women resulting from exercise bouts of different intensity. *J. Am. Coll. Nutr.* 16:140–146.

Poehlman, E.T., T.L. McAuliffe, D.R. Van Houten, and E. Danforth, Jr. (1990). Influence of age and endurance training on metabolic rate and hormones in healthy men. *Am. J. Physiol.* 259:E66–E72.

Poehlman, E.T., C.L. Melby, S.F. Badylak, and J. Calles (1989). Aerobic fitness and resting energy expenditure in young adult males. *Metabolism* 38:85–90.

Poehlman, E.T., C.L. Melby, and M.I. Goran (1991). The impact of exercise and diet restriction on daily energy expenditure. *Sports Med.* 11:78–101.

Radhu, E., and S.P. Bessman (1983). Effect of exercise on protein degradation: 3–methylhistidine and creatinine excretion. *Biochem. Med.* 29:96–100.

Ravussin E., and B.A. Swinburn (1993). Metabolic predictors of obesity: cross-sectional versus longitudinal data. *Int. J. Obesity* 17(suppl. 3):S28–S31.

Ravussin E., K.J. Acheson, O. Vernet, E. Danforth, and E. Jecquier (1985). Evidence that insulin resistance is responsible for the decreased thermic effect of glucose in human obesity. *J. Clin. Invest.* 76:1268–1273.

Reger, W. E., T. A. Allison, and R. L. Kurucz (1984). Exercise, post-exercise metabolic rate and appetite. *Sport Health Nutr.* 2: 117–123.

Rennie, M.J., R.H.T. Edwards, C.T.M. Davies, S. Krywawych, D. Halliday, J.C. Waterlow, and D.J. Millward (1980). Protein and amino acid turnover during and after exercise. *Biochem. Soc. Trans.* 8:499–501.

Rennie, M.J., R.H.T. Edwards, S. Krywawych, C.T. Davies, D. Halliday, J.C. Waterlow, and D.J. Millard (1981). Effect of exercise on protein turnover in man. *Clin. Sci.* 61:627–639.

Richard, D. (1995). Exercise and the neurobiological control of food intake and energy expenditure. *Int. J. Obes.* 19(S4):S73–S79.

Richard, D., J. Arnold, and J. Leblanc (1986). Energy balance in exercise-trained rats acclimated at two environmental temperatures. *J. Appl. Physiol.* 60:1054–1059.

Rimm, E.B., M.J. Stampfer, E. Giovannucci, A. Ascherio, D. Spiegelman, G.A. Colditz, and W.C. Willett (1995). Body size and fat distribution as predictors of coronary heart disease among young and older US men. *Am. J. Epidemiol.* 141:1117–1127.

Rohner-Jeanrenaud F., I. Cusin, A. Sainsbury, K.E. Kakrzewska, and B. Jeanrenaud (1996). The loop system between neuropeptide Y and leptin in normal and obese rodents. *Horm. Metab. Res.* 28:642–648.

Richard, D. (1995). Exercise and the neurobiological control of food intake and energy expenditure. *Int. J. Obes.* 19 (S4): S73–S79.

Romijn, J.A., E.F. Coyle, J. Hibbert, and R.R. Wolfe (1993a). Comparison of indirect calorimetry and a new breath $^{13}C/^{12}C$ ratio method during strenuous exercise. *Am. J. Physiol.* 263:E64–E71.

Romijn, J.A., E.F. Coyle, and L. Sidossis (1993b). Regulation of endogenous fat and carbohydrate metabolism in relation to exercise intensity. *Am. J. Physiol.* 265:E380–391.

Romijn, J.A., E.F. Coyle, L.S. Sidossis, X.J. Zhang, and R.R. Wolfe (1995). Relationship between fatty acid delivery and fatty acid oxidation during strenuous exercise. *J. Appl. Physiol.* 79:1939–1945.

Romijn, J.A., S. Klein, E.F. Coyle, L.S. Sidossis, and R.R. Wolfe (1993c). Strenuous endurance training increases lipolysis and triglyceride-fatty acid cycling at rest. *J. Appl. Physiol.* 75:108–113.

Sainsbury A., I. Cusin, P. Doyle, F. Rohner-Jeanrenaud, and B. Jeanrenaud (1996). Intracerebroventricular administration of neuropeptide Y to normal rats increases obese gene expression in white adipose tissue. *Diabetologia* 39:353–356.

Salmon, D.M.W., and J.P. Flatt (1985). Effect of dietary fat content on the incidence of obesity among ad libitum fed mice. *Int. J. Obes.* 9:443–449.

Saltin, B., and P.D. Gollnick (1983). Skeletal muscle adaptability: significance for metabolism and performance. In L.D. Peachy, R.H. Adrian, and S.R. Greiger (eds.). *Handbook of Physiology. Section 10: Skeletal Muscle.* Baltimore: Williams and Wilkins, pp. 555–561.

Saris, W. H. M. (1991). Exercise, nutrition and weight control. In: F. Brouns (ed.) *Advances In Nutrition And Top Sport.* Basel: Karger, pp. 200–215.

Saris, W.H.M. (1995). Exercise with or without dietary restriction and obesity treatment. *Int. J. Obes.* 19:S113–S116.

52 *PERSPECTIVES IN EXERCISE SCIENCE*

Satabin, P., E. Auclair, E. Servan, C. Larue-Achagiotis, and C. Y. Guezennec (1991). Influence of glucose, medium- and long-chain triglyceride gastric loads and forced exercise on food intake and body weight in rats. *Physiol. Behav.* 50:147–150.

Schrauwen, P., W.D. vanMarken Lictenbelt, W.H.M. Saris, and K.R. Westerterp (1997). The effect of glycogen lowering exercise and diet composition on fat oxidation. *Med. Sci. Sports Exerc.* 29:S199 (Abstract).

Schulz, L.O., and D.A. Schoeller (1994). A compilation of total daily energy expenditures and body weights in healthy adults. *Am. J. Clin. Nutr.* 60:676681.

Schulz, L.O., B.L. Nyomba, S. Alger, T.E. Anderson, and E. Ravussin (1991). Effect of endurance training on sedentary energy expenditure measured in a respiratory chamber. *Am. J. Physiol.* 260:E257–261.

Schutz, Y. (1995). Macronutrients and energy balance in obesity. *Metabolism* 44(suppl. 3): 7–11.

Schutz, Y., J.P. Flatt, and E. Jequier (1989). Failure of dietary fat intake to promote fat oxidation: a factor favoring the development of obesity. *Am. J. Clin. Nutr.* 50:307314.

Schutz, Y., A. Tremblay, R.L. Weinsier, and K.M. Nelson (1992). Role of fat oxidation in the longterm stabilization of body weight in obese women. *Am. J. Clin. Nutr.* 55:670–674.

Schwartz M.W., D.P. Figlewicz, D.G. Baskin, S.C. Woods, and D. Porte (1994). Insulin and the central regulation of energy balance: update 1994. *Endocr. Rev.* 2:109–113.

Schwartz M.W., D.G. Baskin, T.R. Budowski, J.L. Juijper, D. Foster, G. Lasser, D.E. Prunkard, D. Porte Jr., S.C. Woods, R.J. Seeley, and D.S. Weigle (1996). Specificity of leptin action on elevated blood glucose levels and hypothalamic neuropeptide Y gene expression in ob/ob mice. *Diabetes* 45:531–535.

Sedlock, D.A., J.A. Fissinger, and C.L. Melby (1989). Effect of exercise intensity and duration on postexercise energy expenditure. *Med. Sci. Sports Exerc.* 21:626–631.

Segal, K.R., and B. Gutin (1983). Thermic effects of food and exercise in lean and obese women. *Metabolism* 32:581–589.

Segal, K.R., L. Blando, F. Ginsberg-Fellner, and A. Edano (1992a). Postprandial thermogenesis at rest and posexercise before and after physical training in lean, obese, and mildly diabetic men. *Metabolism* 41:868–878.

Segal, K.R., A. Chun, P. Coronel, and V. Valdez (1992b). Effects of exercise mode and intensity on postprandial thermogenesis is lean and obese men. *J. Appl. Physiol.* 72:1754–1763.

Sharp, T.A., G.W. Reed, M.Sun, N.N. Abumrad, and J.O. Hill (1992). Relationship between aerobic fitness level and daily energy expenditure in weight stable humans. *Am. J. Physiol.* 263:E121–128.

Shetty, P.S., A.M. Prentice, G.R. Goldberg, P.R. Murgatroyd, A.P.M. McKenna, R.J. Stubbs, and P.A. Volschenk (1994). Alterations in fuel selection and voluntary food intake in response to isoenergetic manipulation of glycogen stores in humans. *Am. J. Clin. Nutr.* 60:534–543.

Simsolo R.B., J.M. Ong, and P.A. Kern (1993). The regulation of adipose tissue and muscle lipoprotein lipase in runners by detraining. *J. Clin. Invest.* 92:21242130.

Simoneau J.A., S.R.Colberg, F.L. Thaete, and D.E. Kelley (1995). Skeletal muscle glycolytic and oxidative enzyme capacities are determinants of insulin sensitivity and muscle composition in obese women. *FASEB J.* 9:273–8.

Slattery, M.L., A. McDonald, D.E. Bild, B.J. Caan, J.E. Hilner, D.R. Jacobs, Jr., and K. Liu (1992). Associations of body fat and its distribution with dietary intake, physical activity, alcohol, and smoking in blacks and whites. *Am. J. Clin. Nutr.* 55:943949.

Staff (1996). Factors associated with prevalent self-reported arthritis and other rheumatic conditions— United States, 1989–1991. *Morbid. Mortal. Weekly Rep.* 45:487–491.

Staten, M. A. (1991). The effect of exercise on food intake in men and women. *Am. J. Clin. Nutr.* 53:27–31.

Stefanick, M.L. (1993). Exercise and weight control. *Exerc. Sport Sci. Rev.* 21:363–369.

Stubbs, R.J., P.R. Murgatroyd, G.R. Goldberg, and A.M. Prentice et al (1993). Carbohydrate balance and the regulation of day-to-day food intake in humans. *Am. J. Clin. Nutr.* 57:897–903.

Stubbs, R.J., C.G. Harbron, P.R. Murgatroyd, and A.M. Prentice (1995a). Covert manipulation of dietary fat and energy density: effect on substrate flux and food intake in men eating ad libitum. *Am. J. Clin. Nutr.* 62:316–329.

Stubbs, R.J., P. Ritz, W.A. Coward, and A.M. Prentice (1995b). Covert manipulation of the ratio of dietary fat to carbohydrate and energy density: effect on food intake and energy balance in free-living men eating ad libitum. *Am. J. Clin. Nutr.* 62:330–337.

Suter, P.M., Y. Schutz, and E. Jequier (1992). The effect of ethanol on fat storage in healthy subjects. *N. Engl. J. Med.* 326: 983–987.

Swinburn, B.A., B.L. Nyomba, M.F. Saad, F. Zurlo, I. Raz, W.C. Knowler, S. Lillioja, C. Bogardus, and E. Ravussin (1991). Insulin resistance associated with lower rates of weight gain in Pima Indians. *J. Clin. Invest.* 88:168–173.

Tarnopolsky, M.A., S.A. Atkinson, J.D. MacDougall, A. Chesley, S. Phillips, and H.P. Schwarez (1992). Evaluation of protein requirements for trained strength athletes. *J. Appl. Physiol.* 73:1986–1995.

Tarnopolsky, M.A., S.A. Atkinson, J.D. MacDougall, B.B. Senor, P.W.R. Lemon, and H.P. Schwarez (1991). Whole body leucine metabolism during and after resistance exercise in fed humans. *Med. Sci. Sports Exerc.* 23:326–333.

Tarnopolsky, M.A., J.D. MacDougall, and S.A. Atkinson (1988). Influence of protein intake and training status on nitrogen balance and lean body mass. *J. Appl. Physiol.* 64:187–193.

EXERCISE, MACRONUTRIENT, AND WEIGHT   53

Thomas, C.D., J.C. Peters, G.W. Reed, N.N. Abumrad, M. Sun and J.O. Hill (1992). Nutrient balance and energy expenditure during ad libitum feeding of highfat and highcarbohydrate diets in humans. *Am. J. Clin. Nutr.* 55:934942.

Thompson, D. A., L. A. Wolfe, and R. Eikelboom (1988). Acute effects of exercise intensity on appetite in young men. *Med. Sci. Sports Exerc.* 20:222–227.

Titchenal, C.A. (1988). Exercise and food intake: what is the relationship? *Sports Med.* 6:135–145.

Todd, K.S., G.E. Butterfield, and D.H. Calloway (1984). Nitrogen balance in men with adequate and deficient energy intake at three levels of work. *Br. J. Nutr.* 114:2107–2118.

Tremblay, A., N. Almeras, J. Boer, E. Klein-Kranenbarg, and J. P. Despres (1994). Diet composition and postexercise energy balance. *Am. J. Clin. Nut.* 59:975–979.

Tremblay, A., N. Lavallee, N. Almeras, L. Allard, J. P. Despres, and C. Bouchard (1991). Nutritional determinants of the increase in energy intake associated with a high-fat diet. *Am. J. Clin. Nutr.* 53:1134–1137.

Tremblay, A., G. Piourde, J.P. Despres, and C. Bouchard (1989). Impact of dietary fat content and fat oxidation on energy intake in humans. *Am. J. Clin. Nutr.* 49:799–805.

Tremblay, A., E. Wouters, M. Wenker, S. St-Pierre, C. Bouchard, and J.P. Despres (1995). Alcohol and a high fat diet: a combination favoring overfeeding. *Am. J. Clin. Nutr.* 62:639–644.

Treuth, M.S., G.R. Hunter, R.L. Weinsier, and S.H. Kell (1995). Energy expenditure and substrate utilization in older women after strength training: 24–h calorimeter results. *J. Appl. Physiol.* 78:2140–2146.

Troiano, R.P., K.M. Flegal, R.J. Kuczmarski, S.M. Campbell, and C.L. Johnson (1995). Overweight prevalence and trends for children and adolescents. The National Health and Nutrition Examination Surveys, 1963 to 1991. *Arch. Pediatr. Adolesc. Med.* 149:1085–1091.

Tuominen, J.A., J.E. Peltonen, and V.A. Koivisto (1997). Blood flow, lipid oxidation, and muscle glycogen synthesis after glycogen depletion by strenuous exercise. *Med. Sci. Sports Exerc.* 29:874–881.

Turcotte, L.P., E.A. Richter, and B. Kiens (1992). Increased plasma FFA uptake and oxidation during prolonged exercise in trained vs. untrained humans. *Am. J. Physiol.* 262:E791–E799.

Van Dale, D., P.F.M. Schoffelen, F. Ten Hoor, and W.H.M. Saris (1989). Effect of adding exercise to energy restriction, 24–h energy expenditure, resting metabolic rate, and daily physical activity. *Eur. J. Clin. Nutr.* 43:441–451.

Verger, P., M.T. Lanteaume, and J. Louis-Sylvestre (1994). Free food choice after acute exercise in men. *Appetite* 22:159–164.

Verger, P., M.T. Lanteaume, and J. Louis-Sylvestre (1992). Human intake and choice of foods at intervals after exercise. *Appetite* 18:93–99.

Vettor R., N. Zarjevski, I. Cusin, F. Rohner-Jeanrenaud, and B. Jeanrenaud (1994). Induction and reversibility of an obesity syndrome by intracerebroventricular neuropeptide Y administration to normal rats. *Diabetol.* 37:1202–1208.

Vogt, M.T., J.A. Cauley, L.H. Kuller, and S.B. Hulley (1993). Prevalence and correlates of lower extremity artery disease in elderly women. *Am. J. Epidemiol.* 137:559–568.

Voigt, L.F., T.D. Koepsell, J.L. Nelson, C.E. Dugowson, and J.R. Daling (1994). Smoking, obesity, alcohol consumption, and the risk of rheumatoid arthritis. *Epidemiol.* 5:525–532.

Wade, A.J., M.M. Marbut, and J.M. Round (1990). Muscle fibre type and aetiology of obesity. *Lancet* 335:805808.

Walberg, J.L., M.K. Keidy, D.J. Sturgill, D.E. Hinkle, S.J. Ritchey, and D.R. Sebolt (1988). Macronutrient content of a hypoenergy diet affects nitrogen retention and muscle function in weight lifters. *Int. J. Sport Med.* 9:261–266.

Weinsier, R.L., K.M. Nelson, D.D. Hensrud, B.E. Darnell, G.R. Hunter, and Y. Schutz (1995). Metabolic predictors of obesity: contribution of energy expenditure, thermic effect of food, and fuel utilization to four-year weight gain of post-obese and never-obese women. *J. Clin. Invest.* 95:980–985.

White, T.P. and G.A. Brooks (1981). [U-14C]glucose -alanine, -leucine oxidation in rats at rest and during two intensities of running. *Am.J. Physiol.* 240:E115–E165.

Willett, W.C., J.E. Manson, M.J. Stamper, G.A. Colditz, B. Rosner, F.E. Speizer, and C.H. Hennekens (1995). Weight, weight change, and coronary heart disease in women: risk within "normal" weight range. *JAMA* 273:461–465.

Williamson, D.F. (1993). Descriptive epidemiology of body weight and weight change in U.S. adults. *Ann. Intern. Med.* 119:646649.

Williamson, D.F., J. Madans, R.F. Anda, J.C. Kleinman, H.S. Kahn and T. Byers (1993). Recreational physical activity and tenyear weight change in a US national cohort. *Int. J. Obes.* 17:279286.

Wilmore, J.H. (1983). Appetite and body composition consequent to physical activity. *Res. Quart.* 54:415–425.

Witt, K.A., J.T. Snook, T.M. O'Dorisio, D. Aivony, and W.B. Malarkey (1993). Exercise training and dietary carbohydrate: effects on selected hormones and the thermic effect of feeding. *Int. J. Sport Nutr.* 3:272–289.

Wolfe, R.R., R.D. Goodenough, M.H. Wolfe, G.T. Royale, and E.R. Nadel (1982). Isotopic analysis of leucine and urea metabolism in exercising humans. *J. Appl. Physiol.* 56:221–229.

Wolfe, R.R. (1992). *Radioactive and Stable Isotope Tracers in Biomedicine.* New York: Wiley-Liss.

Wolfe, R.R., S. Klein, F. Carraro, and J.M. Weber (1990). Role of triglyceride-fatty acid cycle in controlling fat metabolism in humans during and after exercise. *Am. J. Physiol.* 258:E382–E389.

Woo, R. and F.X. Pi-Sunyer (1985). Effect of increased physical activity on voluntary intake in lean women. *Metabolism* 34:836–841.

Woo, R., J.S. Garrow, and F.X. Pi-Sunyer (1982a). Effect of exercise on spontaneous calorie intake in obesity. *Am. J. Clin. Nutr.* 36:470–477.

Woo, R., J.S. Garrow, and F.X. Pi-Sunyer (1982b). Voluntary food intake during prolonged exercise in obese women. *Am. J. Clin. Nutr.* 36:478–484.

Zachwieja J.J., S.L. Hendry, S.R. Smith, and R.B.S. Harris (1997). Voluntary wheel running decreases adipose tissue mass and expression of leptin mRNA in Osborne-Mendel rats. *Diabetes* 46:1159–1166.

Zarjevski N., I. Cusin, R. Vettor, F. Rohner-Jeanrenaud, and B. Jeanrenaud (1994). Intracerebroventricular administration of neuropeptide Y to normal rats has divergent effects on glucose utilization by adipose tissue and skeletal muscle. *Diabetes* 43:764–769.

Zhang, Y., R. Proenca, M. Maffei, M. Barone, L. Leopold, and J.M. Friedman (1994). Positional cloning of the mouse obese gene and its human homologue. *Nature* 372:425–431.

Zheng D., M.H Wooter, Q. Zhou, and G.L. Dohm (1996). The effect of exercise on ob gene expression. *Biochem. and Biophys. Res. Comm.* 225:747–750.

Zurlo, F., S. Lillioja, A. Esposito-Del Puente, B.L. Nyomba, I. Raz, M.F. Saad, B.A. Swinburn, W.C. Knowler, C. Bogardus, and E. Ravussin (1990). Low ratio of fat to carbohydrate oxidation as a predictor of weight gain: study of 24–h RQ. *Am. J. Physiol.* 262:R684–688.

Zurlo, F., P.M. Nemeth, R.M. Choksi, S. Sesodia, and E. Ravussin (1994). Whole body energy metabolism and skeletal muscle biochemical characteristics. *Metabolism* 43:481–486.

DISCUSSION

MAUGHAN: When most people decide they're going to embark on an exercise program, they do it to lose weight rather than to get fit, and of course they simultaneously decide not only to exercise as hard as they possibly can, but to reduce their energy intake and, indeed, often their carbohydrate intake. Have there been any studies in which people have deliberately attempted to increase energy intake and carbohydrate intake in the early phase of training? In my experience, what often happens to most people who start a weight loss program is that they give up after 3–4 d of hard exercise and a low carbohydrate diet. Supplementation with carbohydrate in the early stages of training may allow these individuals to overcome these early problems.

MELBY: I think such persons usually try to decrease the fat intake more than the carbohydrate intake. However, there are some diets that have become popular that emphasize low carbohydrate intake and liberal amounts of fat and protein. There is very little scientific evidence to support these types of diets, specifically, the Zone Diet®. There are many misconceptions about this diet. If people follow the Zone Diet, they will be in an energy deficit situation and will lose weight. However, the weight loss that occurs is more likely attributed to the low energy content of the diet and not its composition. Individuals will often see some rapid weight loss on the Zone Diet, which you might expect given the fact that the energy and carbohydrate contents are low. However, the exercise isn't much fun because the glycogen stores tend to be low, and in this situation, there is a tendency for people to drop out. But I don't know of any long-term studies that have actually addressed this sort of diet coupled with exercise. But we would expect that on a diet that is low in energy and higher in fat, the fat oxidation is going to increase. The key, though, is not just to look at fat oxidation or to look at fat intake, but to look at fat balance, and in this situation fat balance probably will be negative for a period of time; the question is, Can they stick with it? I doubt it.

MAUGHAN: Wagenmakers has shown that the increase in protein breakdown during exercise seen when leucine is used as a tracer is not observed when phenylalanine is used as a tracer, so perhaps the whole question about how exercise affects protein breakdown will need to be revisited.

MELBY: Even when estimated with leucine turnover, when we look at total energy balance, the contribution of amino acid oxidation during exercise is pretty small.

M. WILLIAMS: Is there any evidence in children that the set point or the settling point might be modified by exercise or diet? Some investigators suggest that there might be a crucial window of opportunity in children to favorably modify the settling point, indicating also that the settling point may be more difficult to modify in adults.

MELBY: I've not seen any studies that have addressed that point, but it is an intriguing hypothesis.

BAR-OR: I am not aware of data that specifically addressed the set-point concept in children. Our clinical experience, however, suggests that 6–12 mo following a 1 y weight-control counseling program, 70–80% of those who did well in the program returned to there baseline body weights. This might suggest the existence of a set point also in children. However, studies by Len Epstein (e.g., Epstein et al., *Health Psychol.* 13:373–383, 1994) have shown that, with proper behavior modification, a select group of obese children can retain their weight loss for as long as 10 y after the completion of a program.

MELBY: It sounds like intervening with overweight kids is not much more successful than with adults. In adults physical activity seems to be the best predictor of whether or not weight loss can be sustained. Those individuals that are able to successfully maintain a physical activity program tend to regain less weight, and that fact is often overlooked when we examine the impact of exercise on body-weight regulation.

GUTIN: Len Epstein feels that you can get something like 75% success in weight control programs when using the most current behavioral techniques with children. So we may have reason to be more optimistic about this thing than if we simply ascribe the results to a metabolic factor of some sort that leads to a set point or a settling point.

We know that as people age they keep gaining fat, even if they don't gain weight. Why do we have to think about a set point or a settling point at all? Why don't we imagine this as a constantly dynamic process that responds to eating and exercise behaviors, along with whatever age-related metabolic changes that might be occurring?

MELBY: Your point is well taken. This is certainly not a static situation; rather it is somewhat dynamic which is the idea behind the settling point rather than a set point. Obviously, because body-fat mass increases with advancing age, regulation does not occur around the same point for one's entire adult life. For many individuals, over the course of years and even several decades, body weight and composition are maintained within a fairly narrow range. This fact, along with the fact that the success rates for weight-loss programs are so small, suggests some regulation around a settling point so that intake and expenditure are somewhat closely matched. Also, there are well-recognized increases and decreases in energy expenditure (RMR, energy cost of physical activity) that accompany overfeeding and underfeeding. These phenomena also lend support to the body's attempt to regulate energy balance.

BAR-OR: Indeed, we have to give credit to Len Epstein for his work; however, his subjects have been an extremely select group of motivated children and have come from highly dedicated families. It is therefore premature to generalize from their findings to all obese children.

Another issue regarding behavior is the extent to which a structured exercise program can modify spontaneous physical activity. Chris has mentioned data on elderly people who have decreased their spontaneous activity when they were given a regimented training program. In contrast, we have data regarding obese boys (Blaak et al., *Am. J. Clin. Nutr.* 55:777–782, 1992), who increased their 24 h energy expenditures (measured by doubly-labeled water) twice as much as would be expected from the intervention program *per se*. In another study (Kriemler et al., *Med. Sci. Sports Exerc.* 28:S12, 1996) we found that averages for spontaneous activity and energy expenditure of obese children increased significantly the day after a visit to the exercise laboratory. It thus seems that there is much still to unravel regarding the relevance of behavioral aspects in the treatment of obesity.

MELBY: We have to recognize that the subjects in the study of Goran and Poehlman were elderly individuals who were exercising at a high intensity—up to about 85% $\dot{V}O_2$max at the end of the study. We might expect that as they become more physically fit over time, they might actually increase their levels of spontaneous activity, which would become relatively easier with improved fitness. But the point is that we really don't know very much about physical activity compensation induced by exercise, and we may very well have individuals that respond entirely differently, with some people increasing their spontaneous activity and some people decreasing it.

BAR-OR: The differences may be cultural as well.

NADEL: You talked about expression of uncoupling protein in the studies of obesity in genetically-prone individuals. I would like to hear some more about how genetic factors affect the control points of metabolism in obese people.

MELBY: UCP-1 seems to be largely expressed in brown adipose tissue which, in adults, seems to be found in negligible amounts. The protein expression increases in response to cold stimulation, leading to an uncoupling of oxidation from phosphorylation, by dissipating the proton gradient in the mitochondrial matrix. The proton gradient then cannot drive ATP synthesis, and more energy must be expended to provide the necessary ATP.

In adult humans, there has been a waning of interest in regard to UCP-1 and obesity. However, UCP-2 seems to be expressed in a variety of tissues, including white adipose tissue and skeletal muscle. It also uncouples oxidation and phosphorylation by dissipating the proton gradient across the inner mitochondrial membrane, thus reducing the phosphorylation-to-oxidation ratio (P:0). The expression of UCP-2 seems to occur in response to fat overfeeding, which may have significant implications for human obesity. If, in fact, some individuals in response to overfeeding are better able to increase thermogenesis, this could possibly explain why they are less prone to become obese and other individuals are more prone to become obese.

The overfeeding studies by Claude Bouchard at Laval University show clearly that one's genotype has a very important influence on risk of weight gain. But we also must recognize that if the environmental (behavioral) factors may counteract the genotypic push so the phenotypic expression of obesity may not actually occur.

WALBERG-RANKIN: How much does the dietary composition, the fat content, for example, matter compared to energy intake in diets designed to reduce body weight? The fat-balance hypothesis suggests that people become obese when they eat a higher fat diet because they can't increase fat oxidation to match fat intake. How, then, can some individuals maintain their weights while eating a high-fat diet without exercise? Why can some individuals adjust to a higher fat diet by increasing fat oxidation, but others cannot?

MELBY: Individuals can eat a high-fat diet and still be weight stable at a low percentage of body fat if they have high rates of fat oxidation. People can even lose weight on a high-fat diet if they are in an energy deficit situation. When they are in energy balance on a high-fat diet, fat oxidation over time will be similar to fat intake. On the higher fat diet, glycogen stores would be maintained at lower levels, and plasma insulin concentrations would drop, resulting in less suppression of lipolysis. This metabolic situation would favor increased fat oxidation on a high-fat diet. In fact, some of the newer diets that are higher in fat imply that this is the reason for their purported effectiveness—lower the insulin concentration to increase fat oxidation. The key, though, is whether or not the individual trying to lose weight is in an energy deficit situation. If the person is in an energy deficit of, say 300–500 kcal/d, over the long haul, whether the composition is higher in fat or lower in fat, the weight loss will most likely be similar.

WALBERG-RANKIN: If someone needs 2,000 kcal/d and I feed them 2,000 kcal of olive oil, shouldn't she maintain her weight?

MELBY: That's a little extreme. Let me put it in these terms. The composition is important primarily because when an individual is on a high-fat diet, he or she tends to overeat. There are many studies that a highly palatable, high-fat diet leads to greater energy intake. So in a real-world situation in which people eat high-fat diets, there is a tendency to overeat. This surplus of dietary energy causes a positive fat balance that over time will lead to fat accretion.

DESPRES: You have just highlighted the major issue, i.e., the greater the fat content of the food, the greater will be the likelihood that the individual will eat more and be in positive energy balance, perhaps as much as 700 kcal/d or more; this should be very much emphasized.

COYLE: On the other hand, people can go to the other extreme of very low-fat diets. The question is, how can they maintain fat balance? Obviously, the American public is not doing a very good job with that because we are gaining fat successively over the years. You mentioned the very important point that when you eat carbohydrate, it has a very potent effect on inhibiting fat oxidation and lowering lipolysis. That may be the theoretical basis for some of these "zone-type" diets that are moderately low in carbohydrate. The premise is that if you lower dietary carbohydrate to a certain level (e.g., 40% of energy), you will raise fat oxidation, but that does not happen very easily. Even small amounts of dietary carbohydrate have a very potent effect of markedly lowering fat oxidation at rest and during exercise. If you eat just 100 g of carbohydrate, you will suppress fat oxidation for 6–8 h. My point is that in order for low-carbohydrate diets to raise fat oxidation, you also have to fast for long periods or you have to exercise for very long periods.

MELBY: It is clear that fat oxidation will be lower on a high-carbohydrate diet. But I don't believe that on such a diet one will have to engage in prolonged fasting or prolonged exercise to oxidize as much fat as is ingested. On the low-fat diet, there is less fat that needs to be oxidized to achieve fat balance, and regular exercise will contribute to oxidation of fat, even on a high-carbohydrate diet. Certainly there are adaptations that occur with exercise training and with the acute effect of exercise that can enhance fat oxidation, but on a high-carbohydrate diet, fat oxidation over 24 h isn't necessarily going to be high.

COYLE: Exactly. So they may not be burning as much fat as they think they are. Would it be fair to make a general statement that for people to be able to maintain fat balance and thus burn as much fat as they are ingesting, they have to perform a certain amount of exercise? The question is how much exercise you need to perform or how much fasting do you have to subject yourself to throughout the day? Typically, we eat some carbohydrate every 8 h with our modern eating patterns and low-activity life-style, and thus suppress fat oxidation to a great extent. To overcome that situation, people have to exercise for what seems to be unreasoningly long periods or fast for long periods.

MELBY: Most free-living individuals can maintain fat balance or achieve negative fat balance over time more readily with a lower fat intake.

HORSWILL: I have a comment on the Zone Diet and the Protein Power Diet. The few clinical studies examining these diets are short-term in nature and do not have strong data to show that changes in fat oxidation lead to reductions in body fat. The rapid weight loss that occurs in association with these diets may be due to the diuretic effect from the urine excretion of ketones and the high urea load; the weight loss is largely from fluid loss.

I have two questions on high whole-body insulin sensitivity as being a risk factor for weight gain or obesity. First, is this risk population specific? Second, is exercise a good therapy for individuals with this condition? If exercise increases insulin sensitivity, exercise would seem to be contraindicated. In fact, insulin resistance would seem preferable for these people since resistance may be a compensatory mechanism allowing the oxidization of more fat and, thus, preventing further obesity.

MELBY: To date, the finding that higher insulin sensitivity is related to greater weight gain is population-specific, identified in the Pima Indians. In this study, there was greater weight gain over 4 y in the most insulin-sensitive individuals, probably reflecting greater carbohydrate and lower fat oxidation. Insulin insensitivity was associated with less weight gain. This would suggest than that is beneficial to be insulin insensitive. However, insulin insensitivity is associated with a number of untoward sequelae, including dyslipidemia, hypertension, and non-insulin dependent diabetes. On the other hand, just because exercise increases insulin sensitivity does not mean that it will indirectly promote weight gain. The association between higher insulin sensitivity and subsequent weight gain was identified in a sedentary population.

2

Assessment of Body Composition and Energy Balance

TIMOTHY LOHMAN, PH.D.
SCOTT GOING, PH.D.

INTRODUCTION

Body composition refers to the absolute and relative amounts of the body constituents. With current methods, body composition can be assessed on elemental (atomic), chemical, cellular, and tissue/system levels (Wang et al., 1992), with the possibility of measuring over 30 components of human composition (Heymsfield, 1996). It is, however, difficult to measure many of these components, so the term *body composition* generally refers to regional or total measures of adipose tissue or body fat, fat-free mass, body water, and bone. Measurement of body composition can be important in the evaluation of health and nutritional status, to formulate dietary guidelines, to monitor changes in body composition with growth, maturation and aging, and to establish optimal weights in athletes. Moreover, accurate assessment of body composition is essential to evaluate the efficacy of exercise, diet, and drug interventions designed to modify body fat, muscle mass, and bone mineral mass and density.

Excess body fat (obesity), particularly an increase in intra-abdominal (visceral) adipose tissue, is associated with greater risks of some cardiovascular and metabolic diseases and may be responsible for increased mortality rates (Seidell, 1996). The relationships between adipose tissue distribution and risk factors for disease develop during pubescence, although the relationships with disease do not become evident until middle age (Baumgartner et al., 1989). Thus, there has been considerable emphasis on obesity screening and assessment of regional adipose tissue in adolescents and adults. Having too little body fat is also risky, and screening for low levels of body fat is important, although not as common as obesity screening.

At the other end of the spectrum are those individuals whose health is already at risk. For example, the contribution of sarcopenia (muscle atrophy) and osteoporosis (bone demineralization) to the decline in functional capacity and increased mortality rates in older adults has recently been given more attention (Roche, 1995) in light of the changing population demographics. For patients in intensive care, low fat-free mass (FFM) is associated with increased mortality rates, perhaps due to an increased risk of infections or to a micronutrient deficiency (Roubenoff & Kehayias, 1991). In patients dying of starvation, malignancy, or chronic infection, the loss of body fat is followed by a loss of fat-free mass (FFM). Death often occurs when FFM is decreased about 40% or when arm muscle area (excluding bone) becomes less than about 12 cm^2 (Heymsfield et al., 1982). Involuntary weight loss in old age is associated with a loss of FFM, particularly in men, and is highly predictive of mortality (Steen et al., 1977). When body mass index (BMI) is low (indicating low FFM), hypertension is less prevalent in both genders, and unfavorable lipid profiles are more common in men (Ramirez et al., 1991; White et al., 1986).

Fractures resulting from falls are important contributors to death in the elderly. The likelihood of falls is increased by the reduction in muscle strength that occurs with aging (Bassey et al., 1992; Myers et al., 1991; Wickham et al., 1989). These falls are more likely to cause fractures when bone mineral content is low. Both bone mineral mass and bone density are decreased when muscle strength and FFM are reduced(Bevier et al., 1989; Marcus et al., 1992; Pocock et al., 1989), and this may be one way in which sarcopenia increases mortality rates.

Recent technological advances combined with new developments in multicomponent models of body composition have improved on traditional models of estimating body composition and have led to better criterion methods. As a result, a great deal of research is currently underway to better describe the healthy changes in body composition that occur with growth, development, and aging. This research should further elucidate the relationships among body composition and health and disease, as well as validate simple methods for screening and for testing interventions with exercise, diet, and drugs, all of which could be designed to modify body composition. The application of these methods and their advantages and limitations in comparison to traditional methods for assessing body composition are described in this chapter.

MULTICOMPARTMENT MODELS: ADVANTAGES AND LIMITATIONS

The traditional approach to estimating body composition is to consider the body as composed of fat and fat-free masses (Figure 2-1). In this two-compartment model, all chemically extractable lipid is defined as "fat." The remaining chemicals, essentially water, protein, mineral, and a small amount of carbohydrate comprise the fat-free mass (FFM). The two-compartment method is a comparatively simple and useful approach because the FFM relates closely with other more physiologically or functionally relevant compartments, such as the lean-body mass (LBM), the body-cell mass, and muscle mass. However, as discussed in the following pages, the assumptions underlying the two-compartment model are not valid for all individuals, and significant errors can occur when certain assumptions are violated. (Note that LBM is often substituted for FFM although, by definition, LBM includes a small amount of essential lipid, usually defined as 3% of FFM. Thus, LBM (FFM × 1.03) and FFM are not equivalent compartments.)

The most common methods for assessing fat and FFM are the body water method (Schoeller, 1996), the body potassium method (Ellis, 1996), and the hydrostatic or underwater-weighing method (Going, 1996). Each method relies on a measurement that is then used to estimate fat mass and FFM based on the two-compartment model (Figure 2-2) (Heymsfield, 1996). The model represents the conceptual basis from

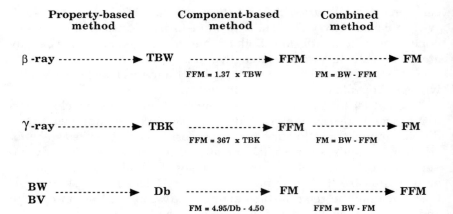

Property-based method		Component-based method		Combined method	

β -ray ················▶ TBW   ················▶ FFM   ················▶ FM

FFM = 1.37 x TBW   FM = BW - FFM

γ -ray ················▶ TBK   ················▶ FFM   ················▶ FM

FFM = 367 x TBK   FM = BW - FFM

BW
BV ················▶ Db   ················▶ FM   ················▶ FFM

FM = 4.95/Db - 4.50   FFM = BW - FM

FIGURE 2-1. *Pathways summarizing the estimation of fat-free mass and fat mass from common laboratory methods.* Abbreviations: BW, body weight; BV, body volume; D_B, body density; FM, fat mass; FFM, fat-free mass; TBK, total body potassium; TBW, total body water. Adapted from Heymsfield, 1996 (p.134).

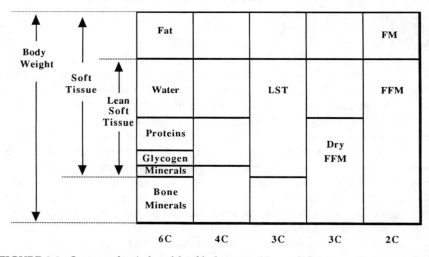

FIGURE 2-2. *Common chemical models of body composition and their respective components.* Abbreviations: FM, fat mass; FFM, fat-free mass; LST, lean soft tissue mass; 2C-6C, two-components through six-components.

which the mathematical estimates of body composition are derived (Table 2-1). Thus, total body water and potassium can be converted to FFM based on their respective concentrations in the FFM, which are known through chemical analysis of human cadavers (Brozek et al., 1963).

In an analogous way, body density from underwater weighing can be converted to percent fat because whole-body density is related to the

TABLE 2-1. *Two-component and multicomponent model equations.*

Number of Components	Model	Methods	Equation
2	BW = FM + FFM	Total body water	FFM = 1.37 × TBW
2	BW = FM + FFM	Total body potassium	FFM = 3.76 × TBK
2	BW = FM + FFM	Densitometry	FFM = $4.95/D_b$ − 4.50
3	BW = FM + TBW + nonfat solids	Total body water, densitometry	FFM = $2.118/D_b$ − 0.78 TBW − 1.354
3	BW = FM + M + LST	DXA, Densitometry	FM = $6.386/D_b$ − 3.961 M − 6.090
4	BW = FM + TBW + M_o + residual	DXA, Total body water, Densitometry	FM = $2.747/D_b$ − 0.714 TBW + $1.146M_0$ − 2.053

Abbreviations: BW = body weight; D_b = body density; DXA = dual energy x-ray absorptiometry; used to measure osseous (bone) mineral; FFM = Fat-free mass; FM = fat mass LST = lean soft tissue; M = total body mineral; Mo = osseous (bone) minerals; TBK = total body potassium; TBW = total body water.

proportions and densities of the body's components (Going, 1996). Based on the two-compartment model,

$$BD = (f + ffm)/[f/d_f + ffm/d_{ffm}]$$

where BD is body density, f and ffm are the fractions of fat and FFM in the whole body, and d_f and dffm are their respective densities. Any number of equations can be derived by solving the above equation for either f or ffm and simplifying using estimates of d_f and d_{ffm}. The Siri equation (f = 4.95/BD-4.50), the most common two-compartment-model equation, was derived using d_f = 0.9 g/mL and d_{ffm} = 1.1 g/mL, which are the assumed densities derived from direct chemical analyses of human cadavers (Brozek et al., 1963; Siri, 1956).

Methods of measuring body composition that are based on the two-compartment model rely upon a known and stable relationship between the compartment of interest (e.g., FFM) and the measured constituent. For example, the validity and accuracy of both the total-body-water method and the total-body-potassium method depend largely on the appropriateness of the conversion constants for the individuals in which they are applied. Similarly, the validity and accuracy of estimating body fat from body density depend on the deviation of the actual d_{ffm} from the assumed d_{ffm} = 1.1 g/mL, which, in turn, depends on variation in the fractional amounts of protein, water, and mineral in the FFM.

It is clear from a number of studies that the composition of the FFM is not constant within or between individuals. Children, for example, have lower protein and mineral concentrations in FFM but a higher water concentration, resulting in a lower d_{ffm} when compared to adults (Lohman, 1986). Also, the loss of muscle and bone mass with aging is reflected in both greater variation and a gradual decline in d_{ffm}, particularly in women (Deurenberg et al., 1989), although the magnitude of the change is controversial (Baumgartner et al., 1991; Going et al., 1995; Heymsfield et al., 1989; Mazariegos et al., 1994; Williams et al., 1993). Gender and racial differences in FFM composition (Gasperino et al., 1995; Ortiz et al., 1992; Schutte et al., 1984) and differences among athletes (Heyward & Stolarczyk, 1996; Modlesky et al., 1996a) have also been described, as have differences between obese men and women compared to their leaner peers (Albu et al., 1989; Deurenberg et al., 1989; Lindsay et al., 1992). As a result of the variation in FFM composition, errors as large as ± 3–5% in estimating body fat can occur, with the magnitude and direction of error dependent on the method and the degree to which the subject's body composition deviates from the assumed FFM composition.

The application of traditional methods in individuals whose composition deviates from the two-compartment model presents two important problems. First, the inflated error confounds interpretation of baseline assessments aimed at screening for excessive fatness or thinness. Second, changes in the water, mineral, and protein fractions of FFM as a result of intervention introduce errors and confound estimates of fat and FFM used to monitor the intervention and assess its efficacy for modifying the composition of the body.

It is difficult to know for whom the two-compartment approach is best suited. In young and middle-aged adults, FFM composition is relatively stable, and percent fat and FFM can be estimated with errors of about 2–3% fat or 2.0–2.5 kg FFM. However, for any given individual, the errors may be greater. Larger errors occur in groups for whom systematic differences have been identified, e.g., certain race/ethnic groups (Schutte et al., 1984), athletes (Modlesky et al., 1996a), obese persons (Deurenberg et al., 1989), children (Lohman, 1986), and the elderly (Going et al., 1995).

MINIMIZING MEASUREMENT ERROR

Three strategies can be adopted for minimizing the errors associated with the measurement of body composition based on the two-compartment model. The ideal approach is to use a measurement technique that does not require the assumption of an invariant fat-free composition. The relatively recent development of dual-energy x-ray absorptiometry (DXA) offers a technique that may satisfy this requirement. Alternatively, it is possible to combine methods and derive estimates of FFM from measurements of several components of the FFM and thus reduce the number of assumptions required by the model. The third alternative, the application of population-specific equations based on multiple-compartment models, is useful when multiple measurements are not possible.

A number of multiple-compartment models have been derived (Heymsfield, 1996). Using total-body neutron activation analysis (Ellis, 1996), one can measure several elements of the FFM simultaneously and derive what may be the most accurate estimate of FFM that is available with current technology (Cohn et al., 1981; Heymsfield & Waki, 1991). However, the expense and radiation exposure to the subjects renders total-body neutron activation analysis impractical except as a research tool. Fortunately, simpler multiple-compartment methods (Figure 2-2) have been developed to estimate FFM from measurements of body density by underwater weighing, body water by isotope dilution, and bone mineral by DXA (Baumgartner et al., 1991; Friedl et al., 1992; Heymsfield et al., 1989; Williams et al., 1993). Recent work has shown that this four-compartment approach yields estimates of FFM that are not different from FFM estimated by a more complex model based on total-body neutron activation analysis (Heymsfield et al., 1990; Heymsfield & Waki, 1991).

It is also possible to reduce the measurement error substantially by using approaches based on three-compartment models (Figure 2-2), which combine measurements of body water or bone mineral with measurements of body density (Table 2-1). Although more accurate than equations based on the two-compartment model, these equations assume a constant mineral-to-protein ratio or protein-to-water ratio. Individual deviation from the assumed ratio introduces error, albeit less than that of the two-compartment model.

The choice of which equation to use depends on which constituent is likely to vary most within the population being assessed. The bone-mineral-body-density equation (Lohman, 1992) is useful when variability in the mineral fraction of FFM (M_{ffm}) is expected to exceed the variability in the water fraction (W_{ffm}), as may occur in perimenopausal (Williams et al., 1993) and older women (Going et al., 1995) and in black males (Schutte et al., 1984). The body-water-body-density equation (Siri, 1963) is useful when the variability in W_{ffm} exceeds variability in M_{ffm}, as may be true during weight loss and when serial measurements are made throughout the menstrual cycle (Bunt et al., 1989; Byrd & Thomas, 1983) (Table 2-1).

Multiple-compartment models have two important limitations. First, additional measurements require additional expense and add to the demands on the subject. Second, with the assessment of multiple compartments comes the potential for increased technical error. Although inflated error is always a possibility when a multiple-compartment model is used,

Friedl et al. (1992) have shown that it is possible to derive more accurate estimates of body composition using the four-compartment model despite the potential problem of "propagation of errors".

Multiple-compartment models are especially useful when following changes in composition and for criterion estimates when validating simpler techniques. As Forbes (1993) has shown, fat and FFM do not change independently. Rather, weight loss and gain are reflected in changes in both compartments, although the contribution of fat and FFM to the overall change varies with the initial level of fatness, severity of dietary energy restriction, and amount and type of physical activity. During very-low-energy diets, FFM decreases along with fat mass because of losses of fluid and muscle mass (Deurenberg et al., 1989; Kushner et al., 1990; van der Kooy et al., 1992). As a result, body density will underestimate fat loss unless an adjustment for the change in the components of FFM is made. Additional studies using multicomponent methods are needed to better characterize the compositional changes that accompany weight loss and the efficacy of the interventions aimed at modifying body composition.

NEW DEVELOPMENTS IN LABORATORY METHODS

Underwater weighing is not possible in persons who are unable or unwilling to be submerged. As a result, an alternative method for accurately estimating body density is needed. Another alternative is to employ a method that does not rely on estimates of body density. The recent development of air-displacement plethysmography for estimating volume and body density and of dual energy x-ray absorptiometry (DXA) for estimating soft-tissue composition makes both of these alternatives possible.

Air Displacement Plethysmography

Dempster and Aitkens (1995) described an instrument called the Bod Pod Body Composition System (Life Measurements Instruments, Concord, CA), for measuring body volume by air- displacement plethysmography. The system consists of a dual-chambered plethysmograph, with a movable diaphragm mounted on the common wall. Volume perturbations, created by computer-controlled oscillations of the diaphragm, create small pressure fluctuations that are analyzed to derive chamber air volume. Using this system, subject volume is estimated from the difference between the empty chamber air volume and the air volume with the subject inside. Body density is calculated from body volume ($D = M/V$).

The Bod Pod has several advantages over underwater weighing

and other attempts at plethysmography (Going, 1996). It is portable and relatively easy to operate, measurement time is short, and it may be better able to accommodate special populations, such as young children and elderly, obese, and disabled persons. Initial results with this system are impressive. The reliability and precision of estimates of volume for an inanimate object are excellent (coefficient of variation (CV%) ≅ 0.025%), corresponding to percent-fat errors of 0.1% fat (Dempster & Aitkens, 1995). Also, precision in human subjects was good (CV% = 1.7% ± 1.1%), and estimates of percent fat from the Bod Pod and underwater weighing in healthy subjects agreed closely (mean %fat difference = −0.3 ± 0.2%) and were highly correlated (r = 0.96) (McCrory et al., 1995). Further research is warranted to assess its precision and accuracy in special populations.

Dual Energy X-Ray Absorptiometry

Dual energy X-ray absorptiometry (DXA) is one of the most promising new methods for estimating body composition. In the past 5 y, several validation studies conducted with this technology have lead to improved software and more-accurate estimates of both total and regional body composition (Lohman, 1996). The introduction of fan-beam technology (Hologic, QDR-2000 and QDR-4500, Waltham, MA) has decreased measurement time and improved resolution, although further validation of estimates of soft tissue composition from this new technology against criterion-referenced multicomponent models is needed. At present, the most widely used equipment employs pencil-beam technology (Lunar DPX, Madison, WI and Hologic QDR-1000, Waltham, MA) combined with newer software (Lunar 1.3y/3.6y extended research mode and Hologic QDR-1000, 1500 and 2000), and this approach has been validated in a number of populations. Several comprehensive reviews of the DXA method have been published (Khort, 1995; Lohman, 1996; Pietrobelli et al., 1996).

The DXA technology has two important advantages over the traditional two-compartment approach. First, DXA is based on a three-compartment model and simultaneously gives estimates of fat, fat-free soft tissue (i.e., lean tissue mass or LTM), and bone. Second, the method provides estimates of regional body composition and total body composition, so that limb and trunk fat can be independently estimated. Regional analysis conducted on spine scans provides estimates of total abdominal fat (subcutaneous plus visceral). There are more than 9,900 operational DXA scanners worldwide capable of body composition assessment, allowing for more body composition/risk factor studies to be conducted. (See Terry et al. (1991) as an example of such a study.) The DXA technology appears ideal for validating other methods of estimating body composition, and for studies of growth, development, and aging. The DXA methodology also allows for multicomponent body composition analysis that is not confounded by variations in bone mineral content.

An important future use of DXA will be to follow the longitudinal changes in bone mineral content and body fat as a result of aging and of various drug, nutritional, and exercise interventions. Beginning in 1998, the contemplated large-scale use of DXA in national probability samples for the National Health and Nutrition Examination Survey (NHANES) should lead to the first-ever reference values for body fatness and to better estimates of the prevalence of obesity among the U.S. population. DXA is currently being used at three Vanguard Centers in the Women's Health Initiative (WHI), the largest clinical trial ever conducted, to follow bone density and body composition changes over a 10 y period. DXA will also be used in the Healthy Aging and Body Composition study (Health ABC) to follow changes in bone and soft tissue composition over 7 y in a cohort of 3,000 men and women age 70–79 y. This study will assess risks related to a variety of weight-related health conditions, functional status, and changes in body composition with aging. At issue in each of these studies is the accuracy of DXA for following changes in body composition. The ability to measure changes in lean, bone, and fat tissues with a single method is an important development, but questions remain regarding the accuracy of DXA given the limitations in other criterion methods.

Regional estimates of body fatness by DXA have been compared to computed tomography and to magnetic resonance imaging (MRI). Early work by Going et al. (1990) showed high correlations between trunk skinfolds and abdominal fat from dual photon absorptiometry (DPA). The high reliability (between-day measurements) of the soft tissue attenuation ratio (R_{ST}) in the abdominal region gave evidence for a high precision of measurement. The combination of trunk skinfolds and abdominal fat from DXA might provide an estimate of intra-abdominal fat (Lohman, 1992). With this approach, individuals with high values for abdominal fat and lower-than-expected trunk skinfolds would have large quantities of intra-abdominal fat, whereas individuals with large trunk skinfolds but less DXA-measured abdominal fat would have less intra-abdominal fat. Lohman (1992) proposed that future research studies include both regional abdominal fat from DXA and trunk skinfolds to evaluate the relation of disease risk factors to body composition.

Terry et al. (1991) measured regional fat by DPA in overweight men and women and showed an inverse relationship between values for abdominal and thigh fat and values for plasma lipid and lipoprotein fractions, especially in overweight women. In general, the ratio of abdominal-to-thigh fat mass was the best predictor of blood lipid levels. The work of these investigators demonstrates the usefulness of DXA in studies of body composition and disease risk.

FIELD METHODS: ANTHROPOMETRY, BIOIMPEDANCE ANALYSIS, INFRARED INTERACTANCE, AND SKINFOLDS

Three of the major field methods for assessing body composition are anthropometry (skinfold and circumference measurements), bioelectrical impedance, and near infrared interactance (Lohman et al., 1988). Heyward and Stolarczyk (1996) reviewed many of the prediction equations developed for these methods. In 1995, The National Institutes of Health sponsored a consensus conference for defining standardized measurements on bioelectrical impedance with major papers on all aspects of BIA research (Foster & Lukaski, 1996). Much less research has focused on infrared interactance.

BODY MASS INDEX (BMI)

Weight and height (stature) can be measured easily in large samples with high precision. Consequently, the body mass index (BMI = $weight/stature^2$; kg/m^2), also known as Quetelet's index, has been used as a proxy for body composition in numerous epidemiological studies and in clinical settings. Somewhat arbitrary BMI standards, based largely on associations with morbidity and mortality, have been suggested as guidelines for desirable weights, and so-called BMI "obesity" standards have been defined (Heyward & Stolarczyk, 1996). Ironically, BMI is only moderately correlated with more direct estimates of body fat and FFM, which undoubtedly contributes to some of the uncertainty regarding the validity of the BMI-mortality relationship.

The major limitation of the BMI is that the numerator (body weight) does not discriminate among muscle, fat, bone, or vital organs; therefore, an individual with greater-than-average FFM relative to stature might have a high BMI value and not be obese. In children and the elderly, where muscle and bone weights in relationship to height are changing, the BMI can be especially difficult to interpret. A similar problem exists when BMI is used to follow weight gain or weight loss, because the composition of the weight change cannot be discerned.

Racial and ethnic differences in the composition of weight per unit height also confound interpretation of the BMI. Several studies have shown significant racial/ethnic differences in body composition, especially in bone and muscle mass. For example, Cohn et al. (1977) showed that total body potassium (TBK) and calcium were 5–10% higher in black women than in white women, suggesting the black women had larger muscle and bone mineral masses. The development of DPA and DXA has made it more feasible to examine race/ethnic differences in bone and soft-tissue composition. The results of studies using this technology have confirmed the higher bone-mineral density in black women and men as well as their greater appendicular skeletal muscle mass compared to weight-matched white controls (Ortiz et al., 1992).

In two studies designed to validate BMI against a direct measure of fatness in different ethnic groups, Asian men and women living in the US had higher percent body fats but lower values for BMI than did white men and women (Wang et al., 1996). Older men and women also have higher percent fats for comparable BMI values compared to younger persons of the same race/ethnicity (Gallagher et al., 1996). Thus, classifying subjects of the same gender into categories of equivalent body composition, independent of age and race/ethnicity, is fraught with error.

In a recent study, Wellens et al. (1996) examined the BMI-body composition relationship in a large number of white men and women using densitometry and the two-compartment model to assess body composition. The age range was limited to 20–45 y because in this age range the density of fat-free mass is close to the assumed value of 1.1 g/mL. In both men and women, the age-adjusted correlations between BMI and percent body fat were higher in the upper third of BMI values compared to the lower third. In the lower third of BMI values, the correlation between BMI and FFM was approximately twice as high as the correlation with percent fat. Using standard criteria (28 kg/m^2 in males and 26 kg/m^2 in women), the BMI correctly identified only 44% of obese women (>33% fat) and 52% of obese men (>25% fat). In contrast, almost 100% of nonobese men and women were correctly classified by BMI. The results of this study and others (Baumgartner et al., 1995) suggest that BMI is an excellent index for classifying the nonobese but is rather insensitive for classifying the obese. Because muscle mass is a major component of body weight, especially at low BMIs, low BMI may be useful as an indicator of muscle mass, although this is not how it is commonly used.

Lower BMI "cut-off" values may be more diagnostic of obesity. For example, Wellens et al. (1996) found that BMI values of 25 kg/m^2 in men and 23 kg/m^2 in women were better criteria for defining obesity. In a similar analysis, Hortobagyi et al. (1994) chose even lower values, 24.5 kg/m^2 in men and 22 kg/m^2 in women, to identify obesity. The difference between the two studies may be due to the broader age range (19–77 y) in the latter study and to the potential errors associated with the two-compartment model in the older subjects.

The insensitivity of the BMI has implications for identifying the obese. Health professionals should be cautious when using BMI as an index of obesity, although the BMI correlates well with percent fat in adults most likely to be identified easily as obese, namely those in the upper BMI range. Other analyses suggest that lower BMI scores than those commonly recommended for white men and women would allow for successful detection of obese adults that would normally be missed by the current standards for obesity (Kuczmarski et al., 1994). These assumptions should be tested in other samples of white adults and in other ethnic groups because the BMI/percent-fat relationship varies with ethnicity.

The issue is whether or not anthropometry, bioelectrical impedence analysis (BIA) and near infrared interactance (NIR) estimate body composition with better accuracy compared to using height and weight to determine body mass index (BMI). In general, research shows that BIA and anthropometry can predict percent body fat with standard errors of estimate (SEE) of 3–4%, whereas NIR and BMI predict percent body fat with standard errors of estimate of 4–5% (Wilmore et al., 1994). Thus, for use in large epidemiological studies, anthropometry and BIA are the methods of choice. Anthropometry and BIA are also appropriate for use in health clubs and weight-loss centers. In comparison to other methods of estimating body composition, these methods are in the "good" range (Table 2-2).

The theoretical limitations in anthropometry and BIA have been well documented. For skinfold measures, only the subcutaneous fat of the body is sampled. Thus, as a measure of total body fatness, skinfolds do not directly estimate intermuscular, intramuscular, or visceral fat. An excellent review of the advantages and limitations of BIA has been published by Foster and Lukaski (1996). They point out that a large proportion of the resistance of the body to a given electric current occurs in the forearm (28%) and the lower leg (33%), whereas the trunk, which contains over 50% of the FFM, contributes only 9% of total body resistance.

TABLE 2-2. *Rating Scale for errors of predicting % fat and fat-free mass (FFM).*

| | Standard Errors of Estimate | | |
| | % Fat | FFM (kg) | |
Rating	Men and Women	Men	Women
Ideal	2.0	2.0	1.5
Excellent	2.5	2.5	1.8
Very Good	3.0	3.0	2.3
Good	3.5	3.5	2.8
Fairly good	4.0	4.0	3.2
Fair	4.5	4.5	3.6
Not recommended	5.0	>4.5	>4.0

Thus, in terms of assessing body composition from BIA, the trunk is underrepresented.

A second application of BIA is in the estimation of the volumes of the intracellular and extracellular fluid spaces and of changes in body fluid status. Early work in the area tested the hypothesis that reactance was more highly related to extracellular space, whereas resistance was related to intracellular space. More recently, the relation between the resistance to low-frequency electrical current and the volume of the extracellular space, and the resistance to high-frequency current to total body water volume has been investigated (Cornish et al., 1992; Van Loan et al., 1995). The development of this multifrequency impedance technique may allow for better estimates of body fluid compartments and the disproportional changes in the resistivities of intra- and extracellular fluids. A recent review demonstrates the theoretical and technical validity of this approach (Lorenzo et al., 1997). Bioelectric impedance spectroscopy (BIS), as this technique is sometimes called, may also be used for estimates of the effect of dehydration on the volume of body fluid compartments and may be applicable in clinical settings, such as in dialysis patients, in whom the ratio of intra- to extracellular fluid varies considerably.

Whereas the majority of evidence favors the increased accuracy of BIA and skinfold estimates over the simpler measures of height and weight, most research with infrared interactance technology shows less promise. Unlike BIA, for which several companies have developed competing technology, only one company has developed infrared interactance for body composition assessment. Most validation studies have used the Futrex-5000, although two other less expensive devices have been developed (Futrex-5000A and Futrex-1000).

The F1000 instrumentation has not been described by manufacturers or in the literature. Using female gymnasts as subjects, Smith et al. (1997) found lower correlations between estimates of percent body fat from underwater-weighing and those from both the F5000A and F1000 ($r = 0.40$–0.63), when compared to those from the F5000 ($r = 0.78$). The SEE for the F5000 has ranged from 4.6% (McLean & Skinner, 1992) to 3.7% (Heyward et al., 1992). In general, only a small gain in the accuracy of the prediction of percent body fat was found using infrared interactance compared to height and weight alone.

POPULATION-SPECIFIC EQUATIONS

The general problem of using skinfolds, circumferences, bioelectrical impedance, height, weight, and body density from underwater weighing to estimate body composition lies in the selection of a valid equation for the subjects being studied. For skinfolds and measures of height and weight, the use of population-specific equations is well established because for a given weight-for-height and for a given skinfold thickness, the relationship to body fatness varies with the population being tested. For example, the work of Jackson and Pollock (1985) clearly shows a different relationship between skinfolds and fatness in men versus women. Though many different bioelectrical impedance equations have been published (Heyward & Stolarcyzk, 1996), the need for specific equations for each population is not as clear because Kushner et al. (1992) showed that one equation could be applied to infants, youth, and adults.

Heyward and Stolarczyk (1996) provided a comprehensive summary of the many population-specific equations. The authors carefully evaluated the hundreds of equations published for different age groups, ethnicities, and levels of activity to provide recommended equations for different methods. Future body composition studies should focus on cross-validation of the major equations for each method to determine which equations are investigator-specific and thus not valid. Often, equations are investigator-specific rather than population-specific because of small sample size, wide age range (sample includes more than one population), and inaccurate measurements of either the criterion variable or the new variable (method) under investigation. These concerns also apply for anthropometry and bioelectrical impedance when validated against body density determined by underwater weighing because of errors introduced by invalid assumptions. Also, if standard measurement procedures are not followed, then the variation across investigations can be substantial. For example, we found that four investigators using four skinfold calipers and the same skinfold equation, but not using the same measurement procedures, recorded a 7% difference in mean fat content of the sample across the 16 combinations of calipers and investigators (Lohman et al., 1984). Finally, if the two-compartment model does not apply to the population under study (e.g., when densitometry is used in prepubescent children), then the equation that is applied will give biased estimates of percent fat.

Population-specific equations for estimating body fat from body density are not available in all age groups (Heyward & Stolarczyk (1996) and have yet to be developed for many ethnic groups and athletic groups. In addition to cross-validation of existing equations, new equations must be developed for these groups.

MEASURING CHANGES IN BODY COMPOSITION USING LABORATORY METHODS

One of the most essential research needs in the field of body composition is to identify improved methods for assessing changes in composition over time. The accuracy with which changes can be detected is reduced by the technical errors that are inherent in a given method, compounded by errors introduced by the investigator and by biological variation in the changes in water and mineral content that accompany changes in fat mass.

The accuracy of DXA compared to densitometry for estimating short-term and long-term changes in body composition has been addressed in recent studies (Going et al., 1993; Nelson et al., 1996). Going et al. (1993) reported that 17 subjects lost an average of 1.50 ± 0.80 kg of body weight after a 24 h dehydration protocol of no food, fluid, or exercise. The mean change in body weight determined by DXA was 1.41 ± 0.92 kg and was in agreement with the mean change in lean tissue mass from DXA (1.47 ± 1.04 kg). There was little change in bone mineral or fat content. In contrast, changes in FFM calculated from underwater weighing averaged 0.98 ± 1.23 kg, a lower mean value than expected and a greater variability than the changes estimated from DXA.

In another study, changes in body composition were measured by DXA and by underwater weighing in both a control and a strength-trained group before and after 9 mo of training (Nelson et al., 1996). While FFM estimated by DXA increased in the control group by 1.4 kg, it increased by only 0.6 kg in the strength-trained group. FFM estimated by densitometry increased by 0.2 kg in the control group and by 1.3 kg in the trained group. Because the changes in FFM estimated by densitometry were in the expected direction, the authors concluded that densitometry provides a sensitive measure of changes in FFM and that further evaluation of the accuracy of DXA was needed. It is possible, however, that changes in the density of the FFM that occur with strength training may confound the estimation of FFM; this conclusion, based on the face validity of the change, must be viewed cautiously. Caution is needed because of discrepancies between directly measured body weight and DXA-derived body weight. For example, in the study by Nelson et al. (1996), DXA overestimated the actual change in body weight in the control group, 2.0 kg vs. 0.4 kg, respectively. In the strength-trained group, DXA-derived body weight increased by 1.4 kg, but actual body weight increased 0.3 kg. These discrepancies are larger than expected based on the results of other studies using DXA (Going et al., 1993).

In contrast to the DXA results reported by Nelson et al. (1996), Nicholas et al. (1993) found a 1.5 kg increase in lean tissue mass by DXA after 6 mo of strength training in women compared to a 0.4 kg increase for controls.

The ability of DXA to detect small changes in soft tissue mass was also examined by Lands et al. (1996). Subjects were measured by DXA before and after a rapid saline infusion. Body weight after saline infusion increased 2.26 kg ± 0.20 while lean tissue mass measured by DXA increased 2.9 kg. In a hemodialysis study in which 2.8 kg of ultrafiltrate was removed from patients, FFM from DXA decreased 2.9 kg (Abrahamsen et al., 1996). Similar accuracy was reported by Woodrow et al. (1996) in DXA estimates of small changes in body composition caused by changes in hydration status.

Theoretical formulas to account for the effect of the variability in body water and bone mineral on percent-fat estimates from body density have been derived by Siri (1956), Selinger (1977), Baumgartner et al. (1991), Lohman (1992), and Heymsfield et al.(1996). These equations are derived from the known densities of water, protein, mineral, and fat in the human body. Assuming that these densities are relatively constant from individual to individual, the following equation can be derived (Lohman, 1992):

$$\% \text{ Fat} = (\frac{2.747}{Db} - 0.714w + 1.146b - 2.0503)\ 100$$

where w = water fraction of body weight, b = osseous mineral fraction of body weight, and D_b = body density. This equation is useful for demonstrating the effects of variation in FFM composition on estimates of body composition. For example, given a body density of 1.040 g/cc, a change in water concentration from 54.3% to 55.3% (holding bone mineral constant at 5.0%) would change the estimated body fatness from 26.0% to 25.3%. For the same body density (1.040 g/cc), a change in bone mineral content from 5.0% to 4.4% (holding water content at 54.3%) alters body fatness values from 26.0 to 25.3%.

Thus, densitometry is a suitable criterion method in the young adult population, in which the variability of water and bone mineral content (± standard deviation) is typically within 1% and 0.6%, respectively. Excellent agreement (i.e., SEE = 2.5–3.5%) between densitometric and DXA-derived estimates of percent fat has been reported (Hansen et al., 1993; Snead et al., 1993; Wellens et al., 1994). In other populations, e.g., elderly men and women, for whom the assumptions underlying densitometry may not be valid, a considerable portion of the disagreement between methods may be due to errors in the criterion method.

Clasey et al. (1997) came to the opposite conclusion, calling into question the validity of DXA in the aging population. They found that DXA-estimated percent fat predicted percent fat using a multicomponent model (density, water, mineral) with a SEE of 5%. The authors concluded that this large SEE was due to DXA. However, their estimated water content of the FFM was considerably higher than expected (78%), with a standard deviation of 5%. In contrast, Hewitt et al. (1993) reported a water content of 72.5 ± 1.4% in older adults. The large variability in the hydration status of FFM in the study by Clasey et al. (1997) may be an artifact of measurement error, that would invalidate the multicomponent model rather than DXA.

DXA estimates of percent fat may also be influenced by variation in body water content and bone mineral content, although the effects are more difficult to assess. Roubenoff et al. (1993), in their critique of DXA assumptions, argued that a subject's hydration status can affect the R_{ST} (soft tissue attenuation ratio) and added that the degree to which variation in hydration status affects DXA estimates of percent fat is currently not well documented (Lohman, 1996), Nord and Payne (1995) estimated that a 5% loss of body water (% of body mass) causes a 2% decrease of body fatness as estimated by DXA.

Other studies have addressed the effects of hydration on DXA estimates of composition. Although Pietrobelli et al. (1996) demonstrated the effect of hydration on the tissue R_{ST} by adding known amounts of fluid to ground beef. The R_{ST} increased in a small but predictable manner. Milliken et al. (1996) added water packets (2.8 kg) to the thigh and abdominal areas of 10 subjects. The addition of the water packets led to an overestimate of percent total body fat of less than 0.5% and an underestimate of the percentage of lean soft tissue of less than 0.5% when total body scans were analyzed using the Lunar software (version 1.3 y, extended research analysis mode). Going et al. (1993) reported that a mean 1.5 kg loss in body weight due to dehydration was estimated by DXA as a loss of 1.47 kg of lean tissue mass (LTM). In comparison, changes in FFM estimated by densitometry in the same study were not as accurately predicted, and there was greater variation within subjects (Going et al., 1993).

Pietrobelli et al. (1996) presented a thorough analysis of the theoretical effects of variability in water content on DXA estimates of composition; they showed that a 1 kg decrease in extracellular fluid would cause a 0.6% error in the estimate of body fat (a 0.07 kg increase in fat). This difference translates into a change of 0.4% in soft tissue as fat or 0.3% in body weight. A 1 kg gain or loss of body water is equivalent to a 1.5% change in the water content of a reference man (67 kg). These theoretical calculations show an even smaller effect of the variability of body water content than that predicted by Nord and Payne (1995). Thus, the concerns of Roubenoff et al. (1993) are not supported by theoretical calculations. These calculations also illustrate that the effect of variation in hydration status on DXA estimates of percent fat is less than that associated with densitometry.

MEASURING CHANGES IN BODY COMPOSITION
USING FIELD METHODS

Assessing changes in body composition as a result of intervention is problematic, particularly when two-compartment models or prediction equations based on two-compartment models are used (Lohman et al., 1988). Total body density is affected not only by losses in fat mass but also by concomitant changes in muscle mass and total body water. Often, fat-free mass (FFM) decreases along with fat mass as a result of reductions in muscle and total body water when obese persons consume very low-energy diets (Derenberg et al., 1989; Kusher et al., 1990; Van den Kooy et al., 1992), and these changes lower the density of the fat-free mass. As a result, measures of body density (converted to FFM and percent fat) will underestimate FFM and fat loss.

Unfortunately, most studies designed to assess whether or not field methods can accurately estimate changes in body composition have used reference methods and prediction equations based on two-compartment models. Thus, there continues to be great debate as to whether anthropometry and bioelectrical impedance can be used to monitor changes in body composition during periods of substantial weight loss and weight gain.

Although skinfold measures provide useful estimates of the change in subcutaneous adipose tissue depots, they do not always reflect changes in the internal fat depots. Moreover, prediction of percent fat from skinfolds assumes that the ratio of internal-to-subcutaneous fat is constant both within and among individuals. However, in obese persons who undergo rapid and substantial weight loss, there may be a disproportionate decrease in internal fat compared to subcutaneous fat (Scherf et al., 1986). Also, the relative decreases in skinfold measures during weight loss may not be the same at all sites (Ross et al., 1991), and change in skinfold thickness is not highly correlated with weight loss (Bray et al., 1978). The ability of changes in skinfold thickness to predict changes in percent fat and FFM has not been established, although it is not likely to be very good, especially when weight loss is substantial (Kushner et al., 1990, Van der Kooy et al., 1992).

Anthropometric equations based upon measures of circumferences often provide more-accurate estimates of body composition in obese individuals than do skinfold measures (Weltman et al., 1987, 1988). Further, changes in circumference measures are more highly related to weight loss (Bray et al., 1978). However, circumference measures cannot distinguish among regional muscle, bone, or fat loss unless combined with other measures such as skinfolds. Moreover, the waist-to-hip circumference ratio (WHR) does not change in response to rapid weight loss in individuals with upper body obesity (WHR > 0.80 for women, WHR > 0.95 for men). Thus, WHR should not be used in clinical settings to assess changes in adipose tissue distribution during acute weight loss (Ross et al., 1991).

There is conflicting evidence regarding whether or not BIA accurately predicts changes in body composition associated with weight loss. Whereas Ross et al.(1989) reported that the equations of Lukaski (1987) and Segal et al. (1988) accurately estimated the average FFM of slightly overweight men before and after weight loss, other investigators found these and other BIA equations either over-estimated (van der Kooy et al., 1992; Vazquez & Janosky, 1991) or under-estimated (Deurenberg et al., 1989) FFM loss in obese men and women. Part of the discrepancy is undoubtedly due to the variance in the criterion measurements. The magnitude of weight loss and whether or not the individual has reached a stable fluid distribution (extracellular-to-intracellular fluid ratio) before post-weight-loss tests are completed are other factors that contribute to the discrepant results. Given the conflicting findings, the validity of the BIA method for assessing changes in body composition should be evaluated more carefully.

ASSESSMENT OF REGIONAL BODY COMPOSITION

Practical field methods for assessment of regional body composition include anthropometry, ultrasonography, segmental bioelectrical impedance analysis, and possibly high-frequency energy absorption. Laboratory methods such as computed tomography (CT), magnetic resonance imaging (MRI), and dual energy x-ray absorptiometry (DXA) provide more direct and more accurate measures of regional composition and are useful for criterion measurements, but they are generally not practical for large-scale screening.

Anthropometry

Skinfolds and circumferences are widely used to estimate regional body composition. Individual skinfolds measure local subcutaneous fat and, when several sites are measured, can be used to reflect fat distribution (Lohman, 1992; Roche, 1996). Although circumference measurements include a variety of tissues (muscle, bone and adipose tissue) and do not, therefore, provide direct information on fat content, they can be useful as ratios. In particular, the waist-to-hip circumference ratio (WHR) is related to risk factors for cardiovascular disease (Seidell, 1996), and standards for WHR have been derived (Bray, 1992). Circumference measures are also used in combination with skinfold data to calculate the cross-sectional areas of adipose tissue and FFM (muscle plus bone) in the limbs. Despite questions of accuracy, these measures correlate well with laboratory measures (Roche, 1996) and are useful in screening for fat and muscle distribution in field and clinical settings.

Anthropometric indices of regional body composition have several limitations that must be considered in their interpretation. Skinfold measures, for example, assess only one of the four major fat depots (subcutaneous fatness), and the contribution of fat distribution to overall variation in skinfold thickness remains controversial (Garn et al., 1988a, 1988b; Mueller & Emerson, 1988), as do the functional differences between subcutaneous adipose tissues at different sites. There is no compelling evidence that waist and hip circumferences accurately predict the levels of fatness in the upper and lower body segments. For example, in the elderly and in obese persons, sagging of the abdominal musculature increases measurement error and confounds interpretation of the waist circumference. Despite these limitations, simple skinfold ratios and the WHR are correlated with risk factors for cardiovascular disease in adolescents (Williams et al., 1993) and adults (Seidell, 1996) and are useful for screening in clinical and field settings until more accurate field methods are developed.

Ultrasound

During the past two decades, B-mode ultrasound instruments have been developed that are capable of constructing cross-sectional images of tissue from reflected ultrasound waves (Roche, 1996). These instruments can measure the thicknesses of subcutaneous adipose tissue (SAT) and muscle, muscle cross-sectional areas, and abdominal depth, making them particularly useful for regional assessments. Equations have also been developed to predict body density and FFM from ultrasound measures of SAT and muscle thicknesses, respectively (Abe et al., 1994). Prediction errors for whole-body composition from regional ultrasound tend to be similar or somewhat larger than the errors associated with other field techniques, such as anthropometry (Abe et al., 1994; Fanelli & Kuzmarski, 1994).

B-mode ultrasound and skinfold-caliper measurements of SAT are about equal in precision (intra- and inter-observer technical errors $\cong 0.2$ mm; r = 0.90–0.99), but ultrasound has the advantages of providing hard copies and avoids the compression of SAT during measurement. Furthermore, ultrasound measurements can be made in obese subjects and at some sites where calipers cannot be applied. The disadvantages of ultrasound are that it is more expensive and less portable.

Ultrasound has been used to measure abdominal depth from the linea alba and from the deep surface of the anterior abdominal SAT to the posterior surface of the abdominal aorta (Roche, 1996). Good precision was reported, with average observer differences equal to 4.5% of the mean (Armellini et al., 1990), although others have failed to replicate these findings (Armellini et al., 1993; Bellisari et al., 1993). Given the strong association of intra-abdominal fat with chronic-disease risk factors, more research is warranted to determine if ultrasound estimates of abdominal depth are reasonable surrogates for the more expensive CT-determined estimates of visceral fat.

Muscle thickness measured in the limbs with B-mode ultrasound are both precise (r > 0.96) and accurate (Fried et al., 1986 Ishida et al., 1992). In addition, B-mode ultrasound with a water-based offset can be used to measure limb-muscle cross-sectional areas, although considerable practice may be necessary to obtain the desired precision (Stokes & Young, 1986). Specialized equipment may also be used to measure the velocity of transmission through a bone and the attenuation of the signal at specific frequencies. These values are related to bone mineral density (Tavakoli & Evans, 1991; Waud et al., 1992) and bone strength, and may be useful in screening for osteoporosis and for risk of bone fracture.

Segmental Bioimpedance Analysis (BIA)

Early studies with segmental BIA (Baumgartner et al., 1989; Going et al., 1987) showed that the sum of body-segment resistance indices was a better predictor of FFM than was the traditional whole-body resistance index (S^2/R). In these studies, the arm index had the highest correlation with whole body FFM (r >0.93) and predicted FFM almost as accurately as S^2/R. The value of this approach is that it can be applied to individuals for whom accurate measurements of stature cannot be made, such as many elderly, chair- and bed-fast patients or amputees.

Segmental BIA may also provide useful estimates of segmental composition independent of whole body composition. For example, height squared-adjusted appendicular (arm and leg) resistance measurements are highly correlated with appendicular skeletal muscle mass (Grammes et al., 1996). Also, the trunk-resistance index significantly improves the prediction of FFM when it is used along with whole-body resistance and reactance (Williams et. al., 1989). Also, the trunk phase angle (arctan of the ratio of reactance to resistance) is a significant predictor of percent body fat. It is possible that trunk impedance may be used to develop more-accurate estimates of intra-abdominal fat than can be obtained through anthropometry (e.g., waist-to-hip ratio), but this possibility has not been explored. Organ et al. (1994) devised a system for electrode placement that allows rapid measurements of resistance in the arms, legs and trunk. Thus, the possibility exists for developing BIA systems for clinical use that not only can estimate total body water, FFM, and body fat but can also provide estimates of segmental body composition.

High Frequency Energy Absorption

High-energy frequency absorption (HFEA) is being developed as a portable, inexpensive, non-invasive procedure for measurement of muscle mass within cross-sections of the limbs. The instrument consists of an adjustable-length, flexible coil 2.5 cm wide. A series of coils of different lengths is used to accommodate limbs with circumferences ranging from 20 to 75 cm. To measure HFEA, a coil of appropriate length is attached to a 9 v battery that, through an oscillator, produces a frequency varying from 15 MHz to 40 MHz. Zero readings, with the coil set at the same circumference as the limb, are obtained before and after HFEA is measured and are used to adjust the observed values. HFEA, in theory, is related to the number of electrolytes beneath the coil. It is assumed that the concentrations of electrolytes in extracellular fluid are near constant and that the ratio of intracellular:extracellular fluid is fixed in the limb musculature. These assumptions are similar to those for total body electrical conductivity (Baumgartner, 1996), which is used to measure total FFM. Because there are few electrolytes in bone and adipose tissue, HFEA could provide accurate estimates of limb muscle mass.

Preliminary results with HFEA are promising. Good precision has been demonstrated, and the instrument has been successfully validated against saline solutions (Roche et al., 1995). Inter-observer error was small (CV~ 4%, n = 5 observers) for thigh and calf HFEA readings but was larger for arm readings (CV = 12.1%). HFEA was a significant predictor of MRI-estimated muscle volume, along with other variables (R^2 = 0.86–0.90), although standard errors of estimate (SEE/$\overline{X}$ ≅ 10–18%) were larger than desirable. Because age and sex were significant in the regression equations for the arm and calf, it is possible that intramuscular adipose tissue, which could vary with age and sex, may have affected the HFEA data but not the MRI data.

PRACTICAL IMPLICATIONS: SCREENING FOR BODY FATNESS, MUSCLE, AND BONE

Given the link between body composition and health, screening programs should be established to identify individuals at risk for obesity, sarcopenia, and osteoporosis. The programs must be based on considerations of which methods are most useful, which components of composition should be measured at different ages, and how frequently serial measurements should be made.

For screening, four constructs of composition must be addressed: 1) total body fatness, 2) fat distribution, 3) bone mineral status, and 4) lean body mass and muscle mass. The importance of measuring these different components varies at different ages (Table 2-3) based on their importance in different life stages. Methods must be selected according to the required accuracy and the training, expense, and time required to collect data.

Methods for estimating body fatness and the factors to consider when selecting a particular method are given in Table 2-4. In general, weight-for-height indices are not useful for assessing body composition. Skinfolds and BIA are the methods of choice for most populations; however, for obese subjects, body circumferences are preferred. Heyward and Stolarzyk (1996) have provided a detailed review of appropriate equations for the different methods of estimating body composition in different populations.

Measurements of fat distribution can begin in adolescence and continue through adulthood, where there is evidence that there is an increased disease risk associated with fat distribution. Circumference measures and the subscapular:triceps skinfold ratio have been identified as practical estimates of fat distribution.

To assess bone mineral status, the only acceptable methods are DXA and ultrasound. Measurements of axial (lumbar spine) and appendicu-

TABLE 2-3. *Screening for body fatness, fat distribution and bone mineral status by life stage (years).*

Variable	Pediatric (1–5)	Childhood (6–11)	Youth (12–17)	Adult (18–40)	Middle age (40–60)	Elderly (>60)
Body fatness	3	3	3	3	3	
Fat distribution			3	3	3	
Bone mineral status				3	3	3
Lean mass					3	3

TABLE 2-4. *Ratings of the Validity and Objectivity of Methods of Estimating Body Composition.*

Method	Precision	Objectivity	Accuracy	Valid Equations	Overall
Body Mass Index	1	1	4,5	4,5	4
Near-Infrared Interactance	1	1,2	4	4	3.5
Skinfolds	2	2,3	2,3	2,3	2.5
Bioelectric Impedance	2	2	2,3	2,3	2.5
Circumferences	2	2	2,3	2,4	3.0

1 = Excellent, 2 = Very Good, 3 = Good, 4 = Fair, 5 = Unacceptable
Precision = reliability within investigators
Objectivity = reliability between investigators
Accuracy = agreement with a criterion method
Valid equations = availability of cross-validated equations

lar (hip) bone mineral density are helpful in assessing fracture risk in middle-aged and elderly populations. Forearm and wrist bone-mineral density are not good predictors of spine and hip bone-mineral density and cost only slightly less to measure than axial bone-mineral density. In the elderly, muscle mass and bone mineral status must be assessed because loss of muscle mass in a major determinant of functional capacity and "failure to thrive."

Body Composition and Bone Health Standards

Recent developments in the assessment of bone mineral density using DXA have brought increased national attention to the costs of osteoporosis and fractures in postmenopausal women. The risk for fracture is greatly increased in this population, with the greatest period of bone loss in femur and spine occurring within the first 10–20 y after menopause (Raun et al., 1994). Furthermore, approximately 12% of postmenopausal women in the study of Raun et al. were two standard deviations or more below the premenopausal level of bone mineral density. Recent estimates indicate that at least 90% of all hips and spine fractures among elderly white women are attributable to osteoporosis (Melton et al., 1997). Ray et al. (1997) recently estimated the total national health care expenditures attributable to osteoporotic fractures in 1995 at 13.8 billion dollars.

Bone mineral density (BMD) standards for bone health have been developed by the World Health Organization. These standards are especially applicable to the lumbar spine and hip regions. Osteopenia has been defined as BMD between 1 and 2.5 standard deviations (SD) below the average BMD for a young adult, and osteoporosis is defined as a BMD greater than 2.5 SD below the young-adult reference value. Women identified with osteoporosis are often treated with hormone replacement therapy or with an antiresorptive drug (e.g., calcitonin). In addition, calcium supplements and exercise are sometimes prescribed, although according to The Surgeon-General's Report for Physical Activity and Health, the best form of exercise to prevent bone loss has not yet been established. The effectiveness of calcium supplementation is also uncertain. In response, the Women's Health Initiative is undertaking a 10 y study to determine the effect of calcium supplementation on BMD and bone fractures.

In the postmenopausal population, the best predictor of risk for bone fracture is the DXA-estimated BMD of the lumbar spine and hip regions. Other risk factors such as small frame size, a body weight below 55 kg, body fat less than 20%, family history of osteoporosis, history of physical inactivity, history of prolonged medication known to reduce BMD (e.g., glucocorticoids), low calcium intake, smoking, and alcoholism account for only 20-40% of the variance in BMD (Lydick et al., 1996; Michaelesson et al., 1996). Thus, because of the relatively low predictive value of other risk factors, and because of the important genetic influence on bone mass, assessment of present BMD status by DXA is the preferred approach for determining fracture risk.

A history of weight loss, chronic dieting, or a history of weight cycling may be other important risk factors for low BMD, although they are not yet well evaluated. A decrease in bone mass with weight loss has been observed by Compston et al. (1992), Jensen et al. (1994), Houtkooper et al. (1995) and Chen et al. (1997). In the study by Jensen et al. (1994), 6.0% of total bone mineral (172 g) was lost over a 15-wk period in a group of obese adults who lost 12.2 kg on a low-energy diet. In one extreme case, an individual who continued to lose weight (45 kg) for 9 mo lost 754 g of bone mineral or 25.4% of her initial bone mineral content. Thus, for obese individuals who do not have high BMD levels, large weight loss may increase the risk for bone fractures. This study suggests that postmenopausal women not on hormone replacement therapy who are identified as having low BMD may lose a significant amount of bone mineral as a result of weight loss and may increase their risk of fracture. In the studies of Houtkooper et al. (1995) and Chen et al. (1997), weight change in pre- and postmenopausal women was significantly correlated with changes in regional and total-body BMD. The reduction in BMD appears to be related to changes in hormonal levels that accompany reductions in body fat, as this association was present after accounting for variation in dietary intake by multiple regression analysis (Houtkooper et al., 1995).

Body Fat Standards for Adults

The role of body fatness as a disease risk factor is limited by the lack of practical and accurate methods for assessing body composition in large epidemiological studies. Thus, for most large-scale databases, only height and weight have been assessed. In national probability samples (NHANES I, II and III), skinfolds have been measured along with height and weight. These data provide the best reference data, resulting in new standards for body fatness (Lohman, et al., 1997). In the past, the recommended amounts of body fat for men and women were 10–20% of body weight for men and 20–30% of body weight for women. These recommendations were based largely on samples of young adult men and women, and no allowance was made for age (Lohman, 1992).

However, median skinfold thickness in large reference samples increase with age. For example, in the NHANES reports, the median skinfolds for young and middle-aged women increase from 31.5 mm (20–24 y) to 46.0 mm (55–64 y). In men, the values increased from 22.0 mm (20–24 y) to 28.0 mm (45–54 y) (Lohman et al., 1997). Converting these skinfold measures to percent fat values provides an improved reference base for implementing body-fat standards for adults (Table 2-5).

Body Fat Standards for Children

Over the past 15 y, body composition standards for children in the USA have been developed by several organizations, e.g., by the American Alliance for Health, Physical Education, Recreation and Dance for the *Health Related Physical Fitness Test* and *Physical Best*, by the state of Texas for *Fit Youth Today*, by the Institute for Aerobics Research for the *Fitnessgram*, and by the YMCA for the *YMCA Youth Fitness Test*. Early standards were based on skinfold thicknesses in children and youth from the NHANES national probability samples that corresponded with adult standards for percent body fat. With the development of skinfold equations based on multicomponent models (Lohman, 1986, 1992; Slaughter et al., 1988), and age-adjusted equations for estimating body density (Lohman et al., 1988; Williams et al., 1992a), valid estimates of percent body fat in children were derived from skinfold measures. These equations for body-fat standards for children are illustrated in the *Fitnessgram* (Figures 2-3 and 2-4).

More recently, health-related fatness standards have been developed that are derived from the relationship between body fatness and cardiovascular-disease risk factors in children and adolescents (Williams et al., 1992b). In the long-running Bogalusa Heart Study, Berenson and colleagues (1980) have shown that large skinfold thicknesses are related to higher levels of blood lipids, lipoproteins, and blood pressure and to lowered glucose tolerance in children and adolescents. Investigators have accumulated a wealth of data from this study that relate body composition in youth to the early development of car-

TABLE 2-5. *Percent Fat Health Standards for Men and Women.*

| | | Recommended Body Fat Levels (% Fat) | | | |
	Not recommended	Low	Mid	Upper	Obesity
Men: age group					
Young adult men	<8	8	13	22	>22
Middle-aged men	<10	10	18	25	>25
Elderly men	<10	10	16	23	>23
Women: age group					
Young adult women	<20	20	28	35	>35
Middle-aged women	<25	25	32	38	>38
Elderly women	<25	25	30	35	>35

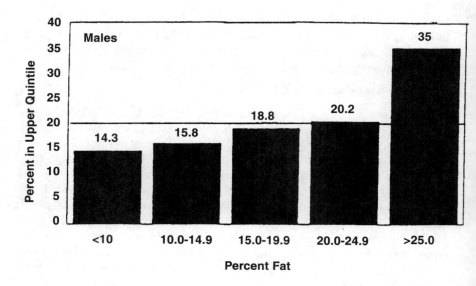

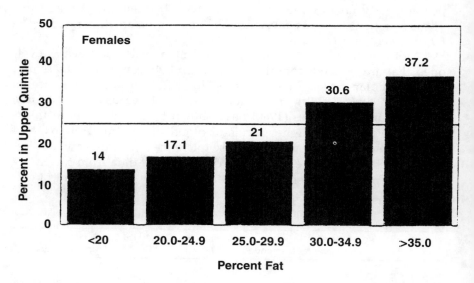

FIGURE 2-3. *Association between percent fat in children and adolescents and cardiovascular risk factors in the Bogalusa Heart Study.* Twenty percent of subjects (solid line) are expected to fall in the upper quintile of cardiovascular risk factors by chance.

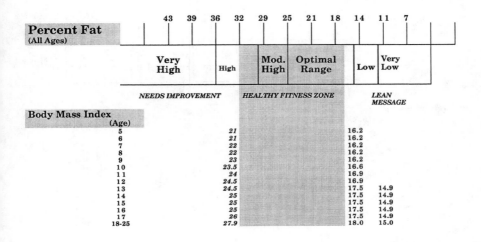

FIGURE 2-4. *Standards for percent fat and body mass index for girls and adolescent females.*

diovascular risk factors (Aristimuno et al., 1984; Berenson et al., 1980, 1982; Smook et al., 1987; Voors et al., 1982). Using blood-lipid and skin-fold data from a subsample of 1667 males and 1653 females aged 5–18 y, Williams et al. (1992b) used age-adjusted, sex- and race-specific equations to estimate the percent body fat from skinfold measurements and to assess the relationship between percent body fat and risk factors for cardiovascular disease. In this analysis, children were divided into intervals of 5% body fat, and odds ratios were calculated for each group that reflected the odds of elevated total cholesterol, unfavorable serum lipoprotein ratios, and elevated systolic and diastolic BP (Williams et al., 1992b). Boys with greater than 25% body fat and girls with greater than 30% body fat had increased risk for higher levels of adverse lipoprotein ratios and elevated blood pressure compared to their leaner counterparts (Figure 2-3). These results became the basis for standards setting the healthy range of body fatness for girls at 17–32% and for boys at 10–25% (Figures 2-4 & 2-5). Table 2-6 contains BMI and skinfold values that can be used to identify children at risk.

Assessment of body composition in children has been the focus of research for the past 30 y. Both anthropometric and bioelectric impedance measures have gained considerable support over the last 15 y. Varied research efforts have contributed to the identification of valid estimates of body composition in youth (Boileau et al., 1984; Foman et al.,

BOYS

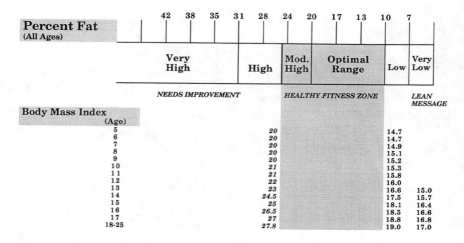

FIGURE 2-5. *Standards for percent fat and body mass index for boys and adolescent males.*

TABLE 2-6. *Percent fat standards for children and adolescents with corresponding cutpoints for BMI and skinfolds.*

Age	Percent Fat	Triceps & Calf (or Subscapular) Skinfolds (mm)	Triceps Skinfold (mm)	Body Mass Index (BMI)
Males				
10	10–25	12–33 (30)[a]	7–19	15.3–21
11	10–25	12–33 (30)	7–19	15.8–21
12	10–25	12–33 (30)	7–19	16.0–22
13	10–25	12–33 (30)	7–18	16.6–23
14	10–25	12–33 (30)	7–18	17.5–24.5
15	10–25	12–33 (30)	7–17	18.1–1–25
16	10–25	12–33 (30)	7–17	18.5–26.5
17	10–25	12–33 (30)	7–16	18.8–27
Females				
10	17–32	20–44 (38)	10–24	16.6–23.5
11	17–32	20–44 (38)	10–24	16.9–25
12	17–32	20–44 (38)	10–24	16.9–24.5
13	17–32	20–44 (38)	10–23	17.5–24.5
14	17–32	20–44 (38)	10–23	17.5–25
15	17–32	20–44 (38)	10–23	17.5–25
16	17–32	20–44 (38)	10–22	17.5–25
17	17–32	20–44 (38)	10–22	17.5–26

[a] Sum of triceps and subscapular skinfolds

1982; Guo et al., 1989; Haschke, 1983; Haschke et al., 1981; Houtkooper et al., 1992; Lohman, 1986; Slaughter et al., 1988). As a result of this work, the densities of the fat-free body mass in infants through adolescents have been defined, and age-specific formulas have now replaced the Siri equation for use in children (Lohman, 1989).

Alternatively, age-adjusted percent body fat can be calculated using the generalized formulas developed by Williams et al. (1992a) as follows.

For females,
% Fat = [(5.69 − (0.038 × Age)) ⎤ D_b] − [(5.31 − (0.4 × age))] × 100.

For males,
% Fat = [(5.68 − (0.041 × Age)) ⎤ D_b] − [(5.31 − (0.45 × age))] × 100.

Body composition can now be accurately estimated in children by use of underwater weighing, skinfold measures, and bioelectrical impedance (Lohman, 1992).

Predictive Value of Body Composition Estimates

If changes in body fatness and other health-related risk factors (e.g., blood pressure, cholesterol, and blood lipoprotein profile) should change in tandem, then early measurements of obesity may be predictive of later morbidity and mortality (Must et al., 1992). For example, it is reasonable to expect obese children and adolescents to become obese adults with the attendant complications associated with obesity, and measurements of body fatness at one time in life may be used to predict fatness later in life (Guo et al., 1994; Roche & Guo, 1994). The ability to accurately predict adult body composition and risk factors from measurements in childhood and adolescence would greatly enhance efforts directed at screening and early intervention.

Tracking from childhood to adolescence and from adolescence to young adulthood is well established (Baumgartner & Roche, 1988). There is also evidence of tracking from adolescence to middle age (Guo et al., 1994) and even to old age (Must et al., 1992). Guo et al. (1994) showed that BMI at age 35 ± 5 y was significantly correlated with BMI at ages 9–18 y in both males and females. Moreover, the prediction of the overweight status of adults (BMI > 28 for men and >26 for women) from BMI measures made at age 18 y was excellent. For 18 year olds with a BMI exceeding the 60th percentile (the cut-off with the best combination of sensitivity and specificity), the prediction of being overweight at age 35 y was 34% fat for men and 37% fat for women. Large BMI (>75th percentile) during adolescence is also predictive of overweight status in later life, with greater morbidity and mortality in men and decreased functional capacity in women (Must et al., 1992).

DIRECTIONS FOR FUTURE RESEARCH

Much of the body composition research in the past has focused on identifying laboratory and field methods of estimating body fatness in different populations. Some of this work has been limited by the two-component model and by assumptions in the criterion method, most often underwater weighing. For example, recent research with weight lifters has shown that body density values used with the two-component model overestimate body fat by 4% in this population (Modlesky et al., 1996a).

Additional research is needed to better define the magnitude of the variation in the composition of FFM, particularly in the water, protein, and bone-mineral fractions. Whether it is the water or bone-mineral component that introduces the most variability in D_{ffm} remains to be resolved among different populations (Lohman, 1992; Williams et al. 1993).

The magnitude of the variability in body water and its effect on longitudinal and cross-sectional studies of body composition has proved particularly difficult to assess. As noted, criterion methods based on the two-compartment model result in inaccurate estimates of FFM. Moreover, when multicomponent models are used to estimate the variation in the water content of the FFM, as in,

$$\text{water}/\text{FFM} = \frac{\text{water (kg)}}{\text{water} + \text{mineral} + \text{protein, (kg)}}$$

technical errors in measuring body water content affect the values for both water and FFM. Using DXA, it is possible to estimate FFM independent of water.

$$\text{water}/\text{FFM} = \frac{\text{water (kg)}}{\text{lean soft tissue} + \text{mineral (kg)}}$$

This approach should be used in future research to quantify the variation in water content of the body.

One approach to multicomponent modeling of body composition is illustrated by the work of Modlesky et al. (1996a). Measurements of body density by underwater weighing, body water content by deuterium dilution, and bone mineral content by DXA were obtained on young-adult male weight lifters and controls. From these measurements, the density of the FFM in the weight lifters was estimated as 1.089 ± 0.005 g/cc. Using the Slaughter and Lohman (1980) formula for estimating FFM from body height, the weight lifters were 4.7 kg above the regression line. The controls were −1.2 kg below the line (Table 2-7). This study is an excellent example of the potential differences in the composition of FFM between athletic and non-athletic populations. The water and mineral components of the FFM vary with the muscle content of the body. An increase in muscle mass results in a greater increase in water content than in bone-mineral content, and the overall density of the FFM is decreased (Lohman, 1992). Therefore, when underwater weighing and the two-component model were used to estimate percent body fat, the weight lifters appeared to be 4.1% fatter than what was predicted by the multicomponent model. In contrast, the same error was only 1.0% for DXA.

In those populations in which the density of FFM differs significantly from the reference value, field equations that were developed and validated using underwater weighing and the two-component model may not provide accurate estimates of FFM. This is an important consideration in the populations of high-school wrestlers and gymnasts for whom equations have been developed using the two-component model to predict minimum wrestling weight (Thorland et al., 1991). These equations may overestimate percent body fat in muscular athletes and allow wrestlers to participate at lower-than-recommended percent body fat levels. Further research is needed to extend this work to other athletic groups and to examine ethnic differences in the composition of FFM.

Another important area for future is better characterization of the relationships among body fatness, health, and disease. The degree to which disease risk is related to whole body fatness independent of fat distribution is not clear. Because the distribution of body fat changes as body fatness increases or decreases, changes in fat distribution are an important concern. The use of DXA to estimate the regional distribution of body fat is a critical research tool for future studies in this area. Combining DXA and skinfold measures, it may be possible to determine the relationships among subcutaneous fat depots in different regions of the body, i.e., thigh, abdomen, chest, arm, and other fat depots, independent

TABLE 2–7. *Body mass and composition of FFM in two populations of adult men (Modlesky et al., 1996a).*

Variable	Controls Mass	% FFM	Weight lifters mass	% FFM
Height, cm	177.4 ± 3.8	—	172.4 ± 6.9	—
Body mass, kg	69.3 ± 5.0	—	89.1 ± 11.2	—
Fat mass, kg	9.9 ± 2.7	—	11.9 ± 5.4	—
Water mass, kg	43.2 ± 3.4	72.6 ± 2.0	57.7 ± 7.4	74.8 ± 1.2
Protein mass, kg	12.7 ± 1.5	21.5 ±1.9	15.4 ± 2.5	19.9 ±1.4
Mineral mass, kg	3.5 ± 0.4	5.9 ± 0.4	4.1 ± 0.6	5.3 ± 0.6

of overall body fatness. Further studies validating DXA as an indirect measure of visceral fat as well as of overall abdominal fat should be conducted using CT and MRI as criterion methods. Further investigations are also needed to develop practical predictors of fat distribution that rely upon simple measures such as waist circumference, various circumference ratios, or other indexes using body size.

The validation of pencil-beam DXA absorptiometers for assessing body composition and for measuring body composition changes has been established. Recent developments in computer software have enabled the estimation of regional body fatness to be more accurate, although differences between instruments are still reported (Modelesky et al., 1996). The application of fan-beam DXA has not been validated for body-composition assessment or for measuring changes in body composition. This technology offers shorter scan times (less than 5 min) and better resolution; however, magnification and positioning effects have yet to be resolved.

The use of multifrequency bioelectrical impedance (BIA) should be further evaluated for use in estimating extracellular fluid volume. Comparisons between single-frequency and multifrequency BIA are essential to determine under what conditions and in which populations the multifrequency approach offers greater predictability.

Better body composition measures of muscle mass are greatly needed, and DXA may prove useful because DXA provides estimates of appendicular muscle mass that are highly correlated with estimates of muscle mass from CT scans (Wang et al., 1996). In the Health ABC study sponsored by the National Institutes on Aging, some of these critical questions will be addressed in a large cohort of elderly subjects.

Along with a greater emphasis on developing accurate measures of bone and muscle-mass, research is needed to determine the long-term effects on intervention programs on delaying or decreasing age-associated losses of bone mineral and muscle mass. The development of effective intervention programs in youth for preventing obesity and assuring adequate bone density also requires more attention.

SUMMARY

Changes in body composition influence health, functional capacity, and physical performance. With recent advances in technology and the development of multiple-component models of body composition, it is now possible to obtain accurate estimates of bone mineral, fat-free mass, appendicular muscle, and body fat in large groups of people. The application of the DXA technology in large-scale studies holds the promise of providing more-definitive descriptions of the changes that occur in total and regional body composition during growth and aging. As a result of improved methods of measurement and better standards, it may soon be possible to screen "at risk" individuals with low bone and muscle mass or to reference those with high levels of total and regional fat and to accurately follow changes during intervention programs designed to increase bone and muscle content and decrease body fat.

BIBLIOGRAPHY

Abrahamsen, B., T.B. Hansen, I.M. Hogsberg, F.B. Pedersen, and H. Beck-Nielsen (1996). Impact of hemodialysis on dual x-ray absorptiometry, bioelectrical impedance measurements, and anthropometry. *Am. J. Clin. Nutr.* 63:80–86.

Aristimuno, G.G., T.A. Foster, A.W. Voors, S.R. Srinivasan, and G.S Berenson (1984). Influence of persistent obesity in children on cardiovascular risk factors: The Bogalusa heart study. *Circulation* 69:895–904.

Bassey, E.J., M.A. Fiatarone, E.F. O'Neill, M. Kelly, W.J. Evans, and L.A. Lipsitz (1992). Leg extensor power and functional performance in very old men and women. *Clin. Sci.* 82:3231–32377.

Baumgartner, R.N. (1996). Electrical impedance and total body electrical conductivity. In: A.F. Roche, S.B. Heymsfield and T.G. Lohman (eds.) *Human Body Composition*. Champaign, IL: Human Kinetics, pp. 79–107.

Baumgartner, R.N, W.C. Chumlea, and A.F. Roche (1989). Estimation of body composition from bioelectric impedance of body segments. *Am. J. Clin. Nutr.* 50:221–226.

Baumgartner, R.N., S.B. Heymsfield S. Lichtman J. Wang, and R.N. Pierson, Jr. (1991). Body composition in elderly people: effect of criterion estimates on predictive equations. *Am. J. Clin. Nutr.* 53:1345–1353.

Baumgartner R.N., S.B.Heymsfield, and A.F Roche (1995). Human body composition and the epidemiology of chronic disease. *Obes. Res.* 3:73–95.

Baumgartner, R.N, and A.F. Roche (1988). Tracking of fat pattern indices in childhood: the Melbourne Growth Study. *Hum. Biol.* 60:549–567.

Baumgartner, R.N., R.M. Siervogel, W.C. Chumlea, and A.F. Roche (1989). Associations between plasma lipoprotein cholesterols, adiposity and adipose tissue distribution during adolescence. *Int. J. Obes.* 13:31–41.

Bellisari, A., A.F. Roche, and R.M. Siervogel (1993). Reliability of b-mode ultrasonic measurements of subcutaneous adipose tissue and intra-abdominal depth: comparisons with skinfold thicknesses. *Int. J. Obes.* 17:475–480.

Berenson, G.S., C.A. McMahon, and A.W. Voors (1980). *Cardiovascular risk factors in children: The early national history of athersclerosis and essential hypertension*. New York: Oxford University Press.

Berensen, G.S., L.S. Webber, S.R. Srinivasan, A.W. Voors, D.W. Harska, and E.R. Dalferes (1982). Biochemical and anthropometric determinants of serum B- and pre-B-lipoproteins in children: The Bogalusa Heart Study. *Arteriosclerosis* 2:325–334.

Bevier, W.C., P.R. Wiswell, G. Pyka, K.C. Kozak, K.M. Newhall, R. Marcus (1989). Relationship of body composition, muscle strength and aerobin capacity to bone mineral density in older men and women. *J. Bone Min. Res.* 4:421–32.

Boileau, R., T.G. Lohman, M.H. Slaughter, T.E. Ball, S.B. Going, and M.K. Hendrix (1984). Hydration of the fat-free body in children during maturation. *Hum. Biol.* 56:651–666.

Bray, G.A. (1992). Pathophysiology of obesity. *Am. J. Clin. Nutr.* 55:488S-94S.

Bray, G.A., F.L. Greenway, M.E. Molitch, W.T. Dahms, R.L. Atkinson, and K. Hamilton (1978). Use of anthropometric measures to assess weight loss. *Am. J. Clin. Nutr.* 31:769–773.

Chen, Z., T.G. Lohman, W.A. Stini, C. Ritenbaugh, and M. Aiken (1997). Fat or lean tissue mass: which one is the major determinant of bone mineral mass in healthy postmenopausal women? *J. Bone Min. Res.* 12:144–157.

Clasey, J., M.I. Hartman, J. Kanaley, C. Wideman, C. Teates, C. Bouchard, and A. Weltman (1997). Body composition by DEXA in older adults: accuracy and influence of scan mode. *Med. Sci. Sports Exerc.* 29:560–567.

Cohn, S.H., C. Abesamis, I. Zanzi, J.F. Aloia, S. Yasumura, and K.J. Ellis (1977). Body elemental composition: comparison between black and white adults. *Am. J. Physiol.* 232:E419–E422.

Cohn, S.H., K.J. Ellis, D. Vartsky, A. Sawitsky, W. Gartenhaus, S. Yasumura, and A.N. Vaswani (1981). Comparison of methods estimating body fat in normal subjects and cancer patients. *Am. J. Clin. Nutr.* 34:2839–2847.

Dempster P., and S. Aitkens (1995). A new air displacement method for determination of human body composition. *Med. Sci. Sports Exerc.* 27:1692–1697.

Ellis, K.J. (1996). Whole-body counting and neutron activation analysis. In: A.F. Roche, S.B Heymsfield and T.G. Lohman (eds.). *Human Body Composition*. Champaign, IL: Human Kinetrics, pp. 45–61.

Foman, S.J., F. Haschke, E.E. Zeiger, and S.E. Nelson (1982). Body composition of reference children from birth to age 10 years. *Am. J. Clin. Nutr.* 35: 1169–1175.

Foster, K.R., and H.C. Lukaski (1996). Whole-body impedance—what does it measure? *Am. J. Clin. Nutr.* 64: 388S–396S.

Friedl, K.E., J.P. DeLuca, L.J. Marchitelli, and J.A. Vogel (1992). Reliability of body-fat estimations from a four-compartment model by using density, body water, and bone mineral measurements. *Am. J. Clin. Nutr.* 55:764–70.

Gallagher, D., M. Visser, D. Sepulveda, R.N. Pierson, T. Harris, and S.B. Heymsfield (1996). How useful is body mass index for comparison of body fatness across age, sex, and ethnic groups? *Am. J. Epidem.* 143:228–239.

Garn, S.M., T.V. Sullivan, and V.M. Hawthorne (1988a). Evidence against functional differences between "central" and "peripheral" fat. *Am. J. Clin. Nutr.* 47:836–839.

Garn, S.M. T.V. Sullivan, and V.M. Hawthorne (1988b). Reply to Mueller and Emerson. *Am. J. Clin. Nutr.* 48:1343–1345.

Gasperino, J.A., J. Wang, R.N. Pierson, and S.B. Heymsfield (1995). Age-related changes in musculoskeletal mass between black and white women. *Metabolism* 44:30–34.

Going, S.B. (1992). Body fatness and the risk for elevated CVD risk factors in children and adolescents: cross-sectional and longitudinal analyses. In: *Assessment and Management of Health. Proceedings of the Korean International Sports Science Seminar*, November, 1992.

Going, S.B. (1996). Densitometry. In: A.F. Roche, S.B. Heymsfield, and T.G. Lohman (eds.). *Human Body Composition*. Champaign, IL: Human Kinetics, pp. 3–23.

Going, S.B., M.P. Massett, M.C. Hall, L. A. Bare, P.A. Root, D.P William, and T.G. Lohman (1993). Detection of small changes in body composition by dual-energy x-ray absorptiometry. *Am. J. Clin. Nutr.* 57:845–850.

Going, S.B., R.W. Pamenter, and T.G. Lohman (1990). Estimation of total body composition by regional dual photon absorptiometry. *Am. J. Hum. Biol.* 2:703–710.

Going, S.B., D.P. Williams, and T.G. Lohman (1995). Aging and body composition: biological changes and methodological issues. In: J.O. Holloszy (ed.) *Exercise and Sport Science Reviews*, Vol. 23. Baltimore: Williams & Wilkins, pp.411–458.

Grammes, J., C. Nunez, D. Gallagher, R. Baumgartner, and S.B. Heymsfield (1996). Arm skeletal muscle estimated by bioelectrical impedance analysis. *FASEB J.* 10:1121.

Guo, S.S., A.F. Roche, W.C. ChumLea, J.D. Gardner, and R.M. Siervogel (1994). The predictive value of childhood body mass index values for overweight at age 37 y. *Am. J. Clin. Nutr.* 59:810–9.

Guo, S., A.F. Roche, and L.B. Houtkooper (1989). Fat-free mass in children and young adults predicted from bioelectric impedance and anthropometric variables. *Am. J. Clin. Nutr.*, 50:435–443.

Hansen, N.J., T.G. Lohman, S.B. Going, M.C. Hall, R.W. Pamenter, L.A. Bare, T.W. Boyden, and L.B. Houtkooper (1993). Prediction of body composition in premenopausal females from dual-energy x-ray absorptiometry. *J. Appl. Physiol.* 75:1637–1641.

Haschke, F. (1983). Body composition of adolescent males. Part I. Total body water in normal adolescent males. Part II. Body composition of the male reference adolescent. *Acta Paed. Scand. Suppl.* 307:1–23.

Haschke, F., S.J. Foman, and E.E. Zeiger (1981). Body composition of a nine-year-old reference body. *Ped. Res.* 15: 847–849.

Hewitt, M.J., S.B. Going, D.P. Williams, and T.G. Lohman (1993). Hydration of the fat-free mass in prepubescent children, young adults and older adults: implications for body composition assessment. *Am. J. Physiol.* 265:E88–E95.

Heymsfield, S.B., and W. Waki (1991). Body composition in humans: advances in the development of multicompartment chemical models. *Nutr. Rev.* 49:97–108.

Heymsfield, S.B., D. Gallagher, M. Visser, C. Nunez, and Z. Wang (1995). Measurement of skeletal muscle: Laboratory and epidemiological methods. *J. Gerontol.* 50A:23–9.

Heymsfield, S.B., S. Lichtman, R.N. Baumgartner, J. Wang, Y. Kamen, A. Aliprantis, and R.N. Pierson, Jr. (1990). Body composition of humans: comparison of two improved four-compartment models that differ in expense, technical complexity, and radiation exposure. *Am.J. Clin. Nutr.* 50:52–58.

Heymsfield, S.B., C. McManus, J. Smith, V. Stevens, D.W. Nixon (1982). Anthropometric measurement of muscle mass: revised equations for calculating bone-fee arm muscle area. *Am. J. Clin. Nutr.* 36:680–90.

Heymsfield, S.B., J. Wang, S. Lichtman, Y. Kamen, J. Kehayias, and R.N. Pierson (1989). Body composition in elderly subjects: a critical appraisal of clinical methodology. *Am. J. Clin. Nutr.* 50:1167–1175.

Heymsfield, S.B., Z.M. Wang, and R.T. Withers (1996). Multicomponent molecular level models of body composition. In: A.F. Roche, S.B. Heymsfield, and T.G. Lohman (eds.). *Human Body Composition*. Champaign, IL: Human Kinetics, pp. 129–147.

Heyward, V.H., and L.M. Stolarzk (1996). *Applied Body Composition Assessment*. Champaign, IL: Human Kinetics.

Heyward, V.H., K.L. Cook, V.L. Hicks, K.A. Jenkins, J.A. Quatrochi, and W. L. Wilson (1992). Predictive accuracy of three field methods for estimating relative body fatness of nonobese and obese women. *Int. J. Sport Nutr.* 2:75–86.

Houtkooper, L.B., S.B. Going, T.G. Lohman, and A.F. Roche (1992). Bioelectrical impedance estimation of fat free body mass in children and youth: a cross-validation study. *J.Appl. Physiol.* 72:366–373.

Houtkooper, L.B., C. Ritenbaugh, M. Aickin, T.G. Lohman, S.B. Going, J.L. Weber, K.A. Greaves, T.W. Boyden, R.W. Pamenter, and M.C. Hall (1995). Nutrients, body composition, and exercise are related to change in bone mineral density in premenopausal women. *J.Nutr.* 125:1229–1237.

Jackson, A.S., and M.L. Pollock (1985). Practical assessment of body composition. *Phys. Sports Med.* 13:77–90.

Jensen, L.B., F. Quaade, and H. Sorensen (1994). Bone loss accompanying voluntary weight loss in obese humans. *J. Bone Min. Res.* 9:459–463.

Kushner, R.F., A. Kunigk, M. Alspaugh, P.T. Andronis, C.A. Leitch, and D.A. Schoeller (1990). Validation of bioelectrical-impedance analysis as a measurement of change in body composition in obesity. *Am. J. Clin. Nutr.* 52:219–223

Kushner, R.F., D.A. Schoeller, C.R. Fjeld and L. Danford (1992). Is the impedance index (ht^2/R) significant in predicting total body water? *Am. J. Clin. Nutr.* 56:835–839.

Lands, L.C., L. Hornby, J. Hohenkerk, and F. Glorieux (1996). Accuracy of measurements of small changes in soft tissue mass by dual-energy x-ray absorptiometry. *Clin. Invest. Med.* 19:279–285.

Lohman, T.G. (1992). *Advances in Body Composition Assessment.* Champaign, IL: Human Kinetics Publishers.

Lohman, T.G. (1986). Applicability of body composition techniques and constants for children and youth. In: K.B. Pandolf (ed.), *Exercise and Sport Sciences Reviews,* Vol. 14. New York:Macmillan, pp. 325–357.

Lohman, T.G. (1989). Assessment of body composition in children. *Ped. Exerc. Sci.* 1:19–30.

Lohman, T.G. (1996). Dual energy x-ray absorptiometry. In: A.F. Roche, S.B. Heymsfield, and T.G. Lohman (eds.) *Human Body Composition.* Champaign, IL: Human Kinetics Publishers.

Lohman, T.G. (1981). Skinfolds and body density and their relationship to body fatness: A review. *Hum. Biol.* 53:181–225.

Lohman, T.G., L.B. Houtkooper, and S.B. Going (1997). Body fat measurement goes high tech. Not all are created equal. *ACSM Health Fit. J.* 1:30–35.

Lohman, T.G., A.F. Roche, and R. Martorell (eds.) (1988). *Anthropometric Standardization Reference Manual.* Champaign, IL: Human Kinetics Publishers, p.186.

Lohman, T.G., M.L. Pollock, M.H. Slaughter, L.J. Brandon, and R.A. Boileau (1984). Methodological factors and the prediction of body fat in female athletes. *Med. Sci. Sports Exerc.* 16:92–95.

Lorenzo, A.D., A. Andreoli, J. Matthie, and P. Withers (1997). Predicting body cell mass with bioimpedance by using theoretical methods: a technological review. *J. Appl. Physiol.* 82:1542–1558.

Lydick, E., J. Turpin, K. Cook, R. Stine, M. Melton, and C. Byrnes (1996). Development and validation of a simple questionnaire to facilitate identification of women with low bone density. *J. Bone Min. Res.* 11(Suppl 1): S368.

Marcus, R., B. Drinkwater, G. Dalsky, J. Dufek, D. Raab, C. Slemenda, C. Snow-Harter (1992). Osteoporosis and exercise in women. *Med. Sci. Sports Exerc.* 24:S301–S307.

Mazariegos, M., Z. Wang, D. Gallagher, R.N. Baumgartner, D.B. Allison, J. Wang, R.N. Pierson, and S.B. Heymsfield (1994). Differences between young and old females in the five levels of body composition and their relevance to the two-compartment chemical model. *J. Gerontol.* 49:M201–M208.

Mazess, R., B. Collick, J. Trempe, H. Barden, and J. Hanson (1989). Performance evaluation of a dual energy x-ray bone densitometer. *Calcif. Tiss. Int.* 44:228–232.

McCrory, M.A., T.D. Gomez, E.M. Bernauer, and P.A. Mole (1995). Evaluation of a new air displacement plethysmograph for measuring human body composition. *Med. Sci. Sports Exerc.* 27:1686–1691.

McLean, K.P., and J.S. Skinner (1992). Validity of Futrex-5000 for body composition determination. *Med. Sci. Sports Exerc.* 24: 253–258.

Melton, L.J., III, M. Thamer, N.F. Ray, J.K. Chan, C.H. Chesnut III, T.A. Einhorn, C.C. Johnston, L.G. Raisz, S.L. Silverman, and E.S. Siris (1997). Fractures attributable to osteoporosis: Report from the national osteoporosis foundation. *J. Bone Min. Res.* 12:16–23.

Michaelesson, K., R. Bergstrom, H. Mallmin, L. Holmberg, A. Wolk, and S. Ljunghall (1996). Screening for osteopenia and osteoporosis: selection by body composition. *Osteoporosis International,* 6:120–126.

Milliken, L.A., S.B. Going, and T.G. Lohman (1996). Effects of variations in regional composition on soft tissue measurements by dual-energy x-ray absorptiometry. *Int. J. Obes.* 20:677–682.

Modlesky, C.M., K.J. Cureton, R.D. Lewis, B.M. Prion, M.A. Sloniger, and D.A. Rowe (1996a). Density of the fat-free mass and estimates of body composition in male weight trainers. *J.Appl. Physiol.* 80(6):2085–2096.

Mueller, W.H., and J.B. Emerson (1988). Functional differences between central and peripheral fat. *Am. J. Clin. Nutr.* 48:1343–1345.

Must, A., P.F. Jacques, G.E. Dallal, C.J. Bajema, and W.H. Dietz (1992). Long-term morbidity and mortality of overweight adolescents: a follow-up of the Harvard growth study of 1922 to 1935. *N. Engl. J. Med.* 327:1350–1305.

Myers, A.H., S.P. Baker, M.L. Van Natta, H. Abbey, E.G. Robinson (1991). Risk factors associated with falls and injuries among elderly institutionalized persons. *Am. J. Epidemiol.* 133:1179–90.

Nelson, M.E., M.A. Fiatarone, J.E. Layne, I. Trice, C.D. Economos, R.A. Fielding, R. Ma, R.N. Pierson, Jr., and W.J. Evans (1996). Analysis of body composition techniques and models for detecting change in soft tissue with strength training. *Am. J. Clin. Nutr.* 64:669–676.

Nord, R.H., and R.K. Payne (1995). A new equation for converting body density to percent fat. *Asia Pacific J. Clin. Nutr.* 4:167–171.

Organ, L.W., G.B. Bradham, D.T.W. Gore, and S.L. Lozier (1994). Segmental bioelectrical impedance analysis: theory and application of a new technique. *J. Appl. Physiol.* 77:98–112.

Ortiz, O., M. Russell, T.L. Daley, R.N. Baumgartner, M.Waki, S. Lichtman, J.Wang, R. N. Pierson, and S.B. Heymsfield (1992). Differences in skeletal muscle and bone mineral mass between black and white females and their relevance to estimates of body composition. *Am. J. Clin. Nutr.* 55:8–13.

Pietrobelli, A., C.Formica, Z. Wang, and S.B. Heymsfield (1996). Dual-energy x-ray absorptiometry body composition model: review of physical concepts. *Am. J. Physiol.,* 271: E941–E951.

Pocock N., J. Eisman, T. Gwinn, P. Sambrook, P. Kelly, J. Freund, M. Yeates (1991). Muscle strength, physical fitness, and weight but not age predict femoral neck bone mass. *J. Bone. Min. Res.* 4:441–8.

Ramirez, M.E., S.C. Hunt, R. Williams (1991). Blood pressure and blood lipids in relation to body size in hypertensive and normotensive adults. *Int. J. Obes.* 15:127–45.

Ray, N.F., J.K. Chan, M. Thamer, and L.J. Melton III (1997). Medical expenditures for the treatment of osteoporotic fractures in the United States in 1995: Report from the national osteoporosis foundation. *J. Bone Min. Res.* 12:24–35.

Roche, A.F. (1995). The significance of sarcopenia in relation to health. *Asia Pacific J. Clin. Nutr.* 4:129–132.

Roche, A.F., and S. Guo (1994). Tracking: Its analysis and significance. *Auxology* 25:465–469.

Roche, A.F., R. Wellens, S.Guo, R.M. Siervogel, M.D. Boska, A. Northeved, and K.F. Michaelsen (1995). High frequency energy absorption and the measurement of limb muscle. *Asia Pacific J. Clin. Nutr.* 4:199–201.

Roubenoff, R., J.J. Kehayias (1991). The meaning and measurement of lean body mass. *Nutr. Rev.* 49:163–75.

Roubenoff, R., J.J. Kehayias, B. Dawson-Hughes, and S.B. Heymsfield (1993). Use of dual-energy x-ray absorptiometry in body composition studies: not yet a "gold standard". *Am. J. Clin. Nutr.* 58:589–591.

Schoeller, D.A. (1996). Hydrometry. In: A.F. Roche, S.B. Heymsfield, and T.G. Lohman (eds.). *Human Body Composition.* Champaign, IL: Human Kinetics, pp. 25–43.

Selinger, A. (1977). The body as a three component system. Unpublished doctoral dissertation. The University of Illinois, Urbana, IL.

Siri, W.E. (1961). Body composition from fluid spaces and density: Analysis of methods. In J. Brozek, and A. Henschel (eds.) Techniques for measuring body composition. Washington, DC: *National Academy of Sciences,* pp. 223–224.

Siri, W.E. (1956). The gross composition of the body. In: C.A. Tobias and J.H. Lawrence (eds.). *Advances in Biological and Medical Physics,* Vol.4. New York: Academic Press, pp. 239–280.

Slaughter, M.H., and T.G. Lohman (1980). An objective method for measurement of the musculo-skeletal size to characterize body physique with application to the athletic population. *Med. Sci. Sports Exerc.* 12:170–174.

Slaughter, M.H., T.G. Lohman, R.A. Boileau, M. VanLoan, C.A. Horswill, and J.H. Wilmore (1988). Influence of maturation on relationship of skinfolds to body density: A cross-sectional study. *Hum. Biol.* 56:681–689.

Smoak, C.G., Burke, D.S. Freedman, L.S. Webber, and Berensen, G.S. (1987). Relation of obesity to clustering of cardiovascular disease risk factors in children and young adults: The Bogalusa heart study. *Am. J. Epidem.* 125: 364–372.

Snead, D.B., S.J. Birge, and W.M. Kohrt. (1993). Age-related differences in body composition by hydrodensitometry and dual-energy x-ray absorptiometry. *J. Appl. Physiol.* 74: 770–775.

Steen, B., A. Bruce, B. Isakkson, T. Lewin, A. Svanborg (1977). Body composition in 70–year old males and females in Gothenburg Sweden. A Population study. *Acta Med. Scand.* (Suppl. 611):87–112.

Terry, R.B., M.L. Stefanick, W.L. Haskell, and P.D. Wood (1991). Contributions of regional adipose tissue depots to plasma lipoprotein concentrations in overweight men and women: possible protective effects of thigh fat. *Metabol. Clin. Exper.* 40:733–740.

Thorland, W.G., C.M. Tipton, T.G. Lohman, R.W. Bowers, T.J. Housh, G.O. Johnson, J.M. Kelly, R.A. Oppliger, and T.K. Tcheng (1991). Midwest wrestling study: Prediction of minimal weight for high school wrestlers. *Med. Sci. Sports Exerc.* 23:1102–1110.

Van Loan, M.D., N.L. Keim, K. Berg, and P.L. Mayclin (1995). Evaluation of body composition by dual energy x-ray absorptiometry and two different software packages. *Med. Sci. Sports Exerc.* 27:587–591.

Voors, A.W., D.W. Harsha, L.S. Webber, B. Rachakishmamurtz, S.R. Srinivasan, and G.S. Berenson (1982). Clustering of anthropometric parameters, glucose tolerance, and serum lipids in children with high and low B- and pre-B- lipoproteins in children: The Bogalusa heart study. *Arteriosclerosis* 2: 346–355.

Wang, Z.M., R.N. Pierson, and S.B. Heymsfield. (1992). The five level model: a new approach to organizing body composition research. *Am. J. Clin. Nutr.* 56:19–28.

Wang, J., J.C. Thornton, S. Burastero, J. Shen , S. Tanenbaum, S.B. Heymsfield, and R.N. Pierson, Jr. (1996). Comparisons for body mass index and body fat percent among Puerto Ricans, Blacks, Whites and Asians living in the New York City area. *Obes. Res.* 4:377–384.

Wellens, R., W.C. ChumLea, S. Guo, A.F. Roche, N.V. Reo, and R.M. Siervogel (1994). Body composition in white adults by dual-energy x-ray absorptiometry, densitometry, and total body water. *Am. J. Clin. Nutr.* 59:547–555.

Wellens, R.I., A.F. Roche, H.J. Khamis, A.S. Jackson, M.L. Pollock, and R.M. Siervogel (1996). Relationships between the body mass index and body composition. *Obes. Res.* 4:35–44.

White, F.M.M., L.H. Pereira, L.H., and J.B. Garner (1986). Associations of body mass index and waist: hip ratio with hypertension. *Can. Med. Assoc. J.* 135:313–20.

Williams, D.P., S.B. Going, T.G. Lohman, et al., (1992a). Estimation of body fat from skinfold thicknesses in middle-aged and older men and women: a multiple component model. *Am. J. Hum. Biol.* 4: 595–605.

Williams, D.P., S.B. Going, T.G. Lohman, D.W. Harska, S.R. Srinivasan, L.S. Webber, and M.D. Berenson (1992b). Body fatness and risk for elevated blood pressure, total cholesterol, and serum lipoprotein ratios in children and adolescents. *Am. J. Pub. Health* 82: 358–363.

Williams, D.P., S.B. Going, M.P. Massett, T.G. Lohman, L.A. Bare, and M.J. Hewitt (1993). Aqueous and mineral fractions of the fat-free body and their relation to body fat estimates in men and women aged 49–82 yr. In: K.J. Ellis and J.D. Eastman (eds.) *Human Body Composition: In Vivo Methods, Models and Assessment.* New York:Plenum Press, pp. 109–113.

Williams, D.P., S.B. Going, L.A. Milliken, M.C. Hall, and T.G. Lohman (1995). Practical techniques for assessing body composition in middle-aged and older adults. *Med. Sci. Sports Exerc.* 27:776–783.

Woodrow, G., J.H. Turney, and M.A. Smith (1996). Influence of changes in peritoneal fluid on body-composition measurements by dual-energy x-ray absorptiometry in patients receiving continuous ambulatory peritoneal dialysis. *Am. J. Clin. Nutr.* 64:237–241.

DISCUSSION

HORSWILL: In the older literature on body composition, some of the investigators measured lean-body mass, whereas others measured fat-free mass. Are these two masses considered the same, or is the subtle difference still worth considering?

LOHMAN: The distinction that Behnke wanted us to make was that lean-body mass has a small amount of essential fat, but fat-free mass has no fat. That concept has been lost; by and large, people are calculating fat-free mass in most of the equations that they are developing rather than lean-body mass. They are not putting in that essential fat, and a lot of people use these terms interchangeably with the subtle distinction lost.

HORSWILL: I am skeptical of the validity of measurements made with the Bod Pod because of potential problems with the effect of the body on raising the temperature in the chamber. A rise in temperature would alter the pressure-volume relationship, which is critical to the principle of the instrument. Does the manufacturer account for temperature, or is that a source of error?

LOHMAN: I do not know how well this method accounts for temperature changes over the 4–5 min required for measurement. I think skepticism is very healthy at this point. Always, we have initial favorable reports on any new method, but subsequent research limitations often show up in later publications.

HORSWILL: In a small plethysmography chamber, infants may generate significant body heat and seriously affect this pressure-volume relationship, so the Bod Pod may not be as effective in some populations as others. What is the current thinking about the acceptability of total body electrical conductivity?

LOHMAN: Total body electrical conductivity (TOBEC) is a good measure of both fat-free body mass and total body water. For this method the subject enters an electromagnetic field, and composition of the body can be estimated by the extent to which that field is disrupted. Because of the limited number of instruments and their relatively high cost, there has not been much research reported in the last 5 y. This technique is probably better than the bioelectrical impedance technique.

HORSWILL: With the use of a multicomponent method to assess body fat in children, body composition estimates are more accurate and mean values for body fat are less likely to be overestimated than was previously the case. Is this likely to be a disservice to the child who is borderline obese but may no longer get treatment?

LOHMAN: What I think is important about these new equations for children is that there are some children that would be incorrectly called obese using underwater weighing as the reference method. Those kids are now better served in a way that is healthy for them; they will no longer be overly concerned about their body composition. Thus, these new equations better serve the kids in the middle of the range as well as the athletic population, and they also help diagnose the kids who are truly obese.

GUTIN: I'm concerned about your suggestion that we should raise the cut point for acceptable body fatness to 35% fat. At about 30% fat in children we see a rather sharp upturn in some of the cardiovascular risk factors. If we were to use disease risk as a criterion, we might suggest 30% as an upper limit for a healthy level of body fatness.

LOHMAN: In the Bogalusa data in children, there is only a slight increase in cardiovascular risk factors for girls over 30% fat; the risk is greater for those over 35% (Smoak et al., 1987). Also, there is some evidence to show that if adults are 40–45% fat, they are not at risk by being slightly fatter than at younger ages. That is why we increased the percent fat standard. It's really at the higher levels of obesity where the risk goes up. What we are trying to do is focus on high levels of obesity rather than being overly concerned about trying to get the entire population to become average or below average in body fat.

BAR-OR: Doesn't the threshold value of body fat for determining obesity really depend on tracking of percent fat? We know that adiposity does track from adolescence to adulthood to a moderate extent, but are there any tracking data that would help us predict what specific levels of adiposity in young people mean for the future? Without this knowledge, I do not see the utility of setting threshold values for young people.

LOHMAN: There are a few tracking studies showing that body composition measured during infancy does not predict adult body composition very well. So if you are singled out as an obese one-year old, you are only slightly at risk for becoming an obese adult. In later childhood, the tracking does a little better, i.e., a 10-year old obese child is more likely to become an obese adult than a child who is not obese, but the relationship is still only a modest one, i.e., correlation coefficients of about 0.4. Adolescent obesity, on the other hand, is much more predictive of adult obesity. If we can keep prepubescent children from becoming obese adolescents, I think this could be crucial to preventing obesity during adulthood. Long-term studies are really needed in this area. This is a great challenge.

GUTIN: This issue of tracking is an interesting one. It seems to me that the Bogalusa data suggest that tracking in childhood is also important because disease risk factors measured in childhood are associated with damage in the arteries during childhood and early adulthood. It may be that an obese child is already suffering damage to the arteries, and that is a good reason to be concerned about obesity.

LOHMAN: Do children with high-risk lipoprotein profiles have evidence of damaged arteries?

GUTIN: Yes, in autopsy studies of people who have died from accidents when they were young adults, lesions in the aorta and the carotid artery were correlated to elevated risk factors that were measured when they were children.

M. WILLIAMS: Are there any data on the proportion of the population that actually knows their body-fat percentage and are using it to practice weight-control methods?

LOHMAN: I don't know of any published surveys to answer that question. In our lab we ask clients before we measure them, "Where do you think your body fat is?" and, "What do you think an ideal body fat is?" We then estimate their body compositions and give them a feedback on where they are on the charts. Some surveys on height and weight show that most people perceive themselves as overweight, but that is not the case at all. Only a small percentage of the general population has been measured for body composition. My dream is that one day we will have body composition centers in each community where people will be accurately assessed for bone, muscle, and fat.

EICHNER: When you say most people view themselves as overweight, isn't there a tremendous gender difference? Most men seem to think they are just fine, while many women view themselves as overweight.

LOHMAN: On the surface, men may report that, but I believe deeper feelings also show a misperception of their ideal weights.

CLARKSON: In using the "bathroom-scale" type of bioelectrical impedance device that the subject stands on, one must input information such as height and activity level. How does activity factor into the equation to determine percent body fat?

LOHMAN: It only factors in because on the average, the more active people in the population tend to be leaner. It's not a theoretical construct in which your conductance is a dependent of your activity levels. If there is more lean tissue in the body, the body is a good conductor with less resistance; with a lot of body fat, the body is not as good a conductor.

WALBERG-RANKIN: You mentioned that much of the resistance in bioelectrical impedance is in the limbs. Since two people could have the same body fat, but different body fat distributed in the legs, how could assessment of only the legs on the "bathroom-scale" device give you an accurate assessment of total body fat?

LOHMAN: What you are thinking of is individual exceptions. The overall prediction error is 3–4%, but there will be one out of 20 where the prediction is 6–8% off. These individuals will be those who indeed have unusual distributions of fat.

WALBERG-RANKIN: Could waist-to-hip ratio be incorporated into the equations to enhance the calculation of body fat with this method?

LOHMAN: That is probably a good idea. There are equations that combine anthropometry and bioelectric impedance and show a greater predictability than either method independently.

HARGREAVES: From a practical standpoint of predicting health outcomes or sport performance outcomes, how accurate do estimates of body composition need to be?

LOHMAN: From a public health standpoint, height and weight predict within 5%, so we need to improve on that. From the standpoint of sports, we did a study in which we measured college women basketball players with four calipers, four investigators, and four skinfold equations. The lowest value we reported was 14% fat for that group of basketball players, which would make them very, very lean, and the highest value was 28% for one investigator working with one set of calipers. Thus, errors accumulate and can get very large for the individual or group, and that is a problem. In the wrong hands with the wrong equation and with the malfunctioning of equipment, we get sizable errors that can mislead people. Recently, I went to a nutrition center where they were doing weight-loss treatments for the public, and they were using a bioelectrical impedance device that was about 15% off.

FIATARONE: I have a question about the use of DXA longitudinal studies, particularly those that are investigating growth hormone and growth hormone secretagogues, in which the intent is obviously to increase the muscle mass. But growth hormone obviously increases water content, skin, connective tissue, and many other tissues that are measured with DXA and not differentiated from muscle. Based on DXA measurements without an independent measure of muscle mass, one can falsely conclude that there is a positive effect of these growth-hormone secretagogues. What is a more appropriate way of looking specifically at muscle mass?

LOHMAN: Muscle mass has been tough to measure in our field. Computed tomography (CT) scans may be the best method presently.

FIATARONE: We have been encouraging commercial supplement suppliers to use CT scans in addition to DXA, but they are very hesitant to do that because they are worried that in fact the DXA results will disappear once specific measures of muscle mass are added.

LOHMAN: Body potassium might be another method that could be useful.

FIATARONE: But an increase in total body potassium could also reflect changes in tissues other than muscle.

BAR-OR: This question is related to the use of segmental bioimpedance analysis for populations whose body proportions are abnormal, e.g., children with cerebral palsy or adults with hemiplegia. One approach might be to measure both sides of the body and then obtain an average value. However, an arithmetic mean may be misrepresenting the reality because of the different size of limbs in the two sides. Is there a better solution to this problem?

LOHMAN: Bioelectrical impedance may not be the method at all for kids with unusual morphologies. You should use some other method, e.g., total body water or anthropometry or DXA.

GISOLFI: Tim, could you expand on the utilization of bioelectrical impedance to measure intracellular and extracellular water?

LOHMAN: The basic idea is that by using a multi-frequency approach where you put several frequencies through the body simultaneously and then plot that spectrum of resistances versus current frequencies, a relationship exists between the extracellular versus the intracellular fluid ratios. The low versus high frequency current will respond differently with changes in extracellular/intracellular volume, and the pattern of the spectral analysis will change if you change the fluid distribution. I am not yet persuaded that this approach can accurately estimate these fluid changes, however, excellent studies are underway.

BAR-OR: To my understanding, the multi-frequency bioimpedance principle is based on the fact that the cell membrane serves as a capacitor. When current passes at a low frequency, the capacitor becomes a barrier, and the measurement reflects only the extracellular volume. However, when the frequency is high enough, this barrier is overcome and then one measures total body water.

How useful is the multi-frequency bioimpedance analysis in determining acute changes in body fluid compartments, e.g., during progressive dehydration? What are the resolution and sensitivity of this method, and what level of acute changes in body fluid compartments can we detect?

LOHMAN: The theory says you ought to be able to pick up changes in fluid distribution. It is the precision of the measurements that might limit the detection of normal variation. A theoretical calculation can be made of how much of a change in frequency spectrum should occur, but the key question is can this be done precisely and sensitively from hour to hour and day to day? My guess is that changes greater than 1% and less than 3% can be detected. How helpful multifrequency analysis is really going to be is just not clear yet.

NADEL: Should people use dehydration as a tool to try to calibrate these systems? We know, for example, that athletes might lose 2–4% body water during prolonged activity, and we can calculate with some degree of accuracy the consequent changes in the extracellular and intracellular fluid compartments. We can calculate the loss of body mass from fuel oxidation rates, so we ought to be able to apply those or estimates to these bioimpedance techniques to determine the extent to which they detect or are fooled by changes in body water.

LOHMAN: That's an excellent idea, and I am not sure whether it has been done that way.

MAUGHAN: There must be some concern as to the reliability of the impedance measures because if you measure body water by BIA and then give the subject 500 mL of water to drink, it is hard to see a consistent difference in whole-body impedance. Having that liquid in the stomach is perhaps not the most appropriate way to appraise whole-body composition, but nonetheless, it should be picked up by the impedance analyzer. Measuring changes in BIA on a time scale of minutes should get rid of most of the other factors that might interfere because there would be no changes in electrode position, subject posture or anything else.

The use of magnetic resonance imaging, of course, is going to be restricted because of the capital cost and the running cost, but nonetheless, it does seem to offer some options. We know that if it is used to measure limb volume, for example, by doing repeated scans along the limb, and this volume is then compared with total limb volume measured by water displacement, the total volume of the limb is estimated very accurately by MRI. The question then is, when you try to estimate the compositions of the limbs or of the whole body, is the limitation going to be in the measurement of the volumes of the different tissues, or in converting those volumes to masses because of the variability in the tissue densities, which, of course, the imaging techniques don't give you?

LOHMAN: The densities of fat, lean, and bone among individuals is fairly constant, but the proportion of each tissue is the main source of variation not accounted for by total limb volume.

ROWLAND: Is there not a very simple method for physicians and others to use to estimate body fat and promote the appropriate public health messages on a broader scale? It seems to me there was a study that suggested that simple visual inspection can produce fairly accurate estimates of body fat.

LOHMAN: I think were one or two such studies published, but they are hard to publish any more because we emphasize technology so much. I believe visual inspection, e.g., in the doctor's office, good give fairly good estimates of body fat, but there is also going to be bias in those estimates based on individual observers. However, I think most could be trained and could do a pretty good job. I would like to see a conference on developing a simple method that would be adopted widely to give the physician and others a useful tool.

SHERMAN: It is my understanding that physical inactivity has been classified as a primary risk factor for heart disease and that obesity is a contributing factor to many of the pathologies associated with heart disease and other diseases such as diabetes. Is there any research that indicates that certain levels of physical activity might ameliorate or reduce the risk factors that are associated with obesity so that some people who might be classified as obese can derive some degree of protection due to the fact that they are physically active.

LOHMAN: It's likely that physical activity is a factor as well as body fat. Reducing risk factors through physical activity would probably ameliorate much of the risk of the relationship between obesity and diabetes and cardiovascular disease. In my judgment, there is evidence for the benefit of physical activity independent of weight loss in the obese, but I still believe that there is an independent risk of obesity as long as it is present. Physical activity is important for all populations, but I think we are missing the boat for the obese as this population is less active. Increasing physical activity levels could definitely reduce their risk factors, independent of fatness.

3

Body Fat Distribution, Exercise and Nutrition: Implications for Prevention of Atherogenic Dyslipidemia, Coronary Heart Disease, and Non-Insulin Dependent Diabetes Mellitus

JEAN-PIERRE DESPRÉS, PH.D

INTRODUCTION

This chapter provides an overview of the critical issues related to the etiology and treatment of visceral obesity and a review of the work conducted in our laboratory in this area of research. In addition to pathophysiological considerations, practical tools for the identification of high-risk, visceral obese patients are provided. Finally, simple exercise recommendations are made with the hope that such exercise prescription will be helpful not only in the treatment of but also in the prevention of the visceral obesity, insulin-resistant dyslipidemic syndrome. Because visceral obesity is highly prevalent in North American and other populations, this information may have important public health implications.

OBESITY AS A RISK FACTOR FOR CARDIOVASCULAR DISEASE: IMPORTANCE OF BODY FAT DISTRIBUTION

Obesity is a prevalent condition in developed as well as in developing countries, and an excess of body fat has been associated with complications such as hypertension, diabetes, and dyslipidemias and with an increased risk of cerebral and vascular diseases (Barrett-Connor, 1985; Bray, 1985; Després, 1994; Kissebah & Peiris, 1989; Kissebah et al., 1989; Manson et al., 1995). Thus, obese patients are more prone to hyperglycemia and hyperlipidemia and are at increased risk for the development of non-insulin dependent diabetes mellitus (NIDDM) and premature coronary heart disease (CHD) (Bray, 1985; Després, 1994; Kissebah et al., 1989). However, the clinician is confronted with the remarkable metabolic heterogeneity found in overweight or obese individuals. Indeed, while some show severe metabolic complications, others have normal blood pressure, euglycemia, and a rather normal lipid-lipoprotein profile, emphasizing the notion that obesity is indeed a heterogeneous condition (Björntorp, 1984).

Research conducted over the last 15 y has emphasized that obesity is heterogeneous not only in its complex etiology but also regarding its complications (Donahue et al., 1987; Ducimetière et al., 1986; Lapidus et al., 1984; Larsson et al., 1984; Ohlson et al., 1985). In 1947, Jean Vague from the University of Marseille was the first to suggest that body fat topography was a more important factor to consider than excess adipose tissue mass per se in the clinical assessment of obese patients (Vague, 1947). Indeed, in a seminal two-page article, Vague (1947) suggested that an excess accumulation of trunk fat, a condition which he referred to as android obesity, was more frequently observed among his overweight patients with hypertension, diabetes or CHD, compared to the typical female type of obesity, which he referred to as gynoid obesity, that was seldom associated with severe metabolic complications. Vague also reported these remarkable ideas in the English literature (Vague, 1956), findings that were confirmed 35 y later by a series of epidemiological and metabolic studies. Among the scientists responsible for the rediscovery of this concept, Kissebah et al. (1982) were the first to suggest that a high proportion of abdominal fat assessed by an elevated ratio of waist-to-hip circumferences (Figure 3-1) was associated with alterations in glucose tolerance as well as with elevated fasting triglyceride levels. Similar conclusions were almost simultaneously reached in a large study in women and men conducted at the University of Göteborg in Sweden (Krotkiewski et al., 1983).

However, the marked enthusiasm and interest of scientists, clinicians, and health professionals for body fat topography was largely stimulated by the publication of results from two prospective studies conducted by Per Björntorp and his colleagues at the University of Göteborg (Lapidus et al., 1984; Larsson et al., 1984). They reported that a high

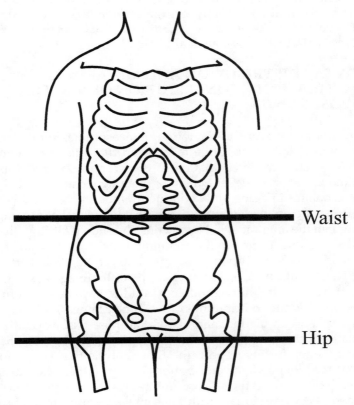

FIGURE 3-1. *Schematic representation of the levels at which waist and hip circumferences should be measured according to the recommendations of the World Health Organization. Waist: midway between the lower rib margin and the iliac crest. Hip: widest over the great trochanters.*

waist-to-hip ratio in men and women was an independent predictor of mortality from cardiovascular disease. In addition, this group also reported that a high waist-to-hip ratio, irrespective of the body mass index (BMI = body weight in kg divided by height in m²), was associated with an increased risk of developing diabetes over a 13.5 y follow-up period (Ohlson et al., 1985). The highest risk was observed among men having both a high body mass index and an elevated waist-to-hip ratio; the increased risk was 30 times the risk of developing diabetes found among non-obese subjects in the lowest tertile of waist-to-hip ratio. Thus, these results emphasize that the crude estimation of total body fatness based on the measurement of the BMI is an unsatisfactory procedure to assess the risk of complications associated with obesity. Following the publication of the results of these prospective studies, several metabolic studies have indicated that an elevated waist-to-hip ratio is associated with insulin resistance, hyperinsulinemia, glucose intolerance, and a dyslipidemic profile that includes hypertriglyceridemia and low HDL cholesterol levels (for reviews, see Björntorp, 1988; Després, 1993, 1994; Després et al., 1990; Kissebah et al., 1989).

BODY FAT DISTRIBUTION AND METABOLIC COMPLICATIONS: CONTRIBUTION OF VISCERAL ADIPOSE TISSUE

Although the waist-to-hip ratio is a measurement of the proportion of abdominal fat, it should be recognized that this variable only provides, at best, a crude estimation of the proportion of abdominal fat. With the more recent development of imaging techniques such as magnetic resonance imaging and computed tomography, it has been possible to measure body fat distribution with a high level of accuracy and to distinguish the amount of subcutaneous abdominal fat from the amount of adipose tissue located in the abdominal cavity, the so-called intra-abdominal or visceral adipose tissue (Borkan et al., 1982; Ferland et al., 1989; Kvist et al., 1988; Sjöström et al., 1986; Tokunaga et al., 1983) (Figure 3-2). Thus, with this methodology, studies have been conducted that have examined the contributions of total body fatness, subcutaneous abdominal fat accumulation, and visceral adipose tissue accumulation as correlates of the common metabolic complications that are observed in obese patients. In this respect, the first analysis that we performed to sort out the independent contributions of total fatness vs. subcutaneous and visceral adipose tissue accumulation was a very simple one. We matched obese individuals with the same amount of total body fat but having either a low or high accumulation of visceral adipose tissue measured by computed tomography (Després, 1991d, 1993; Després et al.,

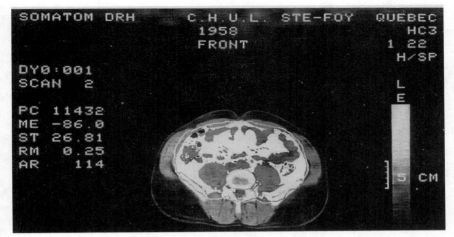

FIGURE 3-2. *Computed tomography scan at the abdominal (L4-L5) level. The visceral adipose tissue area, which is delineated by drawing a line within the muscle wall surrounding the abdominal cavity, is highlighted.*

1990; Pouliot et al., 1992). We then compared these two subgroups of overweight subjects to a group of lean controls. In both genders, we found that obesity per se was associated with metabolic alterations that included moderate increases in fasting plasma insulin levels and slight elevations in plasma triglyceride concentrations (Després, 1991d, 1993; Després et al., 1990; Pouliot et al., 1992). However, in both men and women, obesity with an excess accumulation of visceral adipose tissue was associated with a cluster of metabolic abnormalities that included hypertriglyceridemia, hypoalphalipoproteinemia, and increased plasma insulin concentrations measured in the fasting state and following a 75 g oral glucose load, as well as a deterioration in glucose tolerance (Després, 1991c, 1993; Després et al., 1990; Pouliot et al., 1992). These results indicated that visceral obesity was a better correlate of the metabolic complications commonly found in obese patients than were excess body weight and body fat per se. Additional measurements of the plasma lipid-lipoprotein profile revealed that the reduction in plasma high-density lipoprotein (HDL) cholesterol levels found in visceral obese men and women resulted from a reduction in the plasma concentration of cardioprotective HDL2 cholesterol levels (Després et al., 1989a). Studies in which we have measured the activity of lipoprotein lipase (LPL) and hepatic triglyceride lipase (HTGL) in heparin-treated plasma revealed that the low plasma HDL cholesterol levels of visceral obese subjects were mainly the results of opposite changes in the activity of these two enzymes (Figure 3-3). That is, plasma LPL activity was reduced in vis-

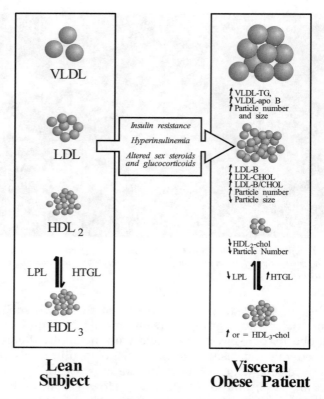

Lean Subject   **Visceral Obese Patient**

FIGURE 3-3. *Main alterations in the plasma lipoprotein-lipid profile observed in abdominal visceral obesity. It is proposed that these changes in plasma lipoprotein-lipid levels increase the risk of premature coronary heart disease in visceral obesity. LPL: lipoprotein lipase; HTGL: hepatic triglyceride lipase. Adapted from Després, 1994*

ceral obesity, whereas HTGL activity was substantially increased in these patients. A highly significant positive correlation was found between visceral adipose tissue accumulation and HTGL activity (Després et al., 1989a). Therefore, the low HDL cholesterol levels noted in visceral obesity are, to a large extent, explained by reciprocal changes in LPL and HTGL activities, especially regarding the cholesterol content of the HDL_2 subfraction.

VISCERAL ADIPOSE TISSUE ACCUMULATION IN MEN AND IN POST-MENOPAUSAL WOMEN

There is a well-known gender difference in abdominal fat accumulation, men being more prone to this condition than women before the latter reach menopause. To examine this phenomenon, we studied the relationship between visceral adipose tissue accumulation and total body fatness in both men and premenopausal women (Lemieux et al., 1993). We found that for any level of total body fat, men had on average twice the amount of visceral adipose tissue found in premenopausal women (Figure 3-4) (Lemieux et al., 1993). As visceral adipose tissue is a highly significant correlate of the cluster of metabolic complications of obesity (Després, 1991b, 1991c, 1991d, 1993, 1994; Després et al., 1989b,

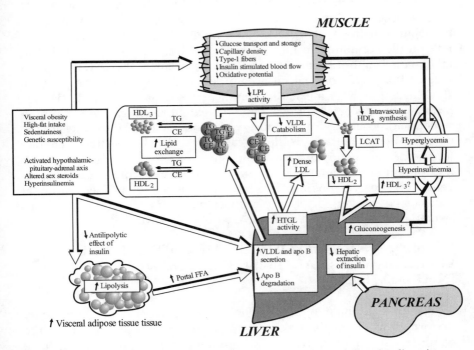

FIGURE 3-4. *Impact of insulin resistance on lipid and lipoprotein metabolism. Insulin resistance may develop as the result of a combination of factors, including a high-fat intake, a sedentary lifestyle, visceral obesity, or in the presence of variants in susceptibility genes. An activated hypothalamic pituitary-adrenal axis, altered sex steroid levels, and a hyperinsulinemic state are also found in visceral obesity. Insulin resistance is frequently associated with an enlarged mass of highly lipolytic visceral adipose tissue, this process being insulin resistant. The increased free fatty acids (FFA) flux to the liver is associated with metabolic impairments such as reduced apolipoprotein (apo)B degradation, leading to increased VLDL and apo B secretion. The hepatic extraction of insulin is reduced, whereas gluconeogenesis is increased. Plasma triglyceride (TG) levels are also elevated as a result of reduced lipoprotein lipase (LPL) activity. Hypertriglyceridemia favors cholesteryl ester (CE)-(TG) exchange among lipoproteins, resulting in a TG enrichment of LDL and HDL. These TG-rich lipoproteins are substrates for the enzyme, hepatic triglyceride lipase (HTGL), which leads to the formation of small, dense LDL particles, and to a reduction in plasma HDL2 concentration. The reduced LPL activity also contributes to the reduction in plasma HDL2 levels. Several alterations in muscle morphology and metabolism may also contribute to exacerbate the dyslipidaemic state. Adapted from Després and Marette, 1994.*

1989d, 1990; Fujioka et al., 1987, 1991a, 1991b; Peiris et al., 1989; Pouliot et al., 1992; Sparrow et al., 1986), we suggested that this greater accumulation of visceral adipose tissue found in men compared to premenopausal women could explain the greater susceptibility of men to the related complications. Indeed, when we matched men and women for the same amount of visceral adipose tissue, a similar cardiovascular disease risk profile was observed in men and women, despite the fact that matched women were characterized by a greater accumulation of subcutaneous fat than men (Lemieux et al., 1994). Thus, we believe that the low accumulation of visceral adipose tissue found in women before menopause helps explain their more favorable cardiovascular disease risk profile compared to men. However, it has been suggested that at menopause, in the absence of hormonal replacement therapy, there is an acceleration of abdominal fat accumulation that parallels the progressive development of metabolic complications (Haarbo et al., 1991). Additional work is needed to examine the extent to which the expanding visceral adipose tissue depot observed at menopause contributes to the deterioration of the risk profile for cardiovascular disease that is characteristic of postmenopausal women. Furthermore, the extent to which this potentially deleterious accumulation of visceral fat can be prevented by lifestyle modifications and, if necessary, by proper hormonal replacement therapy or other pharmacological treatment remain unanswered questions of great relevance to public health.

PLASMA CHOLESTEROL AND LDL-CHOLESTEROL LEVELS IN VISCERAL OBESITY: MISLEADING INFORMATION

The measurement of plasma cholesterol concentration is commonly performed to assess the risk of coronary heart disease, this procedure being largely justified by several epidemiological studies that have shown a positive relationship between plasma cholesterol concentrations and mortality from CHD (Keys, 1970; NIH, 1985; Stamler et al., 1986; WHO, 1982). However, it should be pointed out that the discriminative power of plasma cholesterol and low-density lipoprotein (LDL)-cholesterol levels is limited. For example, Genest et al. (1991) reported that almost 50% of patients with CHD had plasma cholesterol levels similar to or even lower than those of healthy subjects. Thus, there is considerable overlap between patients with coronary artery disease and healthy subjects regarding the distribution of plasma cholesterol levels (Sniderman & Silberberg, 1990). These results suggest that the value of plasma cholesterol measurements alone is of limited clinical use in the assessment of the risk of CHD. Therefore, additional lipid variables should be measured to more precisely assess risk. In this regard, despite the presence of an insulin-resistant hyperinsulinemic state, visceral obese patients are often characterized by nearly normal total cholesterol and LDL-cholesterol levels (Després, 1991b, 1991c, 1993, 1994; Després et al., 1989b). However, this apparently normal lipid profile is often characterized by a high proportion of small, dense cholesterol-ester-depleted LDL particles, which cannot be adequately assessed on the basis of cholesterol and LDL-cholesterol levels (Tchernof et al., 1996b). However, because there is one apolipoprotein (apo)-B molecule per LDL particle, irrespective of its cholesterol ester content, it has been suggested that the measurement of apo-B in the total plasma or in the LDL fraction could provide a better estimate of the number of atherogenic particles than cholesterol or LDL-cholesterol levels in visceral obesity (Després et al., 1995). Indeed, by using rocket immunoelectrophoresis, we have detected a 15-to-20% increase in plasma apo-B or LDL apo-B concentrations in visceral obese patients, despite the fact that these subjects were characterized by apparently normal cholesterol or LDL-cholesterol levels (Després et al., 1995).

It appears that visceral obese men and women are characterized by an increased LDL particle concentration that cannot be adequately assessed by cholesterol or LDL-cholesterol measurements. We have also studied LDL particle size in visceral obesity by using a 2-16% polyacrylamide gel electrophoretic procedure (Tchernof et al., 1996b). Using this methodology, we have assessed the LDL peak particle diameter as well as the LDL particle score that is calculated as a continuous variable using the migration distance of each LDL subspecies found on the gel multiplied by the relative respective area of each peak. The LDL peak particle size and the LDL particle score were highly correlated variables, the shared variance (r^2) between these two measurements reaching almost 60%. The proportion of small, dense LDL particles in the plasma was a very weak correlate of plasma cholesterol and LDL apo-B levels (Tchernof et al., 1996b). However, LDL peak particle diameter was positively correlated with the LDL apo-B over the LDL-cholesterol ratio as well as with plasma triglyceride levels and with the cholesterol-to-HDL-cholesterol ratio. Additional analyses revealed that the high-triglyceride-low HDL-cholesterol dyslipidemic state found in visceral obese, insulin-resistant patients was the best correlate of the proportion of small, dense LDL particles (Tchernof et al., 1996b). Thus, it should be emphasized that measurements of cholesterol and LDL-cholesterol levels are unsatisfactory procedures to assess potential changes in LDL particle concentration associated with an altered body fat distribution and to examine the effects of weight loss on LDL concentration. Additional techniques must be used to identify the 15-to-20% increase in the LDL particle concentration as well as the increased proportion of small, dense LDL particles that can be found in the plasma of visceral obese, insulin-resistant patients. It should also be kept in mind that visceral obesity is highly prevalent, and we have suggested that up to 25% of the sedentary male population could be characterized by this condition (Després, 1991c, 1993; Després et al., 1995). Visceral obesity is also highly prevalent among postmenopausal women, although no study has precisely quantified the prevalence of excess visceral adipose tissue accumulation in this subgroup of women. Additional studies in this area are clearly warranted.

ESTIMATION OF VISCERAL ADIPOSE TISSUE ACCUMULATION FROM ANTHROPOMETRY: THE WAIST CIRCUMFERENCE CONCEPT

As most health professionals do not have access to imaging techniques to assess visceral adipose tissue accumulation, there is an obvious need to identify simple anthropometric correlates of visceral obesity. First, we have attempted to identify whether there is a threshold of visceral adipose tissue accumulation above which there would be a greater likelihood of finding the cluster of metabolic abnormalities reflecting the features of the insulin-resistance syndrome. To do so, we have performed a simple procedure in which men and women were divided into quintiles of visceral adipose tissue accumulation measured at the level of the 4th and 5th lumbar vertebrae (L4-L5) (Després & Lamarche, 1993). Our analyses revealed that men and women with cross-sectional areas of abdominal visceral adipose tissue below 100 cm^2 were characterized by a rather normal metabolic profile, whereas men and women with an accumulation of visceral adipose tissue greater than 130 cm^2 were characterized by the typical cluster of metabolic abnormalities predictive of an increased risk of NIDDM and premature CHD (Després & Lamarche, 1993). Thus, an accumulation of visceral adipose tissue above 130 cm^2 measured at L4-L5 could be predictive of an increased risk of finding an altered cardiovascular disease risk profile.

The frequently used waist-to-hip ratio showed a common variance with visceral adipose tissue accumulation that did not reach 50% in either men or women (Pouliot et al., 1994). However, when we examined the relationship between waist circumference alone and visceral adipose tissue accumulation, the variance shared between waist circumference and visceral adipose tissue was 70-to-75% of the total variance in adipose tissue accumulation (Pouliot et al., 1994). Addition of further anthropometric variables failed to improve the prediction of visceral fat based upon waist circumference. Thus, we concluded that the waist circumference appears to represent the best anthropometric correlate of visceral adipose tissue accumulation (Figure 3-5). Furthermore, adjustment for height failed to substantially improve the prediction of visceral fat based upon waist circumference. Thus, we believe that the measurement of waist circumference has substantial implications from a public health standpoint. Indeed, health professionals should focus on implementing diet and exercise strategies to help people reduce their waistlines rather than concentrate upon normalizing body weight.

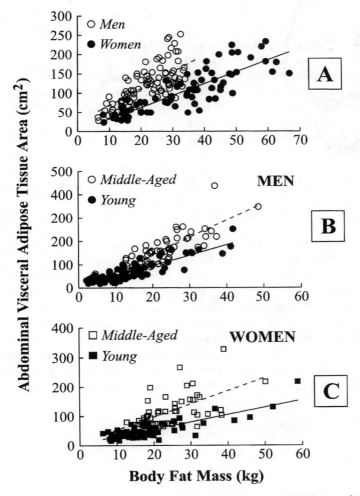

FIGURE 3-5. *Relations of body mass obtained by densitometry to abdominal visceral adipose tissue area measured by computed tomography in men and women (panel A), middle-aged and young men (panel B), middle-aged and young women (panel C).*

Reciprocal changes in muscle mass (increase) and adipose tissue (decrease) could result in no change in body weight following an exercise training program, yet a mobilization of abdominal visceral adipose tissue could still be revealed by a reduction in waist circumference. Thus, a reduction of a few centimeters of waistline without any change in body weight could still indicate a significant mobilization of visceral adipose tissue in response to exercise training. In addition, we reported that the relationship of waist circumference to visceral adipose tissue accumulation is influenced by age (Lemieux et al., 1996a). Indeed, a selective accumulation of visceral adipose tissue occurs with age that cannot always be adequately described by changes in the waistline. We have suggested that among men and women below 40 y of age, a waistline above 1 m would be associated with a high likelihood of finding levels of visceral adipose tissue accumulation above 130 cm^2 as well as the related cluster of metabolic abnormalities. However, among men and women between 40 and 60 y of age, a waist line above only 90 cm is associated with an increased probability of finding more than 130 cm^2 of visceral fat and the expected metabolic complications (Table 3-1) (Lemieux et al., 1996a).

To further examine the impact of the progressive increase in visceral adipose tissue with age, we recently conducted a prospective study in which visceral adipose tissue was measured initially and 7 y later in a group of 32 initially premenopausal women (Lemieux et al., 1996b). Over the 7 y follow-up period, the women did not show any significant increase in total body fat mass assessed by the underwater weighing technique. However, visceral adipose tissue was elevated by more than 30% over 7 y, a finding that was accompanied by a 4-cm increase in waist circumference. The increase in waist circumference showed a highly significant correlation with the change in visceral adipose tissue accumulation assessed by computed tomography (Lemieux et al., 1996b). The increased visceral adipose tissue accumulation was also associated with deterioration in the glycemic response to an oral glucose load. Furthermore, two subgroups of women matched for total body fat mass but varying visceral adipose tissue mass were compared. In the

TABLE 3-1. *Critical waist values. VAT = visceral adipose tissue area.*

	Men and Women Waist Circumference (cm)	
	<40 y	40-60 y
Excess Risk (130 cm^2 VAT)	100	90
Desirable (< 100 cm^2 VAT)	< 90	< 80

women whose visceral adipose tissue did not change over 7 y, there was no deterioration in their glycemic response to a glucose load. However, the women who gained a substantial amount of visceral adipose tissue (increase of about 50%) were characterized by a significant deterioration in the glycemic response to the oral glucose load, despite the fact that the level of total body fat remained unchanged over the 7 y follow-up period (Lemieux et al., 1996b). Thus, results of this longitudinal study emphasize the importance of the increase in visceral adipose tissue often noted with age as a correlate of the age-related deterioration in the metabolic profile, suggesting that prevention of visceral adipose tissue accumulation with age should receive more consideration from a public-health standpoint.

THE HYPERINSULINEMIC, INSULIN-RESISTANT, DYSLIPIDEMIC STATE OF VISCERAL OBESITY: A HIGHLY ATHEROGENIC CONDITION

It is commonly accepted that visceral obesity is associated with an insulin resistant, hyperinsulinemic state that may lead to glucose intolerance, this condition potentially converting to non-insulin dependent diabetes mellitus in the presence of genetic factors that are presently poorly understood (Björntorp, 1988; Kissebah & Peiris, 1989; Lemieux & Després, 1994). In addition, this insulin-resistant hyperinsulinemic condition is associated with a typical dyslipidemic profile that includes hypertriglyceridemia, high apo-B levels, low HDL-cholesterol levels, and an increased proportion of small, dense LDL particles (Després, 1991a, 1991b, 1993, 1994; Després & Marette, 1994; Després et al., 1990, 1995). Prospective studies have shown that this dyslipidemic profile is associated with an increased risk of ischemic heart disease (Assmann & Schulte, 1992; Manninen et al., 1992).

We have also examined this issue in a prospective study conducted in Québec City, the Québec Cardiovascular Study (Lamarche et al., 1995). We had the opportunity to study a sample of 2103 men initially free from ischemic heart disease, who were followed from 1985 to 1990. Over this period, 114 cases of ischemic heart disease were noted, including myocardial infarction, effort angina, and mortality from CHD (Lamarche et al., 1995). When we first compared the prevalence of various dyslipidemic phenotypes in men who developed ischemic heart disease to those who remained healthy, we found that about 50% of the 1989 men who remained free from ischemic heart disease had a normal lipid profile, while only less than one-third of the 114 men who developed ischemic heart disease had a normal lipid profile (Lamarche et al., 1995). Thus, the various dyslipidemic phenotypes were more prevalent in those who developed ischemic heart disease compared to men who remained healthy. Multiple regression analyses revealed that diabetes, apolipoprotein-B levels, age, smoking, and elevated systolic blood pressure were the best predictors of the risk of ischemic heart disease in this cohort (Lamarche et al., 1996). Therefore, apolipoprotein-B, and not cholesterol nor LDL-cholesterol, was the best metabolic predictor of ischemic-heart-disease risk in this sample of French-Canadians (Lamarche et al., 1996). In fact, after inclusion of apo-B in the prediction model, no other lipoprotein lipid variable could further explain the risk of ischemic heart disease, emphasizing the critical importance of assessing apo-B in the estimation of the risk of ischemic heart disease in men.

The Québec Cardiovascular Study also gave us an opportunity to examine the potential relationship between hyperinsulinemia and ischemic heart disease by measuring fasting insulin concentrations in non-diabetic men who eventually developed ischemic heart disease, and matching them for age, body mass index, smoking, and alcohol consumption with non-diabetic men who remained healthy over the 5 y follow-up period (Després et al., 1996). Using an insulin assay that did not cross react with pro-insulin, we found fasting insulin concentrations to be 18% higher in men who developed ischemic heart disease compared to men who remained healthy (Després et al., 1996). An increase of one standard deviation in fasting insulin concentrations was associated with a 70% elevation in ischemic heart disease risk, this association being independent from the concomitant variation in plasma triglyceride, apo-B, and HDL-cholesterol levels. Thus, our study suggests that hyperinsulinemia is an independent risk factor for ischemic heart disease in men. In addition, as visceral obesity is associated with both hyperinsulinemia and elevated apo-B levels, we tested for the potential synergy between hyperinsulinemia and hyperapo-B in the modulation of ischemic heart disease risk. We divided the sample into tertiles of fasting insulin levels and used the 50th percentile of the apo-B distribution to classify subjects with either low or high apo-B concentrations. Among subjects with low apo-B concentrations, hyperinsulinemia was associated with a 3-fold increase in the risk of ischemic heart disease. However, the combination of hyperinsulinemia (upper insulin tertile) and elevated apo-B concentrations (above the 50th percentile) was associated with more than a 10-fold increase in the risk of ischemic heart disease, emphasizing the tremendous impact of the hyperinsulinemic-hyperapo-B state of visceral obesity as a modulator of ischemic heart disease risk. Indeed, this combination of metabolic alterations is specifically found in visceral obese patients even in the prediabetic state and in the absence of a marked elevation in cholesterol and LDL-cholesterol levels. Thus, results of the Québec Cardiovascular Study emphasize that the hyperinsulinemic-hyperapo-B state of visceral obesity is associated with a tremendous increase in the risk of ischemic heart disease, the impact on risk being much more important than the impact of hypercholesterolemia.

Thus, the metabolic abnormalities found in visceral obesity substantially increase the risk of NIDDM and of ischemic heart disease. Furthermore, as visceral obesity is associated with an increased proportion of small, dense LDL particles (Tchernof et al., 1996b), we have measured LDL peak-particle diameter in men of the Québec Cardiovascular Study (Lamarche et al., 1997), and stratified our subjects on the basis of apo-B concentrations (using the 50th percentile of the distribution) and LDL peak particle diameter to identify subjects with small, dense LDL particles. Among men with normal apo-B concentrations, we found that small, dense LDL particles were not associated with an increased risk of ischemic heart disease (Lamarche et al., 1997). However, men with both small, dense LDL particles and elevated apo-B concentrations were characterized by more than a five-fold increase in the risk of ischemic heart disease, indicating that the concentration of the small, dense LDL particles was a major risk factor for ischemic heart disease (Lamarche et al., 1997). Once again, it should be emphasized that visceral obesity is not only associated with a reduction in LDL peak particle diameter, but also with an increased concentration of LDL particles (Després, 1994).

Finally, we have been very interested in examining the risk associated with the simultaneous presence of hyperinsulinemia, hyperapo-B, and small, dense LDL particles. To examine this issue, we have used the 50th percentile of the distribution of each of the three variables in order to identify men who simultaneously had hyperinsulinemia, elevated apo-B levels, and an increased proportion of small, dense LDL particles (B. Lamarche et al., unpublished observations). We found that the simultaneous presence of hyperinsulinemia, hyperapo-B, and small, dense LDL particles was associated with more than a 20-fold increase in the risk of ischemic heart disease, this increase in risk being essentially unaffected by controlling for fasting plasma triglyceride, LDL-cholesterol and HDL-cholesterol levels (Lamarche B. et al., unpublished observations). Thus, it appears that this new triad of metabolic risk factors found in the insulin-resistant state of visceral obesity (Table 3-2) substantially increases the risk of ischemic heart disease. This increased risk is such that this cluster of metabolic alterations may represent the main cause of coronary heart disease in affluent societies.

TABLE 3-2. *Critical metabolic factors associated with visceral adiposity and increased risk of coronary heart disease (CHD).*

⇑ insulin level

⇑ apoliprotein-B

small, dense LDL (or ⇑ TG, ⇓ HDL-C)

⇑ waist circumference

IS THERE A CAUSAL RELATIONSHIP BETWEEN VISCERAL OBESITY, INSULIN RESISTANCE, AND THE DYSLIPIDEMIC STATE?

Visceral adipocytes, which display a high lipolytic activity, are poorly inhibited by insulin and contribute to a greater flux of free fatty acids towards the liver through the portal circulation (Figure 3-6) (Björntorp, 1988, 1990; Després, 1991b; Després et al., 1990). This is why visceral obese patients are frequently characterized by liver steatosis and a fatty liver (Kral et al., 1993). High levels of free fatty acids in the hepatic portal system contribute to reduce hepatic insulin extraction (Hennes et al., 1990; Svedberg et al., 1990), exacerbating systemic hyperinsulinemia. Furthermore, increased esterification of those portal fatty acids into triglycerides would lead to an increased synthesis of very-low-density lipoproteins (VLDL) and to a reduced hepatic degradation of apo-B, leading to an overproduction of apo-B-associated lipoproteins (Björntorp, 1990; Després, 1994). Furthermore, the increased lipid oxidation in the liver is associated with impaired glycolysis (Randle et al., 1963; Taylor et al., 1975), whereas a decrease in glycogen synthase activity is noted in skeletal muscle (Felber, 1972). The increased lipid oxidation provides precursors for gluconeogenesis (Jahoor et al., 1992), contributing to the increased hepatic glucose output, which is a major factor in the glucose intolerance of visceral obesity. Thus, in vivo insulin action is altered in subjects with visceral obesity, and a compensatory hyperinsulinemia is required to regulate glucose levels in these subjects.

Lipoprotein lipase (LPL), the enzyme responsible for the catabolism of triglyceride-rich lipoproteins, also appears to be affected by the insulin-resistant state of visceral obesity. Indeed, in visceral obesity LPL activity is reduced, whereas the activity of hepatic triglyceride lipase (HTGL, an enzyme with high affinity for small, triglyceride-rich lipoproteins) is substantially increased (Després et al., 1989a). Thus, these reciprocal changes in LPL and HTGL activity could reduce the catabolic rate of large triglyceride-rich lipoproteins and increase the catabolism of HDL particles by hepatic triglyceride lipase, leading to their

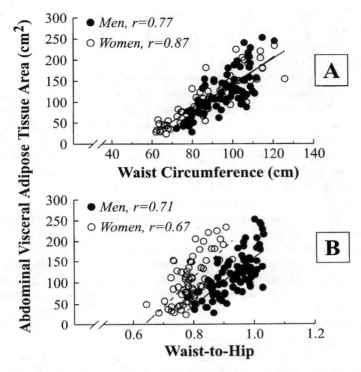

FIGURE 3-6. *Relationships between waist circumference (panel A) and waist-to-hip ratio (panel B) and abdominal visceral adipose tissue area measured by computed tomography in men and women.*

increased conversion to HDL3 which are smaller HDL particles than HDL2 (Després, 1991b, 1994; Després et al., 1989a, 1990).

In this regard, Pollare et al. (1991) reported that skeletal muscle LPL activity is reduced in insulin-resistant subjects and that in vivo insulin sensitivity is positively correlated with skeletal muscle LPL activity. The hypertriglyceridemia resulting from an increased hepatic VLDL production and a decreased degradation due to reduced LPL activity also contributes to an increased transfer of triglycerides from VLDL to LDL and HDL particles in exchange for cholesterol esters from LDL and HDL, ultimately leading to the triglyceride enrichment of LDL and HDL (Després et al., 1989a, 1989c). Such triglyceride enrichment is associated with a reduced cholesterol content of HDL, partly explaining the low HDL cholesterol levels in visceral obesity (Després et al., 1989c). In addition, triglyceride-rich LDL particles represent an unusual but good substrate for hepatic triglyceride lipase, generating atherogenic small, dense LDL particles (Després, 1991b). Thus, reciprocal changes in LPL and HTGL activity are probably important determinants of the dyslipidemic state found in visceral obesity.

The etiology of the insulin-resistant state of visceral obesity is not fully understood, although it is known that an impaired insulin action can be found in both obese and nonobese subjects (Reaven, 1988). Studies conducted among insulin-resistant or NIDDM patients have shown that a family history of diabetes alters the relationship of abdominal fat accumulation to indices of plasma glucose-insulin homeostasis (Fujimoto et al., 1990; Lemieux et al., 1992). We have reported that among subjects with similar deteriorations in plasma glucose-insulin homeostasis, those with a family history of diabetes had lower levels of abdominal fat than did subjects without a family history of diabetes (Lemieux et al., 1992). These results suggest that the presence of genetic susceptibility factors could reduce the threshold of abdominal fat above which metabolic complications predictive of an increased risk of NIDDM could be observed. In summary, from a metabolic standpoint, the high free fatty acid concentrations (increased lipolysis of the visceral depot) found in visceral obesity, combined with a decreased LPL activity and a reduced insulin sensitivity, may lead to alterations ultimately involved in the development of glucose intolerance, hyperinsulinemia, dyslipidemia, NIDDM, and cardiovascular disease.

In addition to the portal circulation hypothesis described above, it has been suggested that abdominal obesity could be a marker of an altered endogenous steroid profile. Studies that have crudely assessed body fat distribution with the waist-to-hip ratio have reported low levels of sex-hormone-binding globulin (SHBG) and high concentrations of free testosterone in women with abdominal obesity (Evans et al., 1983; Peiris et al., 1987). Furthermore, the altered steroid concentrations observed in abdominal obese women have been associated with an impaired in vivo insulin action (Kissebah & Peiris, 1989; Kissebah et al., 1985). Studies have also indicated that the hyperinsulinemic state of abdominal obesity could be attributed to a reduction in hepatic insulin extraction, this phenomenon being associated with low SHBG concentrations and high free testosterone levels in women (Peiris et al., 1987). Thus, the association of steroid levels with metabolic disturbances could be partly independent of the concomitant variation in body fat distribution. In this regard, it has been suggested that although there is an association between visceral obesity and metabolic complications, the dyslipidemic state found among abdominal obese women could partly reflect the concomitant alteration in the sex steroid profile (Kissebah & Peiris, 1989; Kissebah et al., 1985).

In men, however, the associations among steroid levels, visceral obesity, and the metabolic profile appear to be different from those noted in women. As opposed to visceral obese women, visceral obese men are characterized by reduced plasma testosterone concentrations (Seidell et al., 1990; Tchernof et al., 1995a). However, it is poorly understood whether these altered levels of androgenic steroids are independently associated with excess abdominal fat accumulation after control for the concomitant variation in total body fat in men (Tchernof et al., 1995a). Furthermore, the alterations in steroid hormone levels were found to be significantly correlated with deterioration in glucose tolerance and with the dyslipidemic state of visceral obesity (Tchnernof et al., 1995b, 1996a). More recently, we found that visceral obesity in men was associated with increased plasma androstane-3β,17β-diol glucuronide (3α-diol glucuronide) levels, a glucuronide conjugated androgen metabolite associated with the excretion of steroids (Tchernof et al., 1997). We have also found that this plasma level of androgen metabolite was an independent risk factor for ischemic heart disease, probably due to its strong relationship with visceral adipose tissue accumulation (Tchernof A. et al., unpublished observations).

Two possibilities have been raised to explain the association of visceral fat with increased androgen metabolism. First, it is possible that the altered hepatic metabolism of visceral obesity could be responsible for the increased glucuronidation found in visceral obese patients. Second, the possibility cannot be excluded that a high expression of the glucuronosyltransferase enzyme in visceral adipose tissue may be found. These issues will require further study, but it is clear at this stage that visceral obesity is associated with marked increases in plasma 3α-diol glucuronide levels, this alteration being an independent predictor of the risk of ischemic heart disease in men.

The potential contribution of glucocorticoids to the dyslipidemic state of visceral obesity should also not be ignored. Indeed, the insulin-resistant state of obese patients with excess visceral adipose tissue accumulation could also be the consequence of altered glucocorticoid levels (Björntorp, 1991; Brindley, 1992; Brindley & Rolland, 1989). Accordingly, environmental stress can activate the hypothalamic-pituitary-adrenal axis, thereby increasing cortisol production (Björntorp, 1991). It has also been shown that visceral adipose cells have a very high density of glucocorticoid receptors compared to subcutaneous adipocytes, this phenomenon helping to explain the greater sensitivity of visceral adipocytes to stressor agents (Pedersen et al., 1994; Rebuffé-Scrive et al., 1985). Furthermore, the metabolic effects of glucocorticoids on skeletal muscle and the liver induce a state of insulin resistance, concordant with the alterations observed in visceral obesity (Brindley, 1992; Brindley & Rolland, 1989). Indeed, glucocorticoids stimulate VLDL and apo-B production, reduce the activity of LDL receptors, and induce in vivo insulin resistance (Brindley, 1992; Brindley & Rolland, 1989). Thus, the dyslipidemic state of visceral obesity results from complex metabolic and hormonal interactions that lead to insulin resistance, dyslipidemia, and to an increased risk of cardiovascular disease (Després, 1994; Després & Marette, 1994; Després et al., 1990, 1992).

VISCERAL OBESITY: THERAPEUTIC IMPLICATIONS

Visceral obesity appears to be a good marker of metabolic abnormalities that may include an activated hypothalamic-pituitary-adrenal axis, leading to increased control of lipid metabolism by glucocorticoids, an altered sex steroid profile and metabolism, *in vivo* insulin resistance and compensatory hyperinsulinemia, glucose intolerance, and an atherogenic dyslipidemic state (Després, 1994; Després & Marette, 1994; Després et al., 1990, 1992). This cluster of metabolic abnormalities is highly prevalent in affluent societies and is likely to represent the most prevalent cause of coronary heart disease (Després, 1991c). It is therefore important to identify therapeutic options in order to prevent the development of or to treat the related atherogenetic profile. As discussed in this chapter, an increased turnover of free fatty acids and high levels of portal free fatty acids may play a major role in the etiology of the metabolic complications of visceral obesity. Thus, a reduced fat intake should at least theoretically reduce the flux of lipids into an already hyperlipidemic, hyperinsulinemic plasma (Després & Lamarche, 1993). However, the literature is very deficient regarding the treatment of the insulin-resistant dyslipidemic syndrome of visceral obesity by a complex carbohydrate, low-fat diet; additional studies are clearly needed in this area.

In addition, it would also be very important to examine approaches that could lead to a selective reduction in visceral adipose tissue mass. From a metabolic standpoint, the mobilization of visceral adipose tissue should be associated with improvements in the metabolic profile. Studies that have been conducted so far have indicated that the loss of visceral adipose tissue induced either by diet or by endurance exercise was associated with improvements in the cardiovascular disease risk profile (Després & Lamarche, 1993; Fujioka et al., 1991b; Leenen et al., 1992).

The contribution of the skeletal muscle to the etiology of the complications found in visceral obesity has recently been emphasized, and an impaired skeletal muscle oxidative potential has been reported (Colberg et al., 1995). It is well known that regular endurance exercise can improve insulin action in skeletal muscle and can increase lipid oxidation (Björntorp, 1981; Björntorp et al., 1970; Burnstein et al., 1985; Costill et al., 1979; Krotkiewski & Björntorp, 1986; Oshida et al., 1989; Technical

Review, Diabetes, 1991). Research regarding the potential contribution of endurance exercise as one approach to treat visceral obesity and insulin resistance are clearly needed (Table 3-3).

The optimal exercise prescription for the treatment of visceral obesity remains to be established. Epidemiological studies have shown that physically active individuals are at lower risk of coronary heart disease and related mortality compared to sedentary subjects (Leon et al., 1987; Morris et al., 1973, 1980; Paffenberger & Hale, 1976; Paffenberger et al., 1978; Salonen et al., 1988), although the exact mechanisms responsible for the impact of physical activity on coronary heart disease risk remain to be fully understood. In addition, the high level of cardiorespiratory fitness found in physically active individuals appears to be another important factor explaining their reduced risk of coronary heart disease (Blair et al., 1989; Ekelund et al., 1988; Lie et al., 1985; Peters et al., 1983; Slattery & Jacobs, 1988). However, whether a physically active lifestyle needs to improve cardiorespiratory fitness in order to reduce the risk of CHD further is an issue that has not been resolved (Figure 3-7A). From the literature available on metabolic risk factors, we have proposed that the improvement in cardiorespiratory fitness may not be required to reduce the risk of cardiovascular disease by regular endurance exercise (Després & Lamarche, 1993, 1994).

DIETARY TREATMENT OF VISCERAL OBESITY

From the epidemiological and metabolic studies available, it is clear that visceral obesity is an important risk factor for the development of Type II diabetes, dyslipidemia, and CHD. However, although several prospective studies have shown that abdominal obesity is associated with an increased mortality rate from CHD (Donahue et al., 1987; Folsom et al., 1993; Lapidus et al., 1984; Larsson et al., 1984; Terry et al., 1992), it is important to emphasize that research has yet to confirm that

TABLE 3-3. *Factors related to the efficacy of endurance exercise training for affecting visceral adipose tissue.*

Gender
Age
Initial fitness level
Energy deficit induced by exercise
Percentage of saturated fat intake
Genetic factors
Neuroendocrine factors

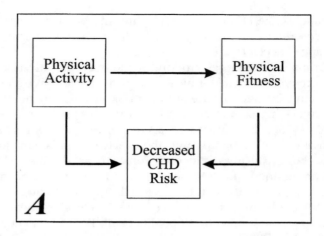

FIGURE 3-7A. *Diagram of critical issues related to the effect of physical activity on the risk of coronary heart disease (CHD). The question of whether or not physical activity requires an improvement in physical fitness to reduce CHD risk is highlighted. It is proposed that a physically active lifestyle may reduce CHD risk through improved metabolic fitness, which does not require improvements in cardiorespiratory fitness.*

intentional weight loss associated with a reduction in abdominal visceral adipose tissue leads to a reduction in mortality from cardiovascular disease (Figure 3-7B). However, it must also be recognized that there is a considerable amount of literature suggesting that reducing body weight and the amount of abdominal fat would indeed be associated with substantial improvements in the cardiovascular disease risk profile, including a reduced blood pressure, improvements in plasma lipoprotein profile, reduction in plasma insulin levels, an improved insulin sensitivity, and improved glucose tolerance (Després & Lamarche, 1993; Fujioka et al., 1991a, 1991b; Leenen et al., 1992). Thus, body weight management, especially among visceral obese patients, appears to be relevant in the prevention of cardiovascular disease. It should also be kept in mind that visceral obesity is likely to represent the most prevalent cause (or correlate) of cardiovascular disease in affluent societies, its prevalence reaching about 25% of sedentary adult males and post-menopausal women (Després, 1991c, 1993).

From the positive association between total adiposity and visceral adipose tissue accumulation, weight loss through dieting should induce a variable mobilization of visceral adipose tissue mass (Lemieux et al., 1993). It is also important to emphasize that some individuals are more susceptible to visceral adipose tissue accumulation than others due to genetic factors that appear to play a major role, although the molecular mechanisms have not been identified (Bouchard et al., 1990). Weight-

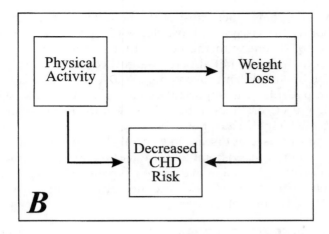

FIGURE 3-7B. *The effect of the related weight loss associated with a physically active lifestyle on CHD risk is emphasized. However, it is suggested that physical activity may reduce CHD risk in a manner that is partly independent of the concomitant variation in body weight and in adipose tissue mass.*

loss studies have generally reported that individuals with the highest initial levels of visceral adipose tissue are generally those showing the most substantial losses of visceral fat in response to a reduced caloric intake (Després & Lamarche, 1993; Fujioka et al., 1991a, 1991b; Leenen et al., 1992). Thus, visceral obese patients are likely to benefit the most from a low-fat diet that induces weight loss. However, very few diet studies have been conducted in patients with the insulin-resistant syndrome of visceral obesity, and further work in this area is urgently needed, considering the important public health implications of such data. However, the available evidence suggests that the magnitude of body fat loss induced by dieting, as well as the magnitude of the reduction in visceral adipose tissue mass, are correlated with the improvements in factors included in the CHD risk profile, such as glucose tolerance and levels of plasma insulin and plasma lipoproteins (Després & Lamarche, 1993; Leenen et al., 1992; Lemieux & Després, 1994).

Another important concept is that normalization of body weight and body fat mass in visceral obese patients is not required to substantially improve the cardiovascular disease risk profile of these patients. Indeed, as there is a preferential mobilization of visceral adipose tissue when visceral obese patients are subjected to a low-energy, low-fat diet, an improvement in the CHD risk profile may be expected, even in the absence of normalization of body weight. Thus, a substantial reduction of visceral fat (up to 40-50%) could be observed with a weight loss of only a few kilograms when most of the body fat loss results from the mobilization of the visceral adipose depot (Després et al., 1995). These results are consistent with the notion that a moderate loss of body weight (up to 5-10% of initial body weight) could be associated with considerable metabolic improvements (Goldstein, 1992). Thus, in visceral obese patients, it is important to keep in mind that a significant mobilization of visceral fat can be observed in the presence of a loss of 5-10% of body weight. Thus, therapeutic approaches aimed at reducing the risk of cardiovascular disease in visceral obese patients should focus on the reduction of the visceral adipose tissue mass rather than on the normalization of body weight in overweight patients, the latter objective being often difficult to achieve and not always clinically justified (Després, 1994; Després et al., 1995).

EFFECT OF EXERCISE TRAINING ON VISCERAL OBESITY AND RELATED METABOLIC COMPLICATIONS

There are currently no data to indicate that voluntary participation in an exercise-training program will reduce the risk of cardiovascular disease mortality in overweight patients with excess visceral adipose tissue accumulation. However, there is considerable literature suggesting that endurance exercise training will promote favorable changes in body composition, in vivo insulin action, and plasma lipoprotein concentrations, all of which would be predictive of a reduced risk of NIDDM and cardiovascular disease (Després & Lamarche, 1993, 1994). Thus, endurance exercise training could be considered as a valuable approach to reduce CHD and diabetes risk in visceral obese patients. Studies that have examined the effects of endurance exercise training in abdominal obese patients have reported substantial improvements in insulin sensitivity, triglyceride levels, HDL-cholesterol concentration, and in the proportion of small, dense LDL particles (Bouchard et al. 1993; Després & Lamarche, 1993, 1994). These metabolic improvements were observed even in the absence of major changes in cardiorespiratory fitness and were rather dependent upon the magnitude of visceral adipose tissue and total body fat mass losses (Després & Lamarche, 1994). It therefore appears that it is not necessary to substantially improve cardiorespiratory fitness (at least as assessed by $\dot{V}O_2max$) in overweight abdominal obese patients to reduce the risks of NIDDM and CHD.

A focus on the duration of exercise rather than on its intensity appears to be more relevant (Després & Lamarche, 1994). When dealing with visceral obesity and related metabolic complications, it is important to emphasize total energy expenditure during exercise rather than exercise intensity. It is difficult to generate a large energy deficit from an exercise training program as opposed to dietary restriction (Bouchard et al., 1993). However, the prognosis for long-term maintenance of reduced body weight after exposure to a hypocaloric diet is very poor as opposed to the relative success associated with being chronically physically active (Bouchard et al., 1993). We have suggested that prolonged endurance exercise training performed at moderate intensity should be the focus of physical activity programs in visceral obese patients; that is, about 50% of VO_2max (which corresponds to a brisk walk performed daily) for at least 45 min. Such an exercise prescription can lead to substantial improvements in the metabolic profile of viscerally obese individual, even in the absence of major changes in body composition (Després & Lamarche, 1993, 1994). In this regard, it is important to emphasize that the traditional approach, in which exercise training is conducted three times a week, 20 min per session, at 70-75% of VO_2max, could lead to a significant improvement in cardiorespiratory fitness (ACSM, 1990), but the rather trivial increase in daily energy expenditure associated with such an exercise prescription is unlikely to lead to major changes in body composition, visceral adipose tissue accumulation, and in CHD-risk variables (Després & Lamarche, 1994).

Although it is fairly well accepted that endurance exercise training has a beneficial effect on the cardiovascular-disease-risk profile, there is some controversy regarding the exercise prescription that should be recommended to optimally reduce cardiovascular disease risk, an issue that is completely unresolved in the visceral obese patients. The American College of Sports Medicine (1990) has recognized that the minimal exercise stimulus to improve cardiorespiratory fitness may not be sufficient to improve health-related fitness, a concept that was emphasized at the Canadian Conference on Exercise, Fitness and Health (Exercise, Fitness and Health, 1990). An exercise program for visceral obese patients should be designed to improve health-related variables rather than to focus on improvements in exercise tolerance (which is, however, a legitimate goal).

The scientific literature indicates that metabolic variables predictive of diabetes and CHD risk are more substantially altered by the volume of exercise than by its intensity (Després & Lamarche, 1993, 1994). Thus, exercise training programs performed at about 70% of VO_2max induce favorable changes in both cardiorespiratory fitness and cardiovascular-disease-risk profile when the net increase in energy expenditure associated with the exercise training program is sufficient (Després & Lamarche, 1994; Haskell, 1984, 1986; Krauss, 1989; Wood & Haskell, 1979; Wood & Stefanick, 1988; Wood et al., 1984). Generally, such exercise programs induce reductions in plasma triglyceride and apo-B levels and an increase in plasma HDL-cholesterol concentrations, although equivocal findings can be found in the literature (ACSM, 1990; Haskell, 1984, 1986; Krauss, 1989; Seals & Hagberg., 1984; Wood & Haskell, 1979; Wood et al., 1984). Among factors that could explain such variation, the subjects' age and their initial cardiovascular disease risk profile, body composition, and gender could help explain the magnitude of metabolic responses induced by these exercise-training programs. In general, the greater is the likelihood of finding significant improvements with regular exercise training when subjects are initially obese, insulin-resistant, and dyslipidemic (Després & Lamarche, 1994). Furthermore, endurance exercise training programs that have not reported substantial changes in the plasma lipoprotein profile may not have been sufficient in duration and frequency of sessions to generate metabolic improvements. It is relevant to point out that studies which have induced large increases in energy expenditure were those that have reported the most substantial weight losses and related improvements in the metabolic profile predictive of CVD risk (Després & Lamarche, 1993, 1994).

In a review of the literature we examined whether it was necessary to improve cardiorespiratory fitness or to generate a large energy expenditure when dealing with the metabolic complications of visceral obese patients (Després & Lamarche, 1994). Generally, the improvement in plasma lipoprotein levels produced by endurance exercise training is poorly predicted by changes in treadmill performance or $\dot{V}O_2$max. This result is consistent with the observations of Williams and colleagues (1982), who have shown that improvements in both $\dot{V}O_2$max and treadmill duration following training were poor predictors of changes in plasma HDL-cholesterol levels. However, they found a highly significant correlation between the increase in plasma HDL concentration and the training volume estimated by the number of miles run per week, a finding consistent with the results of Kokkins et al. (1995). Thus, these studies suggest that the improvements in the metabolic profile predictive of CHD risk observed with endurance training are more related to the volume of exercise than to its intensity. Moderate intensity, prolonged endurance exercise training is associated with improvements in plasma lipoprotein levels when the energy expenditure associated with the exercise prescription is adequate: reductions in body weight, body fat, plasma insulin levels, LDL-cholesterol concentrations, and an increase in HDL-cholesterol levels—particularly the cardioprotective HDL_2 subfraction—have been reported (Figure 3-8) (Després & Lamarche, 1993, 1994). Because exercise is also associated with an acute metabolic response, it is likely that optimal results may be obtained by using prolonged exercise performed on an almost daily basis. By this ap-

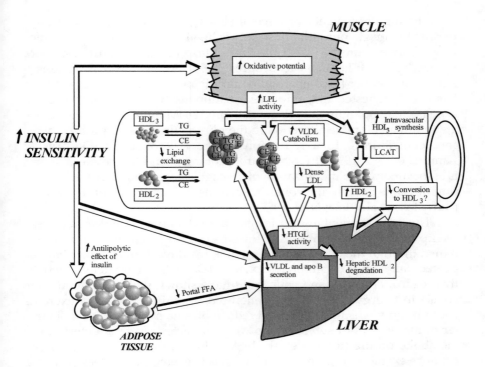

FIGURE 3-8. *Overview of some potentially important factors involved in the adaptation of lipid transport and plasma lipoprotein levels to endurance-exercise training. An important correlate of the lipoprotein changes is the improved in-vivo insulin sensitivity that is observed in endurance-trained individuals. This adaptation improves the antilipolytic effect of insulin on adipose tissue as well as the insulin-stimulated glucose transport in the skeletal muscle. The resulting reduction of plasma insulin levels, combined with reduced portal delivery of free fatty acids (FFA) to the liver, leads to decreased hepatic secretion of very-low-density lipoproteins (VLDL) and apolipoprotein B (apoB) molecules. Furthermore, the reduced fasting plasma triglyceride (TG) levels of endurance-trained subjects also appear to result from a more efficient catabolism of TG-rich lipoproteins because lipoprotein lipase (LPL) is elevated in adipose and muscle as well as in post-heparin plasma. The resulting reduced VLDL level is associated with a decreased exchange of VLDL-triglyceride for high-density lipoprotein (HDL) and low-density lipoprotein (LDL) cholesterol esters. The reduced TG levels observed in trained subjects also favor a decrease in the formation of small, atherogenic LDL particles. Furthermore, the elevated LPL activity of endurance-trained subjects increases the production of HDL precursors, and a high lecithin: cholesterol acyltransferase activity may also be an important correlate of elevated HDL_2 levels. Finally, endurance training markedly reduces hepatic triglyceride lipase activity (HTGL), which is high in sedentary obese individuals. Adapted from Després and Lamarche, 1993.*

proach, the considerable increase in energy expenditure associated with a prolonged endurance exercise training session will generate a negative energy balance that will lead to a beneficial acute metabolic response in addition to the chronic metabolic adaptation found when these sessions are repeated on a regular basis (Després & Lamarche, 1993, 1994).

The high prevalence of visceral obesity, insulin resistance, and hyperinsulinemia in our affluent society is likely to be related to our sedentary lifestyle combined with the high intake of dietary fat (Després & Lamarche, 1993; Lemieux & Després, 1994). As insulin resistance is a major correlate of the dyslipidemic profile of visceral obese patients, it has been suggested that improved insulin sensitivity through regular exercise may not only reduce the risk of NIDDM but may also be associated with a favorable alteration in the plasma lipoprotein profile, therefore contributing to a reduction in the risk of CHD (Després & Lamarche, 1993, 1994). In this regard, prolonged endurance exercise that is associated with a mobilization of glycogen stores and increased oxidation of lipids acutely improves in vivo insulin action for up to 48-72 h (Burnstein et al., 1985; NIH, 1987).

The improvement in the plasma lipoprotein profile of visceral obese dyslipidemic patients involved in an exercise program could be obtained through the daily improvement in insulin action generated by repeated daily bouts of prolonged exercise (Després & Lamarche, 1993). In this regard, Holloszy and colleagues have shown that a substantial increase in energy expenditure generated by daily prolonged exercise could improve insulin action and reduce plasma insulin levels in a matter of a few days in subjects who were characterized by a deteriorated metabolic profile (Rogers et al., 1988). Thus, a moderate-intensity endurance exercise program in which subjects exercise for at least 1 h on a daily basis could improve insulin sensitivity, leading to an improvement in plasma lipoprotein levels. These favorable changes include reductions in plasma triglyceride and apo-B levels, increases in HDL-cholesterol concentrations, and reciprocal changes in the activity of enzymes that play an important role in the modulation of plasma lipoprotein levels, namely plasma post-heparin lipoprotein lipase (LPL is low in visceral obesity but can be increased with endurance exercise training) and hepatic triglyceride lipase (HTGL is very high in visceral obesity, but its activity can be markedly reduced in exercise training) (Figure 3-9) (Després & Lamarche, 1993, 1994). The reciprocal changes in post-heparin LPL and HTGL activities are important determinants of the increased proportion of plasma HDL-cholesterol found in visceral obese patients with endurance training (Després et al., 1991).

These metabolic adaptations are dissociated from changes in cardiorespiratory fitness, and they appear to be related to the degree of weight loss and visceral fat mobilization that results from the increased energy expenditure associated with an endurance exercise program (Després et al., 1991). Oshida and colleagues (1989) have shown that a moderate-intensity jogging program inducing no significant increase in $\dot{V}O_2$max could produce substantial improvements in insulin action. In a

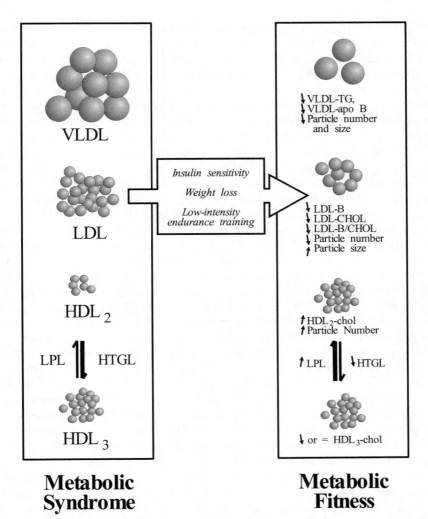

VLDL

Insulin sensitivity

Weight loss

Low-intensity
endurance training

LDL

HDL $_2$

LPL   HTGL

HDL $_3$

↓VLDL-TG,
↓VLDL-apo B
↓Particle number
   and size

↓ LDL-B
↓ LDL-CHOL
↓ LDL-B/CHOL
↓ Particle number
↑ Particle size

↑HDL $_2$-chol
↑Particle Number

↑LPL   ↓HTGL

↓ or = HDL $_3$-chol

Metabolic
Syndrome

Metabolic
Fitness

FIGURE 3-9. *Summary of the effects of prolonged endurance-exercise training in initially seden-tary, overweight individuals. If excess abdominal fat is present, insulin resistance, dyslipoproteine-mia, and hypertension may be found (metabolic syndrome). Daily, prolonged, low-intensity en-durance exercise decreases fasting plasma triglyceride (TG) levels as a result of reductions in the number and size of very-low-density lipoprotein (VLDL) particles, which are the main TG carriers in the fasting state. No change or a slight reduction in plasma low-density-lipoprotein cholesterol (LDL-C) levels may be observed, but this apparently small reduction may mask more important changes in LDL particle size and composition. Finally, two enzymes that are important correlates of plasma high-density-lipoprotein cholesterol (HDL-C) levels show reciprocal responses to en-durance-exercise training. Lipoprotein lipase (LPL) activity, which is positively correlated with plasma HDL$_2$ levels, is increased, whereas hepatic-triglyceride lipase (HTGL) activity, which is negatively correlated with plasma HDL$_2$-C concentration, is reduced after prolonged endurance-ex-ercise training. The right panel presents a metabolic profile predictive of a low CHD risk which we have described as "metabolic fitness." Adapted from Després and Lamarche 1993.*

large randomized study, Peter Wood and colleagues (1988) reported that diet-induced weight loss produced similar increases in plasma HDL-cholesterol levels, compared to weight loss produced by exercise training alone. They therefore emphasized the importance of weight loss and of producing a negative energy balance by exercise in order to improve the cardiovascular-disease risk profile, a concept that has been further supported by a randomized trial of weight loss versus aerobic exercise training (Katzel et al., 1995).

Finally, it is important to point out that although the hyperinsuline-mic-dyslipidemic state of visceral obesity substantially increases the risk of ischemic heart disease, no prospective study has quantified the contribution of improved metabolic and cardiorespiratory fitness to the expected reduction in CHD events in these high risk patients. However, the evidence available is convincing enough to suggest that the improvement in the metabolic condition of the dyslipidemic visceral obese patient could be more effective than the improvement in cardiorespiratory fitness in reducing CHD risk. Thus, 20-30 min of endurance exercise, performed three times a week, at 50-70% of $\dot{V}O_2$max may improve cardiorespiratory fitness, but the increase in energy expenditure associated with such an exercise program is relatively trivial and is not likely to induce substantial weight loss and attendant metabolic improvements unless a reduced-energy diet is employed. However, reducing the intensity of exercise and increasing its duration (e.g., a daily brisk walk of 45-60 min) is likely to generate a larger increase in energy expenditure and substantial improvements in insulin action and in other metabolic risk variables. We have therefore proposed that daily moderate-intensity exercise may be the most relevant form of exercise from a clinical standpoint for many high-risk, sedentary, insulin-resistant, visceral obese patients (Després & Lamarche, 1993, 1994). This suggestion is consistent with the benefits of regular walking on reducing CHD risk factors (Hardman et al., 1989; Leon et al., 1979; Tucker & Freeman, 1990). However, a prospective randomized study on endurance exercise training in insulin-resistant dyslipidemic patients must be conducted to test the hypothesis that exercise can indeed reduce the incidence of NIDDM and CHD. Furthermore, considering the importance of diet in the management of insulin resistance and of the related dyslipidemia in these patients, and taking into account the very high prevalence of this metabolic syndrome in the population, it is hoped that more adequate exercise-diet studies aimed at the management of visceral obese patients will be conducted in the future. The deficiency in the literature in this area is rather amazing considering the critical public health importance of this question.

SUMMARY

Visceral obesity is a prevalent condition in our affluent, sedentary societies. The metabolic complications associated with visceral obesity are such that this condition is probably the most prevalent correlate of coronary heart disease in many populations. The hazard of visceral obesity is currently not fully appreciated by physicians and health professionals. Simple variables such as the waist circumference, as well as metabolic data, including fasting plasma levels of insulin, apo B, triglyceride and HDL-cholesterol could help identify these high risk individuals.

Visceral obesity patients may benefit from the weight loss produced by a reduced-fat, increased complex-carbohydrate diet, but further research on the impact of such diet on the metabolic risk profile of visceral obese patients is needed. Accordingly, large, randomized, exercise-training studies in visceral obese patients are needed. Studies available suggest that moderate intensity but prolonged exercise, performed on an almost daily basis, is a relevant prescription for the treatment of visceral obese patients.

Finally, as long as the increased energy expenditure produced by exercise training is sufficient, the intensity of exercise does not appear to be a critical factor for inducing the beneficial effects of endurance exercise training in visceral obese patients. Thus, from a practical standpoint, it is proposed that a 45-min brisk walk performed on an almost daily basis is an effective exercise prescription for the prevention and treatment of visceral obesity.

FOOTNOTE

Results from the author's laboratory presented in this review have been obtained with the financial support of the Natural Sciences and Engineering Research Council of Canada, the Medical Research Council of Canada, the Canadian Diabetes Association and the Heart and Stroke Foundation of Canada.

BIBLIOGRAPHY

American College of Sports and Medicine (1990). Position stand on "The recommended quantity and quality of exercise for developing and maintaining cardiorespiratory and muscular fitness in healthy adults." *Med. Sci. Sports Exerc.* 22:265–274.

Assmann, G., and H. Schulte (1992). Relation of high-density lipoprotein cholesterol and triglycerides to incidence of atherosclerotic coronary artery disease (The PROCAM Experience). *Am. J. Cardiol.* 70:733–737.

Barrett-Connor, E. (1985). Obesity, atherosclerosis, and coronary artery disease. *Ann. Int. Med.* 103:1010–1019.

Björntorp, P. (1988). Abdominal obesity and the development of non-insulin dependent diabetes mellitus. *Diabetes Metab. Rev.* 4:615–622.

Björntorp, P (1981). Effects of exercise on plasma insulin. *Int. J. Sports Med.* 2:125–129.

Björntorp, P. (1984). Hazards in subgroups of human obesity. *Eur. J. Clin. Invest.* 14:239–41.

Björntorp, P. (1990). "Portal" adipose tissue as a generator of risk factors for cardiovascular disease and diabetes. *Arteriosclerosis* 10:493–496.

Björntorp, P. (1991). Visceral fat accumulation: The missing link between psychosocial factors and cardiovascular disease? *J. Int. Med.* 230:195–201.

Björntorp, P., De Jounge, K., Sjöström, L., and L. Sullivan (1970). The effect of physical training on insulin production in obesity. *Metabolism* 19:631–638.

Blair, S.N., Kohl, H.W. III, Paffenbarger, R.S., Clark, D.G., Cooper, K.H., and L.W. Gibbons (1989). Physical fitness an all-cause mortality. A prospective study of healthy men and women. *JAMA* 262:2395–2401.

Borkan, G.A., Gerzof, S.G., Robbins, A.H., Hults, D.E., Silbert, C.K., and J.E. Silbert (1982). Assessment of abdominal fat content by computed tomography. *Am. J. Clin. Nutr.* 36:172–177.

Bouchard C., Després J.P., and A. Tremblay (1993). Exercise and obesity. *Obesity Research* 1:40–54.

Bouchard C., Tremblay A., Després J.P., Nadeau A., Lupien P.J., Thériault G., Dussault J., Moorjani S., Pinault S., and G. Fournier (1990). The response to long-term overfeeding in identical twins. *N. Engl. J. Med.* 322:1477–1482.

Bray, G.A. (1985). Complications of obesity. *Annals of Internal Medicine* 103:1052–1062.

Brindley, D.N. (1992). Neuroendocrine regulation and obesity. *Int. J. Obes.* 16:S73–S79.

Brindley, D.N., and Y. Rolland (1989). Possible connections between stress, diabetes, obesity, hypertension, and altered metabolism that may result in atherosclerosis. *Clin. Sci.* 77:453–461.

Burnstein, R. Polychronakos, C., Toews, C.J., MacDougall, J.D., Guyda, H.J., and B.I. Pasner (1985). Acute reversal of the enhanced insulin action in trained athletes: association with insulin receptor changes. *Diabetes* 34:756–760.

Colberg, S.R., Simoneau, J.A., Thaete F.L., and D.E. Kelley (1995). Skeletal muscle utilization of free fatty acids in women with visceral obesity. *J. Clin. Invest.* 95:1846–1853.

Costill, D.L., Fink, W.J., Getchell, L.H., Ivy, J.L., and Witzman F.A. (1979). Lipid metabolism in skeletal muscles of endurance-trained males and females. *J. Appl. Physiol.* 47:787–791.

Després, J.P. (1993). Abdominal obesity as an important component of insulin resistance syndrome. *Nutrition* 9:452–459.

Després, J.P. (1994). Dyslipidemia and obesity. *Ballière's Clinical Endocrinology and Metabolism* 8:629–660.

Després, J.P. (1991a). Lipoprotein metabolism in visceral obesity. *Int. J. Obes.* 15:45–52.

Després, J.P. (1991b). Obesity and lipid metabolism: relevance of body fat distribution. *Curr. Opin. Lipidol.* 2:5–15.

Després, J.P. (1991c). Visceral obesity: A component of the insulin resistance-dyslipidemic syndrome. *Can. J. Cardiol.* 10:17B–22B.

Després, J.P. (1991d). Visceral obesity, insulin resistance, and related dyslipoproteinemias. In: H. Rifkin, J.A. Colwell and S.I. Taylor (eds.). *Diabetes*. Amsterdam: Elsevier Science Publ., pp. 95–99.

Després, J.P., and B. Lamarche (1993). Effects of diet and physical activity on adiposity and body fat distribution: Implications for the prevention of cardiovascular disease. *Nutr. Res. Rev.* 6:137–159.

Després, J.P., and B. Lamarche (1994). Low-intensity endurance exercise training, plasma lipoproteins and the risk of coranary heart disease. *J. Intern. Med.* 236:7–22.

Després, J.P., and A. Marette (1994). Relation of components of insulin resistance syndrome to coronary disease risk. *Curr. Opin. Lipid.* 5:274–289.

Després, J.P., Ferland, M., Moorjani, S., Nadeau, A., Tremblay, A., Lupien, P.J., Thériault, G., and C. Bouchard (1989a). Role of hepatic-triglyceride lipase activity in the association between intra-abdominal fat and plasma HDL-cholesterol in obese women. *Arteriosclerosis* 9:485–492.

Després, J.P., Lamarche, B., Mauriège, P., Cantin, B., Dagenais, G.R., Moorjani, S., and P.J. Lupien (1996). Hyperinsulinemia as an independent risk factor for ischemic heart disease. *N. Engl. J. Med.* 334:952–957.

Després, J.P., Lemieux, S., Lamarche, B., Prud'homme, D., Moorjani, S., Brun, L.D., Gagné, C., and P.J. Lupien (1995). The insulin resistance-dyslipidemic syndrome: contribution of visceral obesity and therapeutic implications. *Int. J. Obes.* 19:S76–S86.

Després, J.P., Moorjani, S., Ferland, M., Tremblay, A., Lupien, P.J., Nadeau, A., Pinault, S., Thériault, G., and C. Bouchard (1989b) . Adipose tissue distribution and plasma lipoprotein levels in obese women: Importance of intra-abdominal fat. *Arteriosclerosis* 9:203–210.

Després, J.P., Moorjani, S., Lupien, P.J., Tremblay, A., Nadeau, A., and C. Bouchard (1992). Genetic aspects of susceptibility to obesity and related dyslipidemias. *Mol. Cell. Biochem.* 113:151–169.

Després, J.P., Moorjani, S., Lupien, P.J., Tremblay, A., Nadeau, A., and C. Bouchard (1990). Regional distribution of body fat, plasma lipoproteins, and cardiovascular disease. *Arteriosclerosis* 10:497–511.

Després J.P., Moorjani S., Tremblay A., Ferland M., Lupien P.J., Nadeau A., and C. Bouchard (1989c). Relation of high plasma triglyceride levels associated with obesity and regional adipose tissue distribution to plasma lipoprotein-lipid composition in premenopausal women. *Clin. Invest. Med.* 12:374–380.

Després, J.P., Nadeau, A., Tremblay, A., Ferland, M., and P.J. Lupien (1989d). Role of deep abdominal fat in the association between regional adipose tissue distribution and glucose tolerance in obese women. *Diabetes* 38:304–309.

Després, J.P., Pouliot, M.C., Moorjani, S., Nadeau, A., Tremblay, A., Lupien, P.J., Thériault, G., and C.

Bouchard (1991). Loss of abdominal fat and metabolic response to exercise training in obese women. *Am. J. Physiol. (Endocrinol. Metab.)* 261:E159–E167.

Donahue, R.P., Abbott, R.D., Bloom, E., Reed, D.M., and K. Yano (1987). Central obesity and coronary heart disease in men. *Lancet* April:822–824.

Ducimetière, P., Richard, J., and F. Cambien (1986). The pattern of subcutaneous fat distribution in middle-aged men and the risk of coronary heart disease: The Paris Prospective study. *Int. J. Obes.* 10:229–240.

Ekelund, L.G., Haskell, W.L., Johnson, J.L., Whaley, F.S., Criqui, M.H., and D.S. Sheps (1988). Physical fitness as a predictor of cardiovascular mortality in asymptomatic North American men: the Lipid Research Clinic Mortality Follow-up Study. *N. Engl. J. Med.* 319:1379–1384.

Evans, D.J., Hoffmann, R.G., Kalkhoff, R.K., and A.H. Kissebah (1983). Relationship of androgenic activity to body fat topography, fat cell morphology, and metabolic aberrations in premenopausal women. *J. Clin. Endocrinol. Metab.* 57:304–310.

Exercise, Fitness, and Health. The consensus statement. (1990). In: C. Bouchard., R.J. Shephard, T. Stephens, J.R. Sutton, B.D. McPherson, (eds.) *Exercise, Fitness, and Health.* Champaign, Ill: Human Kinetics, pp. 3–28.

Felber J.P. (1972). From obesity to diabetes. Pathophysiological considerations. *Int. J. Obes.* 16:937–952.

Ferland, M., Després, J.P., Tremblay, A., Pinault, S., Nadeau, A., Moorjani, S., Lupien, P.J., Thériault, G., and C. Bouchard (1989). Assessment of adipose tissue distribution by computed axial tomography in obese women: Association with body density and anthropometric measurements. *Brit. J. Nutr.* 61:139–148, 1989.

Folsom A.R., Kaye S.A., Sellers T.A., Hong C.P., Cerhan J.R., Potter J.D., and R.J. Prineas (1993). Body fat distribution and 5–year risk of death in older women. *JAMA* 269:483–487.

Fujimoto W.Y., Leonetti D.L., Newell-Morris L., Shuman W.P., and P.W. Wahl (1990). Relationship of absence or presence of a family history of diabetes to body weight and body fat distribution in type 2 diabetes. *Int. J. Obesity* 15:111–120.

Fujioka, S., Matsuzawa, Y., Tokunaga, K., Kano, Y., Kobatake, T., and S. Tarui (1991a). Treatment of visceral obesity. *Int. J. Obes.* 15:59–65.

Fujioka, S., Matsuzawa, Y., Tokunaga, K., Kawamoto, T., Kobatake, T., Keno, Y., Kotani, K., Yoshida, S., and S. Tarui (1991b). Improvement of glucose and lipid metabolism associated with selective reduction of intra-abdominal visceral fat in premenopausal women with visceral fat obesity. *Int. J. Obes.* 15:853–859.

Fujioka, S., Matsuzawa, Y., Tokunaga, K., and S. Tarui (1987). Contribution of intra-abdominal fat accumulation to the impairment of glucose and lipid metabolism in human obesity. *Metabolism* 36:54–59.

Genest J.J., McNamara J.R., Salem D.N., and E.J. Schaefer (1991). Prevalence of risk factors in men with premature coronary heart disease. *Am. J. Cardiol.* 67:1185–1189.

Goldstein D.J. (1992). Beneficial health effects of modest weight loss. *Int. J. Obes.* 16:397–415.

Haarbo, J., Marslew, U., Gotfredsen, A., and C. Christiansen (1991). Post-menopausal hormone replacement therapy prevents central distribution of body fat after menopause. *Metabolism* 40:1323–1326.

Hardman, A.E., Hudson, A., Jones, P.R., and N.G. Norgan (1989). Brisk walking and plasma high-density lipoprotein cholesterol concentration in previously sedentary women. *Br. Med. J.* 299:1204–1205.

Haskell, W.L. (1984). Exercise-induced changes in plasma lipids and liporpteins. *Prev. Med.* 13:23–36.

Haskell, W.L. (1986). The influence of exercise training on plasma lipids and lipoproteins on health and disease. *Acta Med. Scand.* 711(Supp):25–37.

Hennes M., Shrago E., and A.H. Kissebah (1990). Receptor and post receptor effects of FFA on hepatocyte insulin dynamics. *Int. J. Obes.* 14:831.

Jahoor F., Klein S., and R. Wolfe (1992). Mechanism of regulation of glucose production by lipolysis in humans. *Am. J. Physiol.* 262(Endocrinol Metab 25):E353–E358, 1992.

Katzel, L.I. Bleecker, E.R., Colman, E.G., Rogues, E.M. Sorkin, J.D., and A.P. Goldberg (1995). Effects of weight loss vs aerobic exercise training on risk factors for coronary disease in healthy, obese, middle-aged and older men. A randomized controlled trial. *JAMA* 274:1915–1921.

Keys A. (1970). Coronary heart disease in seven countries. *Circulation* 41(suppl.1):I1–I211.

Kissebah, A.H., and A.N. Peiris (1989). Biology of regional body fat distribution: Relationship to non-insulin-dependent diabetes mellitus. *Diabetes Metab. Rev.* 5:83–109.

Kissebah, A.H., Evans, D.J., Peiris, A., and C.R. Wilson (1985). Endocrine characteristics in regional obesities: Role of sex steroids. In: J. Vague, P. Björntorp, B. Guy-Grand et al (eds.) *Metabolic complications of human obesities.* Amsterdam: Elsevier Science Publ., pp. 115–130.

Kissebah, A.H., Freedman, D.S., and A.N. Peiris (1989). Health risks of obesity. *Med. Clin. N. Am.* 73:111–138.

Kissebah, A.H., Vydelingum, N., Murray, R., Evans, D.J., Hartz, A.J., Kalkhoff, R.K., and P.W. Adams (1982). Relation of body fat distribution to metabolic complications of obesity. *J. Clin. Endocrinol. Metab.* 54:254–260.

Kokkins, P.F., Holland, J.C. Narayan, P., Colleran J.A., Dotson, C.O., and V. Papademetriou (1995). Miles run per week and high-density lipoprotein cholesterol levels in healthy, middle-aged men. *Arch. Inter. Med.* 155:415–420.

Kral, J.G., Schaffner, F., Pierson, R.N., and J. Wang (1993). Body fat topography as an independent predictor of fatty liver. *Metabolism* 42:548–551.

Krauss, R.M. (1989). Exercise, lipoproteins and coronary heart disease. *Circulation* 79:1143–1145.

Krotkiewski, M., and P. Björntorp (1986). Muscle tissue in obesity with different distribution of adipose tissue: Effects of physical training. *Int. J. Obes.* 10:331–341.

Krotkiewski, M., Björntorp, P., Sjöström, L., and U. Smith (1983). Impact of obesity on metabolism in men and women. Importance of regional adipose tissue distribution. *J. Clin. Invest.* 72:1150–1162.

Kvist, H., Chowdhury, B., Grangard, U., Tylén, U., and L. Sjöström (1988). Total and visceral adipose tissue volumes derived from measurements with computed tomography in adult men and women: Predictive equations. *Am. J. Clin. Nutr.* 48:1351–1361.

Lamarche, B., Després, J.P., Moorjani, S., Cantin, B., Dagenais, G., and P.J. Lupien (1995). Prevalence of dyslipidemic phenotypes in ischemic heart disease (Prospective results from the Québec Cardiovascular Study). *Am. J. Cardiol.* 75:1189–1195.

Lamarche, B., Moorjani, S., Lupien, P.J., Cantin, B., Dagenais, G.R., and J.P. Després. (1996). Apolipoprotein A-I and B levels and the risk of ischemic heart disease during a five-year follow-up of men in the Québec Cardiovascular Study. *Circulation* 94(3):273–278.

Lamarche, B., Tchernof, A., Moorjani, S., Cantin, B., Dagenais, G.R., Lupien, P.J., and J.P. Després (1997). Small, dense low-density lipoprotein particles as a predictor of the risk of ischemic heart disease in men. Prospective results from the Québec Cardiovascular Study. *Circulation* 95:69–75.

Lapidus, L., Bengtsson, C., Larsson, B., Pennert, K., Rybo, E., and L. Sjöström (1984). Distribution of adipose tissue and risk of cardiovascular disease and death: a 12 year follow-up of participants in the population study of women in Gothenburg, Sweden. *Brit. Med. J.* 289:1261–1263.

Larsson, B., Svardsudd, K., Welin, L., Wilhemsen, L., Björntorp, P., and G. Tibblin (1984). Abdominal adipose tissue distribution, obesity and risk of cardiovascular disease and death: 13 year follow-up of participants in the study of men born in 1913. *Brit. Med. J.* 288:1401–1404.

Leenen, R., Van der Kooy, K., Deurenberg, P., Seidell, J.C., Weststrate, J.A., Schouten, F.J.M., and J.G.A.J. Hautvast (1992). Visceral fat accumulation in obese subjects: Relation to energy expenditure and response to weight loss. *Am. J. Physiol. (Endocrinol Metab)* 263:E913–E919.

Lemieux, S., and J.P. Després (1994). Metabolic complications of visceral obesity: contribution to the etiology of type 2 diabetes and implications for prevention and treatment. *Diabète et Metab.* 20:375–393.

Lemieux, S., Després, J.P., Moorjani, S., Nadeau, A., Thériault, G., Prud'homme, D., Tremblay, A., Bouchard, C., and P.J. Lupien (1994). Are gender differences in cardiovascular disease risk factors explained by the level of visceral adipose tissue? *Diabetologia* 37:757–64.

Lemieux, S., Després J.P., Nadeau A., Prud'homme D., Tremblay A., and C. Bouchard (1992). Heterogeneous glycaemic and insulinaemic responses to oral glucose in non-diabetic men: Interactions between duration of obesity, body fat distribution and family history of diabetes mellitus. *Diabetologia* 35:653–659.

Lemieux, S., Prud'homme, D., Bouchard, C., Tremblay, A., and J.P. Després (1996a). A single threshold value of waist girth to identify non-obese and overweight subjects with excess visceral adipose tissue. *Am. J. Clin. Nutr.* 64:685–693.

Lemieux, S., Prud'homme, D., Bouchard, C., Tremblay, A., and J.P. Després (1993). Sex differences in the relation of visceral adipose tissue accumulation to total body fatness. *Am. J. Clin. Nutr.* 58:463–467.

Lemieux, S., Prud'homme, D., Nadeau, A., Tremblay, A., Bouchard, C., and J.P. Després (1996b). Seven-year changes in body fat and visceral adipose tissue in women. Associations with indexes of plasma glucose-insulin homeostasis. *Diabetes Care* 19:983–991.

Leon, A.S., Connett, J., Jacobs, D.R. Jr, and R. Rauramaa (1987). Leisure-time physical activity levels and risk of coronary heart disease and death. The Multiple Risk Factor Intervention Trial. *JAMA* 258:2388–2395.

Leon, A.S., Conrad, J., Hunninghake, D.B., and R. Serfass (1979). Effects of vigorous walking program on body composition, and carbohydrate and lipid metabolism of obese young men. *Am. J. Clin. Nutr.* 32:1776–1787.

Lie, H., Mundal, R., and J. Ericksson (1985). Coronary risk factors and incidence of coronary death in relation to physical fitness: Seven years follow-up study of middle-aged and elderly men. *Eur. Heart J.* 6:147–157.

Manninen, V., Tenkanen, L., Koskinen, P., Huttunen, J.K., Manttari, M., Heinonen, O.P., and M.H. Frick (1992). Joint effects of serum triglyceride and LDL-cholesterol and HDL-cholesterol concentrations on coronary heart disease risk in the Helsinki Heart study. Implications for treatment. *Circulation* 85:37–45.

Manson, J.E., Willett, W.C., Stampfer, M.J., Colditz, G.A., Hunter, D.J., Hankinson, S.E., Hennekens,

C.H., and F.E. Speizer (1995). Body weight and mortality among women. *N. Engl. J. Med.* 333:677–685.

Morris, N., Chave, P.W., Adam, C. et al (1973). Vigorous exercise in leisure-time and the incidence of coronary heart disease. *Lancet* 1:333–339.

Morris, J.N., Everitt, M.G., Pollard, R. et al (1980). Vigorous exercise in leisure-time: Protection against coronary heart disease. *Lancet* 2:1207–1210.

National Institutes of Health (1985). Consensus conference: Lowering blood cholesterol to prevent heart disease. *JAMA* 253:2080–2086.

National Institutes of Health (1987). Consensus development conference on diet and exercise in non insulin-dependent diabetes mellitus. *Diabetes Care* 10:639–644.

Ohlson, L.O., Larsson, B., Svärdsudd, K., Welin, L., Eriksson, H., Wilhelmsen, L., Björntorp, P., and G. Tibblin (1985). The influence of body fat distribution on the incidence of diabetes mellitus—13.5 years of follow-up of the participants in the study of men born in 1913. *Diabetes* 34:1055–1058.

Oshida, Y., Yamamouchi, K., Hayamizy, S., and Y. Saton (1989). Long-term mild jogging increases insulin action despite no influence on body mass index or V̇O$_2$max. *J. App. Physiol.* 66:2206–2210.

Paffenbarger, R.S. Jr, and W.E. Hale (1976). Work activity and coronary heart mortality. *N. Engl. J. Med.* 292:545–550.

Paffenbarger, R.S., Wing, A.L., and R. Hyde (1978). Physical activity as an index for heart attack risk in college alumni. *Am. J. Epidemiol.* 108:161–175.

Pedersen S.B., Jonler M., and B. Richelsen (1994). Characterization of regional and gender differences in glucocorticoid receptors and lipoprotein lipase activity in human adipose tissue. *J. Clin. Endocrinol. Metab.* 78:1354–1359.

Peiris, A.N., Mueller, R.A., Struve, M.F., Smith G.A., and A.H. Kissebah (1987). Relationship of androgenic activity to splanchnic insulin metabolism and peripheral glucose utilization in premenopausal women. *J. Clin. Endocrinol. Metab.* 64:162–169.

Peiris, A.N., Sothmann, M.S., Hennes, M.I., Lee, M.B., Wilson, C.R., Gustafson, A.B., and A.H. Kissebah (1989). Relative contribution of obesity and body fat distribution to alterations in glucose insulin homeostasis: predictive values of selected indices in premenopausal women. *Am. J. Clin. Nutr.* 49:758–764.

Peters, R.K., Cady, L.D. Jr, Bischoff, D.P., Bernstein, L., and M.C. Pike (1983). Physical fitness and subsequent myocardial infarction in healthy workers. *JAMA* 249:3052–3056.

Pollare T., Vessby B., and H. Lithell (1991). Lipoprotein lipase activity in skeletal muscle is related to insulin sensitivity. *Arterioscler. Thromb.* 11:1192.

Pouliot, M.C., Després, J.P., Lemieux, S., Moorjani, S., Bouchard, C., Tremblay, A., Nadeau, A., and P.J. Lupien (1994). Waist circumference and abdominal sagittal diameter: Best simple anthropometric indexes of abdominal visceral adipose tissue accumulation and related cardiovascular risk in men and women. *Am. J. Cardiol.* 73:460–468.

Pouliot, M.C., Després, J.P., Nadeau, A., Moorjani, S., Prud'homme, D., Lupien, P.J., Tremblay, A., and C. Bouchard (1992). Visceral obesity in men. Associations with glucose tolerance, plasma insulin, and lipoprotein levels. *Diabetes* 41:826–834.

Randle P.J., Garland P.B., Hales C.N., and E.A. Newsholme (1963). The glucose fatty-acid cycle; its role in insulin sensitivity and the metabolic disturbances of diabetes mellitus. *Lancet* 1:785–789.

Reaven, G.M. (1988). Role of insulin resistance in human disease. *Diabetes* 37:1595–1607.

Rebuffé-Scrive M., Lundholm K., and P. Björntorp (1985). Glucocorticoid binding in human adipose tissue. *Eur. J. Clin. Invest.* 15:267–271.

Rogers, M.A., Yamamoto, C., King, D.S., Hagberg, J.M., Ehsani, A.A., and J.O. Holloszy (1988). Improvement in glucose tolerance after 1 wk of exercise in patients with mild NIDDM. *Diabetes Care* 11:613–618.

Salonen, J.T., Slater, J.S., Tuomilehto, J., and R. Rauramaa (1988). Leisure-time and occupational physical activity: Risk of death from ischaemic heart disease. *Am. J. Epidemiol.* 127:87–94.

Seals, D.R., and J.M. Hagberg (1984). The effect of exercise training on human hypertension: A review. *Med. Sci. Sports Exerc.* 16:207–215.

Seidell, J.C., Björntorp, P., Sjöström, L., Kvist, H., and R. Sannerstedt (1990). Visceral fat accumulation is positively associated with insulin, glucose and C-peptide levels, but negatively with testosterone levels. *Metabolism* 39:897–901.

Sjöström, L., Kvist, H., Cederblad, A., and U. Tylen (1986). Determination of total adipose tissue and body fat in women by computed tomography, ^{40}K, and tritium. *Am. J. Physiol. (Endocrinol. Metab.)* 250:E736–E745.

Slattery, M.L., and D.R. Jacobs Jr. (1988). Physical fitness and cardiovascular disease mortality: The US railroad Study. *Am. J. Epidemiol.* 127:571–580.

Sniderman A.J., and J. Silberberg (1990). Is it time to measure apolipoprotein B? *Arteriosclerosis* 10:665–667.

Sparrow, D., Borkan, G.A., Gerzof, S.G., and C.K. Wisniewski (1986). Relationship of body fat distribution to glucose tolerance. Results of computed tomography in male participants of the normative aging study. *Diabetes* 35:411–415.

Stamler J., Wentworth D., and J.D. Neaton (1986). Is relationship between serum cholesterol and risk of premature death from coronary heart disease continuous or graded? Findings in 356 222 primary screenees of the Multiple Risk Factor Intervention Trial (MRFIT). *JAMA* 256:2823–2828.

Svedberg J., Björntorp P., Smith V., and P. Lonnroth (1990). FFA inhibition of insulin binding, degradation, and action in isolated rat hepatocytes. *Diabetes* 39:570.

Taylor S.I., Mukherjee C., and R.L. Jungas (1975). Regulation of pyruvate dehydrogenase in isolated rat liver mitochondria. *J. Biol. Chem.* 250:2028–2035.

Tchernof, A., Després, J.P., Bélanger, A., Dupont, A., Prud'homme, D., Moorjani, S., Lupien, P.J., and F. Labrie (1995a). Reduced testosterone and adrenal C19 steroid levels in obese men. *Metabolism* 44(4):513–519.

Tchernof, A., Després, J.P., Dupont, A., Bélanger, A., Nadeau, A., Prud'homme, D., Moorjani, S., Lupien, P.J., and F. Labrie (1995b). Relation of steroid hormones to glucose tolerance and plasma insulin levels in men: Importance of visceral adipose tissue. *Diabetes Care* 18:292–299.

Tchernof, A., Labrie, F., Bélanger, A., and J.P. Després (1996a). Obesity and metabolic complications: contribution of dehydroepiandrosterone and other steroid hormones. *J. Endocrinol.* 150:S155–S164.

Tchernof, A., Labrie, F., Bélanger, A., Prud'homme, D., Bouchard, C., Tremblay, A., Nadeau, A., and J.P. Després (1997). Androstane-3 , 17 -diol glucuronide as a steroid correlate of visceral obesity in men. *J. Clin. Endocrinol. Metab.*; in press.

Tchernof, A., Lamarche, B., Prud'homme, D., Nadeau, A., Moorjani, S., Labrie, F., Lupien, P.J., and J.P. Després (1996b). The dense LDL phenotype: association with plasma lipoprotein levels, visceral obesity, and hyperinuslinemia in men. *Diabetes Care* 19(6):629–637.

Technical Review. Exercise and NIDDM (1991). *Diabetes* 14(Supp):52–56.

Terry R.B., Page W.F., and W.L. Haskell (1992). Waist/hip ratio, body mass index and premature cardiovascular disease mortality in US army veterans during a twenty-three year follow-up study. *Int. J. Obes.* 16:417–423.

Tokunaga, K., Matsuzawa, Y., Ishikawa, K., and S. Tarui (1983). A novel technique for the determination of body fat by computed tomography. *Int. J. Obes.* 7:437–445.

Tucker, L.A., and G.M. Freeman (1990). Walking and serum cholesterol in adults. *Am. J. Publ. Health* 80:1111–1113.

Vague, J. (1956). The degree of masculine differentiation of obesities: a factor determining predisposition to diabetes, atherosclerosis, gout and uric-calculous disease. *Am. J. Clin. Nutr.* 4:20–34.

Vague, J. (1947). La différenciation sexuelle, facteur déterminant des formes de l'obésité. *Presse Médicale* 30:339–340.

WHO Expert Committee on the Prevention of Coronary Heart Disease, *World Health Organization Technical Reports* Series 678. Geneva, Switzerland, World Health Organization, 1982.

Williams, P.T., Wood, P.D., Haskell, W.L., and K. Vranigan (1982). The effect of running mileage and duration on plasma lipoprotein levels. *JAMA* 247:2674–2679.

Wood, P., and W. Haskell (1979). The effect of exercise on plasma high-density lipoproteins. *Lipids* 14:417–427.

Wood, P.D., and M.L. Stefanick (1988). Exercise, fitness and atherosclerosis. In: Bouchard, C., Shephard, R.J., Stephens, T., Sutton, J.R. and B.D. McPherson (eds.). *Exercise, fitness and health. A consensus of current knowledge.* Champaign, IL: Human Kinetics, pp.. 409–420.

Wood, P.D., Stefanick, M.L., Dreon, D.M., Frey-Hewitt, B., Garay, S.C., Williams, P.T., Superko, R.S., Fortmann, S.P., Albers, J.J., Vranizan, K.M., Ellsworth, N.M., Terry, R.B., and W.L. Haskell (1988). Changes in plasma lipids and lipoproteins in overweight men during weight loss through dieting as compared with exercise. *N. Engl. J. Med.* 319:1173–1169.

Wood, P.D., Williams, P.T., and W.L. Haskell (1984). Physical activity and high-density lipoproteins. N.E. Miller and G.J. Miller (eds.) *Clinical and metabolic aspects of high-density lipoproteins.* Amsterdam: Elsevier Science Publishers, pp. 133–165.

DISCUSSION

GISOLFI: Dr. Despres, could you speculate on the mechanisms by which visceral obesity—as opposed to fat in other areas of the body—may lead to coronary heart disease?

DESPRES: I'm not convinced that excess visceral adipose tissue is an independent risk factor for coronary heart disease if the intermediate metabolic abnormalities are controlled. There are people who have suggested that excess visceral fat might be a marker of a more primary neuroendocrine alteration. Visceral obesity has been related to an increased fat intake. This could lead to concomitant alterations in steroid metabolism and in the sex-steroid profile, which may contribute to selective deposition of visceral fat as opposed to subcutaneous fat. Obviously, there is a large genetic effect on where fat is deposited, and my colleague, Claude Bouchard, has studied this effect. However, it is one thing to say there is a genetic component, but discovering the molecular mechanism responsible for the genetic component is much more complicated. I believe that Per Bjorntorp's hypothesis is quite compelling. He suggests that excess visceral fat accumulation might be a marker of a civilization syndrome or of our inability to cope with stress, which may lead to an activated hypothalamic-pituitary-adrenal (HPA) axis and to an increased release of glucocorticoids. They induce a deleterious state of insulin resistance, and the visceral adipocytes have high concentrations of glucocorticoid receptors, i.e., 4–6 fold greater than in subcutaneous fat. Perhaps this explains the selective accumulation of lipid in the visceral fat cells. But this might be a marker of a more primary neuroendocrine abnormality, whatever it is.

However, once this excess visceral fat has accumulated, because of the peculiar metabolic profile of these intra-abdominal fat depots and the fact that the venous outflow is through the portal vein, even a high concentration of circulating insulin will not be able to shut down lipolysis. This hyperlipolytic state continues to expose the liver to high concentrations of fatty acids, leading to a cascade of additional metabolic abnormalities. Also, David Kelly at the University of Pittsburgh has suggested that excess visceral fat is associated with metabolic and morphological alterations in skeletal muscle, and these changes could lead to other metabolic abnormalities that affect CHD risk.

So, is excess visceral adipose tissue accumulation causally related to the cluster of metabolic abnormalities that increases the risk of NIDDM and coronary disease? I think the answer is, yes, but it is not the full answer; I believe that visceral fat is also partly a marker of additional abnormalities.

GISOLFI: Claude Bouchard suggests that total body fat, not visceral fat, is most indicative of coronary heart disease risk.

DESPRES: That is Claude's opinion; history will tell 30 y from now who was right. Maybe I'm totally wrong. We'll see.

EICHNER: Besides cortisol, is the visceral fat also more sensitive to epinephrine than is subcutaneous fat?

DESPRES: Yes.

EICHNER: Then let me propose that it is not a civilization syndrome but a pre-civilization syndrome that dates back to the dawn of humanity; men were designed to have five pounds of visceral fat for ready fuel to engage in combat with saber-toothed tigers and other enemies.

DESPRES: I fully agree with that.

EICHNER: But men were not designed to have 50 pounds of visceral fat. In ancient times, visceral fat conferred a survival benefit, because tribal elders were aged 35 years; those men did not die of coronary heart disease.

DESPRES: It is a great hypothesis; five pounds of visceral fat would not substantially impair locomotion. Gluteal femoral fat, on the other hand, is very hard to mobilize in women except during lactation.

SPRIET: It is difficult to understand why the body would store fat in visceral depots, given the way the fat gets into the body. I think it is easier to understand why it would be there in times when it needs to be broken down. Is there anything we need to know about the relative amount of visceral adipose tissue that is drained by the portal circulation?

DESPRES: A fairly large proportion of omental and mesenteric fat is drained by the portal vein. Is it necessary from an evaluation standpoint to distinguish non-portal fat from portal fat? Well, when the total visceral fat depot is enlarged, it is mainly the portally-drained fat depots that are increased in size. Thus, there is no need to selectively distinguish portal from non-portal fat if the CHD risk in a given individual is to be estimated. This fact also makes it simpler to use imaging techniques to measure visceral fat.

SPRIET: This point is important for people who are not familiar with the anatomy. Also, is there anything that has been learned from the data on men and women who have similar amounts of abdominal fat that may explain the selective deposition of visceral adipose tissue?

DESPRES: The first papers on this topic were published in the 80's and were mainly conducted in women. Endocrinologists knew that abdominally-obese women tended to have higher plasma concentrations of free testosterone concentration and that there was a contribution of glucocorticoids to the metabolic alterations found. Also, sex-hormone-binding globulin levels were lower in women with excess abdominal fat, so a more "androgenic" profile was associated with insulin resistance and dyslipidemia. We first thought that similar phenomena would occur in men. However, we and others have published studies indicating, the higher the testosterone levels in men, the lower is the amount of visceral fat and the more favorable was the metabolic risk profile. Further work will be necessary to better understand which are the primary factors involved.

Adipose tissue is a very active tissue for the interconversion of steroid hormones. Thus, in visceral obese women it is possible that there is an increased conversion of steroid precursors and estrogens by the fat tissue into androgens. In men, on the other hand, it could be the other way around, i.e., testosterone may be converted in the fat tissue to estrogens.

MURRAY: It is possible for two individuals with the same waistline to have widely varying degrees of abdominal fat, and if so, then is "waist management" the best way to address this challenge?.

DESPRES: The shared variance between waist circumference and visceral adipose tissue is not greater than 70–75%, so there will be some people who will be misclassified by measuring only waist circumference. Having said that, in practice, after measuring a large waistline, one should suggest further testing of the metabolic risk profile, including triglycerides, HDL-cholesterol, and the ratio of total cholesterol to HDL-cholesterol—all simple variables to measure. If the metabolic risk profile is favorable, there is a very low likelihood that this individual has too much visceral fat. But, if a large waistline is associated with the cluster of metabolic abnormalities that we have described, this individual probably has too much visceral fat.

We have conducted longitudinal studies indicating that the change in waist circumference observed over several years is closely correlated with the change in visceral fat. I clearly recognize that the waist circumference has limitations—there will be individuals misclassified—but if this measurement is combined with simple metabolic variables, at-risk individuals can be detected with good accuracy, and their responses to therapeutic treatments can be monitored.

NADEL: Is a person who has been relatively lean for most of his/her life but who then becomes viscerally obese at lower risk for disease than the person who stored visceral fat and has higher plasma triglyceride concentration throughout those middle years?

DESPRES: The earlier one begins to accumulate excess visceral fat, the longer will be the "incubation" period, and the worse will be the risk for cardiovascular disease 15 years down the road.

KENNEY: You have reported very compelling data suggesting that we should use waist circumference rather than waist-to-hip ratio as a marker of heart disease risk. From a public health perspective, while it sounds like a very simple straightforward technique to do waist-to-hip ratio measurements, in practice it is fraught with error as people try to determine in people of different obesity levels what is the waist and what is the hip, even though there are clear guides for measurement sites. Measuring circumference of the waist rather than waist-to-hip ratio seems to reconcile differences between men and women in terms of the slope of the response between circumference and health risk. Would you comment, please?

DESPRES: First of all, to make the measurement more reliable, we use bone landmark references to standardize the position of the waist circumference. We use the mid-distance between the bottom of the rib cage and the top of the iliac crest to standardize the waist circumference measurement.

The waist-hip ratio may be quite misleading if you're monitoring changes over time. For example, in the 7–year longitudinal study we conducted with women, the waist-hip ratio was a very poor predictor of the change in visceral fat. These women increased their waistline and also gained some hip fat. The computer tomography imaging technique revealed a 30% increase in visceral fat—much greater than the relatively small change in waist-hip ratio. The waist-hip ratio was a very misleading indicator of visceral fat.

I disagree with the use of waist-to-hip ratio cutoff points without first classifying the subjects on the basis of total body fat. For example, some people have suggested that a waist to hip ratio above 0.8 in women and above 1.0 in men would be associated with excess abdominal visceral fat. However, if we compare a lean woman with a waist to hip ratio of 0.8 and a body mass index of 22 with an obese women who also has a 0.8 waist to hip ratio but a body mass index of 35, it is clear that the obese woman has a much greater absolute amount of visceral fat than the lean woman. That is why the use of the waist to hip ratio is very misleading.

MELBY: Some of Gerald Reaven's work suggests that a higher carbohydrate intake in individuals with this syndrome is really inappropriate. His group reports better apparent success in improving the dyslipidemic profile with a higher fat, lower carbohydrate intake than is often recommended.

DESPRES: If one is clinically successful in clamping the energy intake and inducing a negative energy balance while adding a slightly higher intake of dietary fat, yes, the patient will lose weight, insulin sensitivity will be enhanced, and the lipid profile will be improved. However, the problem that we have in practice is that freely eating individuals will eat more and gain weight when they are exposed to a high-fat diet. That is the concern we have with that approach.

MELBY: What about the hypertriglyceridemia associated with high-fat or high-carbohydrate diets?

DESPRES: In the Quebec Cardiovascular study, we found that hypertriglyceridemia is not a risk factor as long as apo B concentration is low.

Why is that so? It is because there are different types of hypertriglyc-eridemia. Hypertriglyceridemia from a high-fat diet may be associated with an overproduction of lipoproteins by the liver and an increased production of apo B because increased lipid availability can reduce apo B degradation in the liver. This type of apo B-rich hypertriglyceridemia is very atherogenic. On the other hand, hypertriglyceridemia induced by a high complex-carbohydrate diet, does not generate an increased production of apo B lipoproteins. Rather, this type of hypertriglyc-eridemia produces triglyceride-rich VLDL particles. We need more study to confirm that this type of hypertriglyceridemia is not athero-genic.

Populations on low-fat diets—vegetarians for example—tend to have slightly higher triglyceride levels and very low HDL cholesterol concentrations. From these lipid variables, we would think they are at risk for heart disease, but in fact, their prevalence of heart disease is rather low.

HORSWILL: In Reaven's studies in which more dietary carbohydrate was not better, was the fiber content of the diet taken into consideration? Fiber can have a beneficial effect on insulin secretion, maybe insulin ac-tion, and can also reduce cholesterol levels. Has the effect of a fiber-rich, high-carbohydrate diet on visceral fat mass been investigated?

DESPRES: This is a poorly documented topic. We should keep in mind that patients don't eat macronutrients; they eat food. We focus on veg-etables, on complex carbohydrates from bread, from rice, and so on. Some low-fat food has a high sugar content that may induce high glycemic response, leading further weight gain. You get the very sharp insulin response when you consume some of these low-fat foods. Thus, we focus on a whole selection of natural foods rather than telling the pa-tients to reduce their intake of fats and to eat fat-free foods, because such advice can be misleading in some cases.

SHERMAN: Is daily exercise needed because of the cumulative effect over a period of time, or because the acute effects persist for only about 24 h?

DESPRES: I emphasize daily activity because it is the only way one can generate an increase in energy expenditure that will be associated with substantial and long-term improvements in insulin sensitivity and in the lipid-lipoprotein profile. It should be a minimum of every other day to benefit from the acute effect.

HARGREAVES: I wonder about the strength of the association between insulin resistance and a potential defect in skeletal muscle that has been shown by the group in Pittsburgh. If the primary problem is in muscle, and it leads to insulin resistance and visceral obesity, then should there be consideration of the optimal exercise prescription to change the profile of skeletal muscle? That may differ from that which might be used to alter adipose tissue metabolism.

DESPRES: Few exercise studies have specifically examined this issue. My exercise recommendation reflects a compromise between what we believe could be a decent prescription and our ability to change life-style habits. As you know, from a public health standpoint, we would like the message to be as simple as possible, but you are absolutely right that we need more data on this problem.

LOHMAN: Jean-Pierre, there is evidence that certain types of fat distribution, e.g., more thigh fat, can have some protective effects. What is your view on that?

DESPRES: Clearly, the accumulation of gluteal femoral fat in women is associated with a more favorable metabolic risk profile. The greater the activity of lipoprotein lipase in femoral adipose tissue, the higher is the HDL-cholesterol level in those premenopausal women. Is there a cause and effect relationship? We believe that gluteal femoral fat accumulation may be only a marker of an endocrine profile that is associated with proper insulin sensitivity and with a favorable lipid-lipoprotein profile.

DAVIS: You have described the selective increase in visceral fat after menopause in women, which seems intuitively to implicate the loss of estrogen as a causative. However, your focus seems to be only on the androgenic hormones like testosterone. How does estrogen fit into your explanation of the relationship between body fat distribution and cardiovascular disease?

DESPRES: There is a two-year intervention study showing that hormonal replacement therapy can slow down the accumulation of abdominal fat in women who passed through menopause. In our cross-sectional studies there is a clear distinction between three groups of women. Women who passed through menopause without hormone replacement therapy have the highest level of visceral fat; those who passed through menopause while on hormone replacement therapy have an intermediate level; and women who have not passed through menopause have the lowest level of visceral fat. The molecular mechanism responsible for the relationship between relative estrogen deficiencies and accumulation of visceral fat is far from being fully understood. Lipoprotein lipase is sensitive to some sex steroids and it is possible that the drop in estrogen causes a reduction in subcutaneous lipoprotein lipase activity. If so, the energy has to go somewhere else. This may lead to a cascade of endocrine alterations contributing to a selective accumulation of visceral fat. Unfortunately, we have more descriptive studies than mechanistic studies on this issue. However, results are consistent with the notion that estrogen deficiency accelerates visceral fat accumulation, and replacement of estrogen slows down this accumulation.

MELBY: African-Americans have a high prevalence of insulin resistance and NIDDM, yet their lipid profiles are not bad. Mexican-Americans with excess abdominal adiposity seem to exhibit less risk for hypertension than do non-Hispanic whites and African- Americans with abdominal obesity. It appears that there are racial differences in the relationship between abdominal adiposity and these untoward sequelae.

DESPRES: You are absolutely right. One should not apply reference values obtained on one population to others because we do not know if the relationships are the same. We need to study more population groups to sort this out.

GUTIN: I like your distinction between $\dot{V}O_2$max on one hand versus metabolic fitness on the other; you say that cardiovascular fitness is one thing and metabolic fitness is another. I wonder whether we should be using $\dot{V}O_2$max as interchangeable with cardiovascular fitness. For example, one would have to strain to find a direct link between the limiting factor for $\dot{V}O_2$max, which is usually thought to be maximal stroke volume, and any of these metabolic changes. Perhaps we should find some other indices of cardiorespiratory fitness, such as physiologic responses measured at a submaximal level, that are more dependent on muscle metabolism. There may be better ways of defining cardiovascular fitness.

DESPRES: One such measure may be submaximal exercise capacity, e.g., number of minutes on a treadmill at say, 70% of $\dot{V}O_2$max. I emphasized $\dot{V}O_2$max because that is the focus of many exercise programs, but your comment is very relevant.

HOUTKOOPER: Jean-Pierre, we've been talking about the big public health problem related to obesity, but there is a subgroup of people who are focused on being extremely lean and having a very low percentage of body fat. What are the minimal levels of acceptable body fat levels, and does it make a difference if someone who has extremely low levels of body fat has a fat distribution pattern that is very visceral? Are there negative health consequences in such lean people?

DESPRES: It would be hard to find an extremely lean person who had enough visceral fat to cause metabolic complications.

HOUTKOOPER: But there certainly would be some metabolic consequences for having entirely too little fat in the body.

DESPRES: Adipose tissue plays an important physiological role. Fat produces cytokines and leptin, and it plays an important role in steroid conversion and so on. It therefore plays an important role in women in determining a certain steroid profile associated with normal metabolic functions.

HOUTKOOPER: Clinicians struggle with advising clients on the minimal levels of body fat that are consistent with good health.

DESPRES: The healthy weight or the healthy body fat content can be very different among individuals. For example, women with 40–45% of their body weight as fat want to lose weight, and we should help them. However, if they have a perfectly normal metabolic risk profile, we certainly do not want to use drugs to accomplish this end. But, obviously, the goal should never be to change them into anorectic fashion models.

COYLE: What is known about what causes changes in the accumulation of visceral fat? Increases in visceral fat content can be due to increased deposition or reduced lipolysis and oxidation, and I assume both are operative. Is one more important than the other?

DESPRES: A hyperlipolytic state exists in visceral adipose tissue, and it is resistant to hyperinsulinemia. Even in the postprandial state lipolysis continues and probably maintains a highly atherogenic condition. A net accumulation of energy in adipocytes requires a high activity of lipoprotein lipase. Thus, the neuroendocrine profile of visceral obesity should contribute to an increased lipoprotein lipase activity rather than to a blunted lipolysis. I favor an emphasis on increased lipogenesis rather than a reduced lipolysis.

COYLE: What is the source of substrate for that greater rate of triglyceride synthesis? Are you assuming it is plasma fatty acids, or have you recognized the possibility of massive de novo lipogenesis from glucose.

DESPRES: I cannot, at this stage, but I think it more likely that the activity of lipoprotein lipase is increased. Also, the acylation-stimulating protein (ASP) is important for modulating the fatty acid accumulation in adipose tissue once lipoprotein lipase activity has broken down the triglyceride core of lipoproteins. Are there regional differences in the responses of adipocytes to ASP? We think so.

GISOLFI: Is it correct that women who breast feed tend to accumulate less femoral and gluteal fat? Also, what have we learned, if anything, about the relationship between the hormonal profile during breast-feeding and the distribution of body fat?

DESPRES: There has been only one study indicating that this fat is mobilized during lactation. There is obviously a different metabolic profile, and the study of lactating women would certainly be a relevant model to explore this issue further. However, there is very little information currently available.

4

Exercise and Eating Disorders

LINDA B. HOUTKOOPER PH.D., R.D.

INTRODUCTION

The image of a taut, lean body so prized by the mass media and contemporary culture has not always excited so much attention. In fact, throughout history plumpness was preferable. A rotund figure proclaimed that a person was affluent and well fed, important considerations during times when famines were common. Over the last three decades in industrialized countries, there has been a cultural trend toward adopting an archetype of physical perfection embodied in a thin, ideal body shape for females (Rodin, 1993; Rodin & Larson, 1992). In the 1960s a model named Twiggy became a symbol of an ideal body type for young women. She was reported to be 5 feet 6½ inches tall, weighed 90 pounds, and had bust, waist, and hip measurements of 31-22-31 inches, respectively (Woscyna, 1991). Twiggy represented the extreme model that served as a turning point in the ever-increasing cultural idolization of slimness. Female models today are still significantly thinner than those in the 1950s.

Thinness has become equated with beauty, acceptance, competence, control, power, and goodness for young women (Mortenson et al., 1993; Root, 1991). Consequently, increasing pressure has been put on adolescent girls and women to restrict food intake to achieve thin physiques (Beals & Manore, 1994). Female athletes are subject not only to the cultural pressure to be thin and to conform to specific aesthetic requirements of their sports but also have added demands to perform well in those sports (Wilmore, 1991). In some sports, a certain physique or a low body weight is considered to be essential for optimal performance, and this has led to a female athlete credo of "get thin and win" (Thornton, 1990). Participation in these sports is associated with a higher risk of eating disorders. These sports are categorized into three groups: 1) "appearance sports," such as dance, diving, figure skating, gymnastics, and synchronized swimming; 2) sports in which low body weight is considered an advantage, such as distance running, swimming, and track; and 3) sports that require weight categories or weigh-ins, such as body building, rowing, weight lifting, and wrestling (Benardot et al., 1994).

Cultural pressures to be thin and attain ideal physiques in order to be attractive or excel in sports can lead females to strive to be thinner than what may be realistically achievable (Leon, 1991; Manore, 1996). Research has clearly demonstrated that biological factors significantly influence body shape and weight (Bouchard, 1992); these factors preclude some individuals from achieving and maintaining a low body weight and culturally determined ideal body shapes.

Attempts to attain a low body weight and ideal physique for aesthetic purposes or to excel in sport performance can lead to disordered thoughts about food and to behaviors aimed at controlling body weight, composition, and body shape such as restricting food intake and using pathogenic weight control practices. These disordered eating and weight control behaviors occur in a spectrum ranging from mild pathological eating practices to severe clinical eating disorders such as anorexia nervosa and bulimia nervosa. Anorexia nervosa and bulimia nervosa are psychological disorders with dysfunctional implications for eating and exercise related practices (American Psychiatric Association, 1994; Beals & Manore, 1994; Brownell, 1995; Sundgot-Borgen, 1993b; Wilmore, 1991). Current estimates indicate that more than 90% of the clinical eating disorders of anorexia and bulimia nervosa occur in females, but the prevalence of these disorders in males and in athletes is unclear (American Psychiatric Association, 1994; Anderson, 1995; Brownell, 1995).

The American Psychiatric Association (1994) reported that the average age for the onset of anorexia nervosa is 17 y, with some evidence indicating bimodal peaks at ages 14 and 18 y. Furthermore, the onset of this disorder rarely occurs in females over age 40 y. Surveys indicate that restricting food intake and "dieting" begin at an early age and continue through adulthood (Emmons, 1994; French et al., 1995; Serdula et al., 1993). The 1990 Youth Risk Behavior Survey indicated that among 11,467 high school students, 44% of female students and 15% of male students were trying to lose weight (Serdula et al., 1993). An additional 26% of female students and 15% of male students reported that they were trying to avoid gaining more weight. These students reported using exercise, skipping meals, taking diet pills, and vomiting as means to help control their weight.

The Behavioral Risk Factor Surveillance System, a random-digit dial survey conducted with 60,861 adults in 1989, provided estimates of the prevalence of weight loss practices of adults. Among these adults, 38% of the women and 24% of the men reported that they were trying to lose weight. These surveys also indicated that about 25% of the female high school students and 20% of the women who considered themselves to be at the "right weight" were still trying to lose weight. Although maintenance of desirable body weight in adults may decrease risk for chronic disease in adulthood, overemphasis on thinness can lead to unhealthy weight loss practices and contribute to the development of eating disorders (Herzog & Copeland, 1985).

There is clearly less widespread cultural reinforcement for thinness and dieting for males than for females. Beginning as early as lower elementary school, boys are less likely than girls to consider themselves overweight or in need of dieting (Anderson, 1995; Serdula et al., 1993). Adult males tend to describe themselves as overweight only at weights 15% higher than ideal body weight (Anderson, 1995). Women generally report feeling thin only when they are below 90% of ideal body weight, whereas men rate themselves as thin until their weight is 105% of an ideal body weight (Anderson, 1995). Dieting in males is often related to participation in certain sports, past obesity, gender identification conflicts, and the avoidance of feared medical illness (Anderson, 1995; DePalma et al., 1993; Steen & Brownell, 1990). In preadolescents with eating disorders, the sex ratio of cases appears to be approximately equal (Bryant-Waugh & Lask, 1995).

Excessive Exercise and Eating Disorders

Dieting to control body weight or shape typically precedes the development of eating disorders. However, in some situations the use of exercise alone or in combination with restricted food intake leads to eating disorders in animals and humans (Anderson, 1990b; Davis & Cowles, 1989; Epling & Pierce, 1988, 1996; Epling et al., 1983). Research with animals has extended the understanding of environment-behavior interactions that affect anorexia and has described the biochemical changes that accompany starvation induced by physical activity. Studies based on an animal model of self-starvation have provided most of the basic information that supports the theory of activity anorexia. Rats placed on a single daily restricted energy feeding run more and more, eventually stop eating, and die of starvation (Epling & Pierce, 1988; Epling et al., 1983). Hyperactivity has been shown to frequently accompany self-starvation in animals (Epling & Pierce, 1996).

A potential link between excessive exercising and eating disorders in humans has been proposed and has aroused considerable controversy (Davis & Cowles, 1989; Davis & Fox, 1993; Weight & Noakes, 1987; Yates et al., 1983; 1994). Yates and colleagues (1983) first proposed that excessive running in middle-aged males (who base their self worth on physical efficacy) was an analog of anorexia nervosa in female patients (who base their self worth on appearance), but their work was harshly criticized as anecdotal and flawed. The three case studies reported in their paper were not specific individual profiles but rather were composites based on clinical observations that the authors thought represented typical subjects. They collected all of their information by interviewing 60 "obligatory" male runners and did not keep precise notes or make tape recordings, the term "obligatory running" was not defined, and raters or blinding procedures were not used to evaluate the interview material. This article painted a very negative picture of habitual male runners and claimed that "athletes with a penchant for profound exertion are at high risk for depression, anorexia, and other disorders." On the basis of the apparent congruence they found between excessive exercise and disordered eating behavior, the existence of a syndrome termed "activity disorder" was postulated (Yates et al., 1983).

Several subsequent studies strongly criticized the methods and the theory proposed by Yates and colleagues (Blumenthal et al., 1984; Davis & Fox, 1993; Nudelman et al., 1988; Weight & Noakes, 1987). However, as a group these subsequent studies did suggest that some "obligatory" female and male runners do have unusual ideas about food, diet, and fat. Unfortunately, these studies used different populations, definitions, methods, questionnaires, and generally small samples, making a morass of this whole new area of investigation. For example, Blumenthal et al. (1984) and Nudelman et al. (1988) compared male "obligatory" runners to female patients with anorexia or bulimia nervosa and found, not surprisingly, that their psychological profiles were quite different. The studies by Davis and Fox (1993) and Weight and Noakes (1987) included 351 adult females and 125 distance runners, respectively, in their investigations. They found marginal evidence to support the idea that excessive exercisers and women with eating disorders share some psychological features. For instance, Weight and Noakes (1987) reported that five (4%) of the runners had a low body weight and history of amenorrhea and stated that the "better athletes" were more likely to exhibit the physical and psychological features of anorexia nervosa. However, they concluded that abnormal eating attitudes and anorexia nervosa were no more common among competitive female runners than they are among the general population.

Yates et al. (1992) extended their earlier work in a study of 66 runners, in which more than half the runners were female and nearly half were classified, using defined criteria, as "obligatory" runners. They used several standard psychological tests and classified runners as "obligatory" based on responses to questionnaire items and interviews. The survey items addressed whether or not the runners continued to run when injured, number and type of injuries sustained, miles run per week, circumstances that could cause them to stop running, and whether or not the commitment to running had jeopardized a job or significant relationship or caused them to be less interested in sex, family life, or work. They concluded that even though obligatory runners were more focused on body weight and more preoccupied with the body, the obligatory and nonobligatory runners were mostly normal and more similar than different.

In a recent review, Yates et al. (1994) indicated that there is little support of the disease model in which "obligatory" exercise is equivalent to anorexia nervosa in women. They put forward a "risk factor model" in which they proposed that given common situational, cultural, psychological, and biological factors, perfectionists can easily be caught up in a diet or exercise program that may escalate to the point of harm. They asserted that excessive dieting and excessive exercise are "sister activities" and that a serious investment in one is likely to be accompanied by a preoccupation with the other. Whether or not excessive exercisers have something in common other than that they exercise a great deal and whether or not they are psychologically or biologically different in significant ways from those who don't exercise are matters for future empirical investigation.

HISTORY, DEFINITIONS, AND CRITERIA FOR EATING DISORDERS

Certain behaviors are deemed to constitute a clinical disorder or illness on the basis of changing and somewhat arbitrary criteria. The key functional requirements for behavior to be clinically defined as an eating disorder are that the behavior must no longer be under personal control and/or must cause significant adverse changes in psychological, social, or physical functioning (Anderson, 1990b). Anderson proposed that the process whereby eating behaviors become a disorder is analogous to the process of a person getting into a canoe some distance above Niagara Falls and then paddling downstream. Initially, the person is in control of the movement of the canoe down the stream, but at some point as the canoe approaches the edge of the water falls, the forces in the stream take over and the person is clearly no longer in control. At a certain point, without outside intervention, the person in the canoe will plunge down the falls with disastrous consequences.

Clinical Eating Disorders

The most severe clinical eating disorders are anorexia nervosa and bulimia nervosa. Both disorders can lead to serious physical damage and even death (American Psychiatric Association, 1994). The American

Psychiatric Association has also established a category for coding eating disorders that do not meet criteria for anorexia or bulimia nervosa as "Eating Disorder Not Otherwise Specified."

Anorexia Nervosa. The first medical description of anorexia nervosa was published in 1689 in London in a textbook of medicine by Richard Morton, a fellow of the College of Physicians (Silverman, 1995). Morton described a condition that he referred to as "nervous consumption" caused by sadness and anxious cares. The descriptions were based on his clinical observations and included both a female and male case. During the 20th century, work by Dr. Hilde Bruch lead to a revolution in the understanding of the psychopathology of anorexia nervosa (Silverman, 1995).

The current diagnostic criteria for anorexia nervosa include the *behavior* of self-induced starvation leading to body weight below a minimal level considered normal for age and height, the *psychopathological* intense fear of becoming fat or gaining weight, and a significant disturbance in the perception of body shape and size that is out of proportion to reality, and, in postmenarcheal females, a *biological* abnormality of reproductive hormone functioning leading to amenorrhea (American Psychiatric Association, 1994). Table 4-1 summarizes the diagnostic criteria for anorexia nervosa defined in the fourth edition of the Diagnostic and Statistical Manual of Mental Disorders (DSM-IV) of the American Psychiatric Association.

TABLE 4-1. *Diagnostic Criteria for Anorexia Nervosa.*

A. Refusal to maintain body weight over a minimal normal weight for age and height, e.g., weight loss leading to maintenance of body weight 15% below that expected; or failure to make expected weight gain during period of growth, leading to body weight 15% below that expected.
B. Intense fear of gaining weight or becoming fat, even though underweight.
C. Disturbance in the way in which one's body weight, size, or shape is experienced, undue influence of body weight or shape on self-evaluation, or denial of the seriousness of the current low body weight.
D. In postmenarcheal females, amenorrhea, i.e., the absence of at least three consecutive menstrual cycles. (A woman is considered to have amenorrhea if her periods occur only following hormone, e.g., estrogen, administration.)

Specify type:

Restricting Type: during the current episode of Anorexia Nervosa, the person has not regularly engaged in binge-eating or purging behavior (i.e., self-induced vomiting or the misuse of laxatives, diuretics, or enemas).
Binge-Eating/Purging Type: during the current episode of Anorexia Nervosa, the person has regularly engaged in binge-eating or purging behavior (i.e., self-induced vomiting or the misuse of laxatives, diuretics, or enemas).

Adapted from the Diagnostic and Statistical Manual of Mental Disorders IV, Washington, DC, American Psychiatric Association, 1994.

These criteria provide guidelines for determining if an individual's body weight is below a minimal normal level. Criterion A for diagnosis of anorexia specifies that a body weight less than 85% of the weight that is considered normal for a person's age and height is the cutoff for a minimal level of body weight. This value for minimal weight is usually calculated using the Metropolitan Life Insurance table values for adults. Growth charts are used for children and youths up to 18 years of age. An alternative guideline for minimal body weight is used in the International Classification of Diseases–10 Diagnostic Criteria for Research; this guideline is a minimal body mass index (weight in kilograms/height in meters^2) of 17.5 kg/m^2 (American Psychiatric Association, 1994). Restriction of food intake is the primary means of weight loss for the Restricting Subtype of anorexia nervosa. Individuals may start dieting by excluding foods perceived to be high in calories and/or fat, but most eventually follow a very restricted diet that is often limited to only a few foods (American Psychiatric Association, 1994). The Binge-eating/Purging Subtype of anorexia nervosa is distinguished by regular use of binge-eating and purging behaviors such as self-induced vomiting to achieve weight loss (American Psychiatric Association, 1994).

Criterion B specifies that the individual with this eating disorder exhibits intense fear of gaining weight or becoming fat, and this fear is not alleviated by weight loss. In fact, distress about weight gain will often increase as weight continues to decrease (American Psychiatric Association, 1994).

The experience and significance of body weight and shape are distorted in individuals with this disorder (Criterion C) (American Psychiatric Association, 1994). Some individuals feel globally overweight, whereas others realize that they are thin but are still concerned that parts of their body are too fat. They are obsessive about weighing themselves and measuring body parts. The self-esteem of individuals with anorexia is highly dependent on their body weight and shape. Weight loss is viewed as a sign of an impressive achievement of self-control, whereas weight gain is perceived as an unacceptable failure of self-control. Although some individuals with this disorder may acknowledge being thin, they typically deny the serious health implications of their condition.

Criterion D stipulates that amenorrhea is present in postmenarcheal females, and menarche is delayed in prepubertal females (American Psychiatric Association, 1994). In postmenarcheal females with this disorder, amenorrhea is related to abnormally low levels of estrogen secretion that result from a decreased secretion of follicle-stimulating hormone and luteinizing hormone.

Bulimia Nervosa. The term "bulimia" is derived from the Greek words for "ox" and for "hunger." The syndrome of bulimia nervosa was only recently defined (Russell, 1979), but the term "bulimia" has been traced in Western European sources for more than 2,000 y, with remarkable consistency of meaning. Bulimia has been defined as a state of pathological voraciousness that leads to ingesting excessive quantities of food (Parry-Jones & Parry-Jones, 1995). Bulimia nervosa is characterized by a history of rapidly ingesting large amounts of food in a discreet time period against a person's initial resistance and is usually followed by purging (American Psychiatric Association, 1994). During these binge-eating episodes the individual has feelings of being unable to stop eating or to control what or how much is eaten. The binge-eating episodes are associated with feelings of being out of control as well as of depression or guilt. There is a continuum of bulimic behaviors between the extremes of the anorectic with mild bulimia, who feels she has binged when she has eaten a salad against her will, and the other extreme of a normal weight bulimic who may ingest large amounts of food containing up to 8–10,000 kcal in a brief time and then purge (American Psychiatric Association, 1994; Anderson, 1990b). Typical purging methods include self-induced vomiting; misuse of laxatives, diuretics, or enemas; fasting; or excessive exercise. The diagnostic criteria for bulimia nervosa, defined by the American Psychiatric Association (DSM-IV), are summarized in Table 4-2.

Eating Disorder Not Otherwise Specified. The Eating Disorder Not Otherwise Specified category of the DSM-IV includes disorders of eating that do not meet the criteria for any specific eating disorder (American Psychiatric Association, 1994). Examples are summarized in Table 4-2.

Subclinical Eating Disorders

Individuals who show signs of disordered eating and distorted concerns regarding body weight or shape, but who fail to meet the strict DSM-IV criteria for eating disorders, exhibit subclinical eating disorders (American Psychiatric Association, 1994; Beals & Manore, 1994). Whereas individuals diagnosed with anorexia nervosa and bulimia nervosa exhibit severe emotional distress and/or specific psychopathologies that go beyond concerns about weight and use of weight reduction methods (American Psychiatric Association, 1994; Leon, 1991), these psychopathological profiles are generally not present in individuals with subclinical eating disorders (Leon, 1991, Sundgot-Borgen, 1993b, Wichmann & Martin, 1993). The concept of subclinical anorexia was first identified in female college students (Button & Whitehouse, 1981) and later in adolescents who had growth failure or delayed puberty due to malnutrition resulting from self-imposed calorie restriction based on a fear of becoming obese (Pugliese et al., 1983).

TABLE 4-2. *Diagnostic Criteria for Bulimia Nervosa & Eating Disorders Not Otherwise Specified.*

Bulimia Nervosa
A. Recurrent episodes of binge eating. An episode of binge eating is characterized by both of the following:
   (1) eating, in a discrete period of time (e.g., within any 2-hour period), an amount of food that is definitely larger than most people would eat during a similar period of time and under similar circumstances
   (2) a sense of lack of control over eating during the episode (e.g., a feeling that one cannot stop eating or control what or how much one is eating).
B. Recurrent, inappropriate, compensatory behavior in order to prevent weight gain, such as self-induced vomiting; misuse of laxatives, diuretics, enemas, or other medications; fasting; or excessive exercise.
C. The binge eating and inappropriate compensatory behaviors both occur, on average, at least twice a week for three months.
D. Self-evaluation is unduly influenced by body shape and weight.
E. The disturbance does not occur exclusively during episodes of Anorexia Nervosa.

Specific type:

Purging Type: during the current episode of Bulimia Nervosa, the person has regularly engaged in self-induced vomiting or the misuse of laxatives, diuretics, or enemas
Nonpurging Type: during the current episode of Bulimia Nervosa, the person has used other inappropriate compensatory behaviors, such as fasting or excessive exercise, but has not regularly engaged in self-induced vomiting or the misuse of laxatives, diuretics, or enemas

Eating Disorder Not Otherwise Specified

This category is for disorders of eating that do not meet the criteria for any specific Eating Disorder. Examples include:

A. For females, all of the criteria for Anorexia Nervosa are met except that the individual has regular menses.
B. All of the criteria for Anorexia Nervosa are met except that, despite significant weight loss, the individual's current weight is in the normal range.
C. All of the criteria for Bulimia Nervosa are met except that the binge eating and inappropriate compensatory mechanisms occur at a frequency of less than twice a week or for less than three months.
D. The regular use of inappropriate compensatory behavior by an individual of normal body weight after eating small amounts of food (e.g., self-induced vomiting after the consumption of two cookies).
E. Repeatedly chewing and spitting out, but not swallowing, large amounts of food.
F. Binge-eating disorder: recurrent episodes of binge eating in the absence of the regular use of inappropriate compensatory behaviors characteristic of Bulimia Nervosa.

Adapted from the Diagnostic and Statistical Manual of Mental Disorders IV, Washington, DC, American Psychiatric Association, 1994.

Athletes and Subclinical Eating Disorders. Athletes with subclinical eating disorders may exhibit some of the psychological traits associated with clinical eating disorders, such as high achievement orientation, obsessive-compulsive tendencies, and perfectionism. That these traits are also generally associated with success in athletic performance has led to the belief that subclinical eating disorders are more common among athletes than among the general population (Leon, 1991). Anecdotal reports and research with methodological limitations have provided indirect evidence suggesting that the prevalence of subclinical eating disorders is quite high in female athletes, particularly among athletes participating in sports that require a low body weight (Beals & Manore, 1994; Brownell & Rodin, 1992; Davis & Cowles, 1989; Gadpaille et al., 1987; Leon, 1991; Stoutjesdyk & Jevne, 1993).

Anorexia Athletica. The term "anorexia athletica" has been used to describe a subclinical eating disorder syndrome characterized by disordered eating and compulsive exercising (Pugliese et al., 1983; Sundgot-Borgen, 1993b). The essential feature of anorexia athletica is an intense fear of gaining weight or becoming fat, even though the individual weighs 5% less than the expected normal weight for age and height. Weight loss is achieved by restriction of food intake, extensive compulsive exercise, or both (Sundgot-Borgen, 1993b). Frequently the athletes also report binging, self-induced vomiting, or the use of laxatives or diuretics.

The criteria for subclinical eating disorders have not been well defined. Thus, more well-designed research is needed to define and determine the prevalence, incidence, and consequences of subclinical eating disorders in athletes.

Diagnostic Criteria in Males

Males who develop eating disorders are more likely than are females to have experienced medically defined, premorbid obesity (Anderson, 1995). Studies of anorexia nervosa indicate that the psychosocial and clinical characteristics are essentially indistinguishable between females and males (Crisp & Burns, 1983; Hsu, 1980). The diagnostic criteria for anorexia in males are similar to those for females (Anderson, 1995). These criteria include self-induced starvation, a morbid fear of fatness, and relentless pursuit of thinness, but they differ in the reproductive hormone abnormalities. Males with anorexia nervosa are characterized by lower testosterone levels that cause decreased sexual drive and performance (Anderson, 1995). The diagnostic criteria for bulimia are gender independent (Anderson, 1995).

Exercise and Primary or Secondary Eating Disorders

In assessing possible links between exercise training and eating disorders, it is important to differentiate between primary and secondary eating disorders (Leon, 1991). For example, the clinical features of both anorexia nervosa and bulimia nervosa often include a strong exercise component expressed by intensive and highly ritualized daily activities, such as performing a specific number of sit-ups or aerobic exercises. For individuals with a primary eating disorder, exercise is a pathway for expression of the disorder, but little is known about the prevalence of "compulsive exercise" in these patients. A recent study reported that in a sample of 113 nonathletic female patients who met the lifetime DSM-III-R criteria for anorexia nervosa, bulimia nervosa, or both disorders, more than 25% of them were identified as compulsive exercisers (Brewerton et al., 1995). Compulsive exercise was defined as exercising at least 60 min or more every day. The Diagnostic Survey of the Eating Disorder (DSED) was the instrument used to obtain the self-reported data regarding the frequency and duration of exercise. The results of this study indicated that the eating disorder patients who were "compulsive exercisers" had significantly greater ratings of body dissatisfaction but were significantly less likely to vomit or use laxatives and binge eat than were the "noncompulsive exercisers."

A study including 1,494 adolescents indicated that physical activity was related to healthier eating patterns and food preferences but was also related to increased eating disorder symptoms (French et al., 1994). However, interpretations of the results of this study are limited because a nonstandardized, self-report instrument was used to assess dieting behavior and physical activity patterns.

A secondary eating disorder may develop as a result of participating in a sport in which low body weight is stressed as ideal for optimal performance (Leon, 1991). During training, some athletes may exhibit excessive concerns about weight and use pathological weight control practices, such as the use of diuretics, laxatives, or self-induced vomiting, with a resolution of these concerns and behaviors after the athletic season is over (Leon, 1991). However, a subset of these athletes may be psychologically vulnerable to the development of an eating disorder; even after the season is over they may continue to have intense concerns regarding body weight and shape, may engage in disordered eating and weight control practices, and may develop a clinically diagnosable eating disorder.

Methods of Diagnosing Eating Disorders

Eating disorders as defined by the DSM criteria of the American Psychiatric Association (American Psychiatric Association, 1994) are difficult to detect and diagnose, even by professionals, because of the complex and secretive nature of these disorders. Typically, the diagnosis of eating disorders includes self reports of eating-related behaviors and utilizes instruments such as questionnaires developed by investigators for use in a study or standardized instruments such as the Eating Attitudes Test (EAT) (Garner & Garfinkel, 1979) or the Eating Disorder Inventory (EDI) (Garner et al., 1984).

Eating Attitude Test. The EAT is the instrument most often used in the assessment of eating disorders (Beals & Manore, 1994; Brownell & Rodin 1992). The original version of the EAT contained 40 items (EAT-40), and a more recent version contains 26 items (EAT-26) (Garner et al., 1982). Individuals report how well the statements in the EAT apply to them by using a 6-point rating scale ranging from "rarely" to "always." Examples of statements include "I like eating with other people," "I am terrified about being overweight," "I feel like food controls my life," "I wake up early in the morning," and "I enjoy trying rich new foods." A score of 30 or higher on the EAT-40 and 20 or higher on the EAT-26 are typical scores obtained for patients diagnosed with clinical anorexia nervosa. Neither of these instruments was originally designed to clinically diagnose anorexia nervosa or bulimia nervosa. Rather, they were developed as screening devices for use in nonclinical settings to assess attitudes and behaviors exhibited by individuals with clinical anorexia nervosa or bulimia nervosa (Garner & Garfinkel, 1979; Garner et al., 1982, Leon, 1991). High reliability and validity have been reported for these instruments when used in non-athletic populations (Garner & Garfinkel, 1979; Garner et al., 1982), but they have not been validated in athletic populations.

Eating Disorder Inventory. The Eating Disorder Inventory (EDI) has also been used to assess the occurrence of eating disorders. This 64-item instrument contains eight subscales (Garner et al., 1984). The first three subscales (Drive for Thinness, Bulimia, and Body Dissatisfaction) assess behaviors and attitudes regarding body image, eating, and dieting. The remaining five subscales (Interpersonal Distrust, Perfectionism, Interoceptive Awareness, Maturity Fears, and Ineffectiveness) assess psychopathology related to individuals with clinical anorexia nervosa. A newer version, the EDI-2, (Garner, 1991) contains 91 items and three additional subscales that assess Asceticism, Impulse Regulation, and Social Insecurity. The EDI has been used for diagnostic screening in both clinical and non-clinical settings (Brownell & Rodin, 1992). However, Garner (1991) has indicated that the total EDI score should not be used to measure disordered eating pathology because each subscale of this instrument is intended to measure a conceptually independent trait. He recommends comparing each subscale score to a standardized patient score. The EDI instruments have been demonstrated to be reliable and valid in primarily non-athletic populations (Garner, 1991).

Diagnosis in Athletes. Reports from validation studies of the EDI in athletes have yielded conflicting results. Sundgot-Borgen (1993b) reported that in one validation study, 48% of the athletes that were classified as "at risk" for having an eating disorder by the EDI actually met the criteria of anorexia nervosa or bulimia nervosa when they completed in-depth clinical interviews designed to assess the eating disorder status in the athletes. However, in another study reported by Wilmore (1991) there was no relationship between results of the EDI and athletes diagnosed with frank eating disorders. Sundgot-Borgen (1994b) attributed the discrepancies in the findings to the different methodologies used in the two studies, including different criteria for classifying the athletes as "at risk" for eating disorders and different numbers of athletes in each study.

Some studies have determined the occurrence of eating disorders in a group of athletes by simply providing descriptions of anorexia and bulimia to study participants and then asking them to report whether or not they have these problems. For example, a recent study reported that 40% of 30 aerobic dance instructors reported having either anorexia nervosa or bulimia nervosa (Olson et al., 1996). Other studies have used questionnaires that assessed dieting practices, preoccupation with weight, and attitudes about eating, but the reliability and validity of these questionnaires was usually not reported (Brownell & Rodin, 1992). An exception is a questionnaire developed by Steen and Brownell (1990) designed to assess eating, dieting, and weight control practices in athletes competing in weight-controlled sports such as wrestling and rowing. Currently this is the only questionnaire that has been developed for use with athletes that has assessed criteria for validity and reliability.

Self-reported information obtained by using nonstandardized or standardized instruments to assess the presence of attitudes and behaviors exhibited by patients with eating disorders has been shown to have questionable validity when used with athletes under some circumstances (Brownell & Rodin, 1992; O'Connor et al., 1995). Methodological differences, such as whether or not athletes believe they can be identified from instrument responses, contribute to decreased validity of the findings. Athletes may not truthfully respond to the items in the instruments if they believe that being identified as having an eating disorder would jeopardize their status or retention on a team. Thus, these instruments may be underestimating the prevalence of eating disorder symptoms among athletes.

Preferred Methods of Diagnosis. Caution must be exercised when drawing conclusions about the presence of eating disorders on the basis of scores on instruments like the EAT or EDI because these instruments primarily assess attitudes and behaviors that coexist with those exhibited by people with eating disorders. Many EAT or EDI scores in the elevated ranges associated with patients with eating disorders have been shown to be false positives when they are compared with information obtained from in-depth clinical interviews conducted to determine if the individuals actually met the criteria for a particular eating disorder

(Sundgot-Borgen 1993b; Szmukler & Russell, 1985). Therefore, these instruments are best used as initial screening devices (Leon, 1991). A self-report check list assessing each of the DSM-IV diagnostic criteria for eating disorders, combined with a psychiatric clinical interview and measures that more specifically assess the presence of diagnostic criteria, appears to be the most effective means of determining the presence of clinical eating disorders (American Psychiatric Association, 1994; Leon, 1991, Sundgot-Borgen, 1993b).

DEVELOPMENT AND PREVALENCE OF EATING DISORDERS

Eating disorders usually begin as a voluntary restriction of food intake but progress by stages in predisposed individuals into a syndrome in which personal control of behavior is lost (Anderson, 1990b). Development of most disordered eating behavior occurs along a continuum without a clear point that indicates where normality ceases and abnormality occurs. Deciding to occasionally skip a meal because of a deadline at work or a hectic schedule or choosing to eat larger than normal amounts of food at holiday meals or parties does not constitute disordered eating behavior. However, repeated unwillingness to eat adequate amounts of food that leads directly to a state of starvation or indirectly to binge eating (and is not a consequence of involuntary deprivation or the result of a primary medical or psychiatric illness) defines the behavior as psychiatrically abnormal (Anderson, 1990b). At the extremes of clinical anorexia nervosa and bulimia nervosa, there are few disagreements about when an eating behavior is abnormal.

Prevalence of Anorexia Nervosa Among Nonathletes

Studies examining the prevalence of clinical eating disorders among females in late adolescence and early adulthood have reported rates of 0.5–1.0% for cases that meet full criteria for anorexia nervosa (American Psychiatric Association, 1994). There are limited data concerning the prevalence of anorexia in males, but some evidence indicates that occurrence may be greater than previously believed (Anderson, 1990a; 1995). Anorexia appears to be more prevalent in industrialized societies, including the United States, Canada, Europe, Australia, Japan, New Zealand, and South Africa, in which there is an abundance of food and in which being considered attractive is linked to being thin (American Psychiatric Association, 1994). Little systematic work has been done to examine the prevalence in other cultures (American Psychiatric Association, 1994).

Prevalence of Bulimia Nervosa Among Nonathletes

The American Psychiatric Association (1994) reported that the prevalence of clinical bulimia nervosa among adolescents and young adult females is approximately 1–3%. The rate of occurrence of this disorder in males is approximately one-tenth of that in females. Bulimia nervosa has been reported to occur in roughly similar frequencies in the same industrialized countries in which anorexia nervosa occurs. Few studies have examined the prevalence of this eating disorder in other cultures.

In clinical studies in the United States, individuals presenting with bulimia nervosa are primarily white, but the disorder has also been reported among other ethnic and racial groups (American Psychiatric Association, 1994; French et al., 1995). Bulimia nervosa usually begins in late adolescence or early adult life. The course may be chronic or intermittent, with periods of remission alternating with recurrences of binge eating and purging.

Individuals make transitions in both directions between having anorexia nervosa and bulimia nervosa. The most common transition is changing from a food-restricting subtype of anorexia nervosa to the bulimia-nervosa subtype or to bulimia nervosa, while maintaining a normal weight (Anderson, 1990b).

Prevalence of Clinical Eating Disorders in Athletes

There has been increasing concern that athletes may be at higher risk than nonathletes for developing eating disorders because of heightened body awareness and pressures in some sports to have a low body weight and certain body shape in order to be competitive. Many athletes also have psychological qualities similar to those of nonathletes with eating disorders. For these reasons, it is often assumed that eating disorders are more common among athletes and that the prevalence of eating disorders is greatest in sports in which low body weight is related to improved performance in the sport. There is some evidence that supports this assumption (Brownell & Rodin, 1992; Sundgot-Borgen, 1994b).

The estimates of the prevalence of eating disorders in athletes range from as low as 1% to as high as 39% (Beals & Manore, 1994; Brownell & Rodin, 1992; Dick, 1991; Sundgot-Borgen, 1994a). The disparity in these estimates is attributed to the differences in methodology used to assess the occurrence of eating disorders. As indicated earlier, some studies used criteria derived from the strict diagnostic definitions of eating disorders established by the American Psychiatric Association. Other studies estimated prevalence using questionnaires or standardized instruments that assessed behaviors and attitudes exhibited by people with clinical eating disorders. These instruments have not been adequately validated in athletic populations.

Definitive estimates of the prevalence of eating disorders among female and male athletes are currently not available because of the limitations of measurement instruments and methods that have been termed a "methodological morass" (Brownell, 1995; Brownell & Rodin, 1992). To date, most studies have typically included participants in only a single sport, have not included appropriate control groups, and have not used the prevailing diagnostic criteria for determination of the presence of eating disorders (Brownell, 1995; Brownell & Rodin, 1992; Sundgot-Borgen, 1993b). These limitations must be considered when interpreting results of studies regarding prevalence of eating disorders.

Some studies have reported a greater than expected prevalence of anorexia in ballet dancers compared to the general population (Brooks-Gunn et al., 1987; Hamilton et al., 1988). In these studies eating disorders were simply described, and the dancers were asked if they had these problems.

Summaries of findings from studies investigating the prevalence of eating disorders among athletes assessed using standardized instruments such as the EAT and EDI have yielded inconsistent results. Some studies have reported a lower prevalence in athletes than in nonathletes, no difference between the two groups, and a higher prevalence in athletes than in nonathletes (Brownell, 1995; Brownell & Rodin, 1992; Sundgot-Borgen, 1994a). These discrepancies may be due to inconsistencies in the definition of eating disorders among studies, differences in nonathletic control groups, and lack of appropriate statistical analyses. For example, one study determined that university athletes have a lower prevalence of eating disorders than do students who were not athletes. The 126 athletes in the study had lower EDI scores than did 590 nonathletic student controls in five comparison groups, but no statistical comparisons among the groups were made (Kurtzman et al., 1989).

Comparisons of Athletes and Nonathletes. Brownell and Rodin (1992) reported in their comprehensive review of studies, in which athletes and nonathletic controls did not differ on overall scores on the EAT or EDI, that it was difficult to determine if there really were no differences between the groups or if the lack of differences was due to weaknesses in the methodology of the studies (Evers, 1987; Frusztajer et al., 1990; Sundgot-Borgen & Corbin, 1987; Warren et al., 1990; Weight & Noakes, 1987). For example, Evers (1987) concluded that there were no significant differences in EAT scores when university dancers were compared to nonathletic controls. However, 33% of the dancers' and 14% of the controls' EAT scores were in the range considered to be symptomatic of anorexia. In another example, a study by Frusztajer et al. (1990) included 30 subjects equally distributed among three groups: ballet dancers with stress fractures, dancers without stress fractures, and nondancer controls. Results of this study indicated that there was a nonsignificant increase in EAT scores in the group of ballet dancers with stress fractures compared to the other two groups, but the small sample sizes made it difficult to draw conclusions about comparisons of prevalence of eating disorders among the groups.

A recent study indicated that there were no differences in EDI-2 subscale scores between collegiate female athletes and nonathletes who had high academic achievement (Ashley et al., 1996). The study included 145 female intercollegiate athletes and a control group of 14 nonathletes who had a high grade-point average in an advanced collegiate program of study. The results indicated that there were no significant differences between the groups in percentage of respondents scoring above the norms for anorexia nervosa on any EDI-2 subscale. Furthermore, the athletes did not have significantly higher scores on any of the EDI-2 subscales, compared to nonathletes, and there were no significant differences among the "lean" athletic group, "other" athletic group, or the control group on any of the EDI-2 subscales. The African-American athletes did have significantly lower scores on the Body Dissatisfaction subscale than did the white athletes, indicating they were more satisfied with their bodies.

Another recent investigation also found no significant differences when comparing average EDI-2 subscale scores between 25 collegiate female gymnasts and 25 nonathletic controls matched for age, height, and weight (O'Connor et al., 1995). In a study comparing EDI-2 scores of 68 male bodybuilders to a control group of 50 male college students, Anderson et al. (1996) found that average scores did not indicate the presence of eating disorder tendencies in either group. The student control group scores were higher than those of bodybuilders on the Body Dissatisfaction subscale.

The most comprehensive study to date on the prevalence of eating disorders in female athletes demonstrated that eating disorders were more prevalent among athletes than among nonathletic controls (Sundgot-Borgen 1993b). This investigation included 522 elite Norwegian female athletes who participated in 35 sports, and 448 nonathletic control subjects. This study compared data obtained using the EDI to results of in-depth clinical interviews. On the basis of EDI scores (greater than or equal to 40), 22% of the athletes and 26% of the control subjects were classified as "at risk" for developing eating disorders. Subsequent clinical evaluations and personal interviews, using the model described by Johnson (1986) with "at risk" athletes, indicated that 18% of the athletes and 5% of the nonathletic controls actually met the criteria for anorexia nervosa, bulimia nervosa, and anorexia athletica. If the diagnosis of anorexia athletica was excluded, only 9% of the "at risk" athletes met the criteria for the frank eating disorders of anorexia nervosa and bulimia nervosa. The athletes who had eating disorders participated in sports in which leanness or maintaining a specific weight was considered important. The results of this investigation also showed that these elite athletes under-reported the use of purging practices such as vomiting and use of diuretics and laxatives and over-reported the use of binge eating. In addition, the athletes who reported having an eating disorder indicated that they had anorexia nervosa; however, most of the athletes actually met the criteria for bulimia nervosa or subclinical eating disorders. Other studies have also shown that athletes have a higher prevalence of eating disorders than do nonathletes, but all of these studies have methodological limitations (Benson et al., 1990; Davis & Cowles, 1989; Loosli & Benson, 1990; Sundgot-Borgen, 1993b; Sundgot-Borgen & Corbin, 1987).

Comparisons Among Sports. Studies that included only athletes have shown that disordered eating practices are prevalent serious problems, irrespective of what practices might occur in a nonathletic comparison group (Dummer et al., 1987; Rosen & Hough 1988; Rosen et al., 1986; Sundgot-Borgen, 1993b). For instance, a study with 42 collegiate gymnasts showed that all of these athletes were dieting and that 62% had used at least one pathogenic weight control method (Rosen & Hough, 1988). In a comparison study of athletes in "thin-build" sports with athletes in "normal-build" sports, Davis and Cowles (1989) reported that there were no overall differences in EAT scores. However, the thin-build athletes (n=64; gymnasts, synchronized swimmers, divers, figure skaters, long distance runners, and ballet dancers) had lower body weights, greater weight concerns, more body dissatisfaction, and more assiduous dieting than did athletes participating in sports that do not stress a thin physique (n=62; basketball, field hockey, sprinting, downhill skiing, and volleyball).

Research investigating the pathogenic eating behaviors of male athletes has focused mainly on the effects of rapid weight loss on body builders (Hickerson et al., 1990; Kleiner, 1990) and wrestlers (Brownell et al., 1987; Tipton & Oppliger, 1984; Webster et al., 1990). Brownell et al. (1987) reported that wrestlers achieved rapid and cyclic weight loss through dehydration and severe restriction of energy intake. A study by Kleiner et al. (1990) indicated that 45% of male body builders used fluid intake restriction or chemical agents, such as steroids, diuretics, or laxatives, to attain a desired weight and physique. A recent study investigated the weight control practices of 131 lightweight male college football players, using the Diagnostic Survey for Eating Disorders (DePalma et al., 1993). The survey results showed a pronounced cycle of binging and then restricting food intake. Results indicated that 74% had experienced binge eating, 17% experienced self-induced vomiting, 66% fasted, 4% used laxatives, and about 3% used diet pills, diuretics and enemas to control their weight. More than 20% reported that "often" or "always" their weight control practices interfered with their thoughts and extracurricular activities. Discriminant factor analysis yielded several variables that in 70–85% of the cases correctly identified individuals in the sample who were at risk for pathogenic eating behaviors. The risk index model developed in this study needs to be cross-validated in other groups of athletes to determine its usefulness for identifying athletes at risk for developing eating disorders.

Comparisons of Female and Male Athletes Within a Sport. The few studies that have compared the prevalence of eating disorders between females and males in a sport show a higher prevalence in females than in males. An investigation of competitive ice skaters (23 females, 17 males) indicated that the mean score on the EAT was 29 for the females and 10 for the males (Rucinski, 1989). Forty eight percent of the females had EAT scores greater than 30, which is the cut point for a screening assessment of anorexia nervosa.

Another study compared female and male athletes in rowing, a sport with and without weight limitations for both females and males (Sykora et al., 1993). The study included 82 heavyweight rowers (56 females, 26 males; no weight limitations) and 80 weight-limited lightweight rowers (17 females and 63 males). The similar athletic training of the two groups allowed the heavyweight rowers to serve as a comparison group for the lightweights. A questionnaire developed by the investigators and the EAT-26 were used to examine eating, weight control, and dieting practices among the four groups. Results indicated that average scores for females and males were greater than 30, the cut-point related to anorexia nervosa, and that the females had higher average EAT scores than did the males. Contrary to expectations, there were no significant differences between the average EAT scores of the lightweights and heavyweights or between the female and male average scores within the lightweight and heavyweight groups. Likewise, lightweights and heavyweights and males and females did not differ significantly in the reported frequency of binge eating. However, a greater percentage of females (20%) than of males (12%) reported binging more than two times per week for three months, which is one diagnostic criterion for bulimia nervosa. The investigators concluded that rowing joins the growing list of sports where eating disorders occur and that male athletes may be more vulnerable to these problems than previously recognized.

Prevalence of Nonclinical Eating Disorders Among Ethnic and Racial Groups

The number of athletes or people in the general population who have disordered eating behaviors and unhealthy weight loss practices is believed to be much greater than the number of those who actually meet the strict DSM-IV diagnostic criteria for anorexia nervosa or bulimia nervosa (Anderson, 1995; Beals & Manore, 1994; Brownell & Rodin, 1992; Sundgot-Borgen, 1993a). The high prevalence of disordered eating and weight control practices among American white adolescent girls is well-documented (American Psychological Association, 1994). A recent review of the limited amount of research literature on eating disturbance among different ethnic and racial groups in the United States concluded that compared with white girls, disordered eating and weight control practices are less frequent among African-American and Asian-American girls, equally common among Hispanic girls, and more frequent among Native American girls (Crago et al., 1996; Story et al., 1997). There are no published reports regarding the prevalence of subclinical eating disorders among adolescent athletes in various ethnic and racial groups.

RISK FACTORS FOR DEVELOPMENT OF EATING DISORDERS IN ATHLETES

Several factors contribute to the development of disordered eating practices and subclinical or clinical eating disorders. The specific factors that precipitate the development of these problems are unique for each person. There is an increased risk of anorexia nervosa and bulimia nervosa among first-degree biological relatives or individuals with these disorders (American Psychiatric Association, 1994). Studies of anorexia nervosa in twins have reported concordance rates for identical twins to be significantly higher than those for fraternal twins (Holland et al., 1988). However, what distinguishes the people who voluntarily start dieting or exercising to control their weight, body composition, or body shape but then go on to develop either anorexia or bulimia nervosa is of great theoretical interest and practical concern.

Psychological Factors

The psychological characteristics associated with eating disorders include perfectionism (Brownell & Rodin, 1992; Davis & Cowles, 1989; Warren et al., 1990; Yates, 1989; 1992), ineffectiveness, guilt, and distrust (Klemchuk et al., 1990), obsessive personality traits (Davis & Cowles, 1989; Yates, 1989), and high achievement expectations (King, 1989; Warren et al., 1990; Yates, 1989; 1992). It has also been postulated that people who develop bulimia instead of anorexia are often more impulsive, feel the psychological distress of hunger more intensely, are less tolerant of continued psychological distress of any kind, and are more likely to have personality disorders in the borderline, narcissistic, or histrionic group rather than in the sensitive, obsessional, perfectionist, and avoidant group (Anderson, 1990b; Piran et al., 1988).

Self-esteem is defined as the extent to which a person feels positive about herself or himself and is also referred to as self-concept, self-worth, and self-image (Lindeman, 1994). The development of self-esteem occurs during childhood and adolescence in a pattern that is similar to the pattern of development of cognitive and motor skills. Low self-esteem is a trait associated with eating disorders (Silverstone, 1992; Thompson & Sherman, 1993) and could be a precipitating factor in the development of eating disorders (Lindeman, 1994). Studies investigating the association between exercise and self-esteem indicate that in general, exercise participation enhances self-esteem (Lindeman, 1994). Little is known about whether athletes have greater self-esteem than do nonathletes. A study comparing self-concepts of male/female, college/high school, nonathlete/athlete matrices reported that only high-school male athletes had lower self-concept scores than did nonathletes (Ibrahim & Morrison, 1976). In all other group comparisons, no differences were found between athletes and nonathletes. Clearly, more research is needed to determine the role of self-esteem and the risk of development of eating disorders.

Exercise Factors

A limited amount of research has investigated exercise participation as a risk factor for developing eating disorders. Wolf and Akamatsu (1994) investigated the relationship between exercise and disordered eating attitudes and behaviors in Caucasian male (n=120) and female (n=168) college undergraduate students. Results showed that females in general, and female exercisers in particular, scored higher on the various measures of disordered eating attitudes and behaviors than did the males and nonexercisers. In the study, "exercisers" were defined as individuals who participated in an organized sport or regular exercise at least three times per week and included activities such as dance, gymnastics, basketball, football, running, swimming, and cross-training (mixed sports activities). Nonexercisers were defined as individuals who did not participate in any organized sport or regular exercise and participated in informal exercise less than three times per week. The participants completed demographic questionnaires and the EDI-64 and EAT-40. Higher scores on the EAT are indicative of more atypical eating patterns and attitudes. In this study, females in general, and female exercisers in particular, scored higher on the various measures of disordered eating attitudes and behaviors than did the males and nonexercisers. Using a cutoff of 30 on the EAT and a criterion of 15 on the EDI Drive for Thinness Scales to identify subjects with disordered eating concerns and behaviors, Wolf and Akamatsu (1994) reported that 22% of the female exercisers exceeded the EAT cutoff, compared with 10% of female nonexercisers, suggesting a higher rate of disordered eating concerns and behaviors among female exercisers. Twenty percent of female exercisers exceeded the cutoff on the EDI Drive for Thinness scale, compared with 8% of the female nonexercisers.

Wolf and Akamatsu (1994) also conducted discriminant function analysis, using the EDI subscale scores as predictor variables, to determine if female exercisers and nonexercisers with EAT scores higher than 30 could be distinguished from each other and from the other females with lower scores. Results indicated that when female exercisers (n=17) and nonexercisers (n=8) who had EAT scores of 30 or greater were compared with females in the remainder of the sample, two discriminant functions were significant. Function 1 included the Drive for Thinness scores, whereas function 2 included three of the EDI personality subscales: Maturity Fears, Interoceptive Awareness, and Interpersonal Distrust. Function 1 discriminated the disordered eating concerns group from the nondisordered group, whereas function 2 discriminated between exercisers and nonexercisers with disordered eating concerns. Altogether, 89% of the study participants were correctly classified into groups. The authors concluded that although female exercisers and nonexercisers with disordered eating concerns were similar in the pursuit of thinness, they differed in regard to personality dimensions characteristic of eating disorders. The exercisers had some characteristics of females with eating disorders (anorectic/bulimic eating attitudes and greater drive for thinness), but they did not have the full behavioral and psychological syndrome common to clinical eating disorders.

Excessive Exercise. Davis and Fox (1993) evaluated the relationship between "excessive exercise" and eating disorders in a nonathletic group. The study included females recruited from a university community and health clubs. Exercise participation was assessed by self-report, and weight preoccupation was measured using the Drive For Thinness subscale of the EDI-64. Excessive exercise was defined as 1 h or more of exercise performed at least six times a week. Study participants were classified as "excessive exercisers" or as sedentary, exercising no more than half an hour per week. The "excessive exercisers" (n=44) reported greater body satisfaction and body focus, were less neurotic, and were more extroverted than nonexercisers (n=46). It is clear that the definition of "excessive exercisers" includes far less daily exercise than is typical for athletes in rigorous training programs. Therefore, the results of this study cannot be extrapolated to athletes who participate in much more rigorous exercise programs.

Sport-Related Factors. In a study of 603 elite female athletes in Norway, the EDI was used to classify individuals at risk for eating disorders (Sundgot-Borgen, 1994b). Athletes defined as at risk (n=103) completed structured clinical interviews, and 92 of these athletes met the criteria for anorexia nervosa, bulimia nervosa, or anorexia athletica. Members of a control group of 30 athletes chosen at random from a pool of not-at-risk athletes matched for age, community of residence, and sport were also interviewed. Compared with controls, athletes with eating disorders began sport specific training and dieting earlier and felt that puberty occurred too early for optimal performance. The athletes with eating disorders reported several key trigger factors that they associated with their development of eating disorders. These factors are listed in Table 4-3. Additional studies are needed to determine if these trigger factors are also identified by female and male athletes in other ethnic or racial groups.

CONSEQUENCES OF EATING DISORDERS ON PERFORMANCE AND HEALTH

A recovering anorectic and member of the team that won the 1986 NCAA cross-country title stated, "For women, eating disorders are like steroids for men. You'll get results, but you'll pay for it" (Noden, 1994). Disordered eating of any degree leads to adverse health consequences, with risk of morbidity, impaired athletic performance, and mortality increasing as the severity of disordered eating increases. The weight loss, food restriction, and purging practices associated with eating disorders have powerful physiological and psychological effects. These effects can

TABLE 4-3. *Trigger Factors Associated with Onset of Eating Disorders In Athletes.*

- Prolonged periods of dieting or weight fluctuations
- Traumatic events such as illness or injury to self or family member, new coach, casual comments about weight, leaving home, failure at school or work, family problems, problems with relationships, death of significant other, sexual abuse, or work transition
- Large increase in training volume and significant weight loss associated with increase in training volume
- Belief that menarche has been reached too early
- Early start of sport-specific training
- Large discrepancy between self-defined ideal weight and actual weight
- Recommendation to lose weight without guidance

include a decrease in exercise capacity, increased risk of injury, and medical complications. These complications include depression, nutrient deficiencies, fluid and electrolyte imbalances, and adverse changes in the cardiovascular, digestive, endocrine, skeletal, and thermoregulatory systems (Brownell et al., 1987; Dueck et al., 1996a; Eichner, 1992; Friday et al., 1993; Johnson, 1994; Kaiserauer et al., 1989; Loucks et al., 1992; Nattiv et al., 1994; Rencken et al., 1996; Rucinski, 1989; Steen & Wilmore, 1987; Stephenson, 1991; Sundgot-Borgen, 1993a; Van De Loo & Johnson, 1995; Walberg & Johnson, 1991). Some of these complications can be fatal.

Female Athlete Triad

Attaining and maintaining unrealistically low body weight through disordered eating and exercise practices can put young women at risk for developing two associated disorders, amenorrhea and osteoporosis (Brooks-Gunn et al., 1987; Nattiv et al., 1994; Putukian, 1994; Yeager et al., 1993). The female athlete triad refers to the interrelations among disordered eating, amenorrhea, and osteoporosis. Alone, each disorder is of medical concern, but when all three components of the triad are present, there is the potential for more serious impacts on health and risk of mortality (American College of Sports Medicine, 1997; De Souza & Metzger., 1991; Nattiv et al., 1994; Putukian, 1994; Yeager et al., 1993).

Amenorrhea. Primary amenorrhea, or delayed menarche, is present when menses has not begun by 16 y of age. Secondary amenorrhea is defined as the absence of at least three to six consecutive menstrual cycles (Nattiv et al., 1994). The prevalence of amenorrhea has been difficult to determine, in part due to variability in definition (Van De Loo & Johnson, 1995). In the general population the prevalence of amenorrhea is estimated to range from 2–5% (Yeager et al., 1993). The reported prevalence is higher in athletes, ranging from 1-66% (Keizer & Rogol, 1990; Yeager et al., 1993). Delayed menarche occurs in athletes who begin training at an early age, but the prevalence of primary and secondary amenorrhea in the young athlete is unknown (Van De Loo & Johnson, 1995).

It is a common misconception among some athletes, coaches, and trainers that amenorrhea is a benign consequence of strenuous exercise, a marker of adequate training, and an indicator that body fat levels are at an optimal level for a sport (Dueck et al., 1996b). However, no causal links have been established between exercise per se and menstrual disorders (Kaiserauer et al., 1989; Loucks, et al., 1992). Rather, exercise-induced menstrual dysfunction can be attributed to overtraining (Keizer & Rogol, 1990). Menstrual dysfunction associated with athletics is related to many factors, including a history of weight fluctuations, rigorous training schedules, social pressures associated with competition, and nutrient deficiencies (Dueck et al., 1996b).

A survey study by Walberg and Johnston (1991) compared menstrual function and EDI scores among 103 recreational and competitive weight lifters and 92 control group females who did not weight train. The results indicated that menstrual dysfunction was present in about 13% of the controls, 30% of the recreational weight lifters, and 86% of the competitive body builders. The study also indicated that all the weight lifters, and particularly the competitive body builders, were more likely to report a history of anorexia nervosa, as well as some current attitudes and behaviors common to eating disorder syndromes. However, the average scores on all EDI subscales for the weight lifters and controls were in the normal range. Weight lifters did have significantly higher scores on the Drive For Thinness subscale than did the controls. There were no significant differences between subscale scores for the recreational and competitive body builders; however, some individual scores were above the average score for diagnosed anorexia nervosa patients.

Several studies have suggested that exercise-associated amenorrhea may be the result of periods of energy deficiency termed an "energy drain" (Loucks, 1990; Otis, 1992; Wilmore et al., 1992). This "energy drain" model is based on evidence indicating that exercise-induced menstrual dysfunction may be initiated in part by negative energy balance, which produces an array of physiological responses that cause amenorrhea. A review by Dueck et al. (1996a) summarized the research related to the role of energy balance and the "energy drain" theory associated with athletic menstrual dysfunction. It is also important to be aware that menstrual dysfunction in female athletes at all levels of competition can be related to genetics or other environmental factors and may not be related to disordered eating practices and eating disorders (Hamilton et al., 1988).

Osteoporosis. Osteoporosis in the young female athlete refers to inadequate formation and premature bone loss, resulting in low bone mineral density and increased risk of fracture (Van De Loo & Johnson, 1995). The prevalence of premature osteoporosis in young female nonathletes and athletes is currently unknown (Snow-Harter, 1994). Studies conducted with female athletes have shown that premature osteoporosis may occur as a result of amenorrhea or oligomenorrhea and may be partially irreversible, despite resumption of menses, estrogen replacement, or calcium supplementation (Cann et al., 1984; Drinkwater et al., 1986; 1990; Rencken et al., 1996). An increase in the risk for stress fractures has been reported in athletes with amenorrhea, and this appears to be related to low bone mineral density (Van De Loo & Johnson, 1995).

One study including a small number of subjects demonstrated that individuals with subclinical and clinical eating disorders have decreased bone mineral density and are at risk for osteoporosis (Joyce et al., 1990). Multiple factors, including body surface area, age of onset of the eating disorder, and length of the disorder, contributed to osteoporosis in this sample. Estrogen deficiency by itself was not a major cause of osteoporosis. Although some studies have indicated that weight gain in females with amenorrhea results in an increase in bone mineral density and often precedes the return of menses, other investigators reported that weight and estrogen exposure have interdependent effects on bone (Van De Loo & Johnson, 1995).

Other evidence suggests that not all groups of competitive athletes with menstrual dysfunction, including elite adolescent ice skaters, gymnasts, and runners, are at risk for developing low bone mineral density (Hetland et al., 1993; Kirchner et al., 1995; 1996; Robinson et al., 1995; Slemenda & Johnson, 1993). In fact, a recent study of college-aged gymnasts showed that despite a lower than recommended energy and calcium intake, as well as a history of menstrual dysfunction, the gymnasts had greater bone density than did female controls matched for age, height, and weight (Kirchner et al., 1995). This same group of investigators also compared 18 former collegiate gymnasts with 15 controls matched for age, height, and weight and found that the former gymnasts had significantly greater bone mineral density (Kirchner et al., 1996). They also reported no bone mineral density differences between the former gymnasts who had regular menstrual cycles versus those who had interrupted menstrual cycles.

Another study comparing collegiate gymnasts, runners, and nonathletic college women showed that gymnasts had greater bone mineral density than did runners, despite a similar prevalence of amenorrhea (Robinson et al., 1995). Presumably, the greater bone density in the gymnasts was the result of the impact loading required in their sport. In a study of a group of 205 recreational and elite female runners and normally active controls, mean ages 29–35 years, there was no significant relationship between running activity and bone mineral density, despite the presence of significant sex hormonal and menstrual dysfunction (Hetland et al., 1993). The sex hormone and menstrual dysfunction paralleled the amount and intensity of running, but almost all of the recreational runners and 89% of the elite runners had normal bone density. Only the runners with amenorrhea had a significantly lower lumbar spine bone mineral density, compared with normally menstruating runners.

No longitudinal studies have compared eating disorder prevalence, menstrual function, and bone mineral density status in large groups of female athletes. Such studies are needed to determine how exercise and eating disorders affect risk and treatment of the female athlete triad disorders. Table 4-4 summarizes current recommended guidelines for the treatment of the female athlete triad (Joy et al., 1997a; 1997b).

PRACTICAL IMPLICATIONS: PREVENTION AND TREATMENT OF EATING DISORDERS

Primary prevention of eating disorders by professionals is limited because they have little control of the many factors that contribute to the development of eating disorders (Thompson & Sherman, 1993). The focus of prevention and treatment of eating disorders by professionals is on secondary interventions. The goals of secondary intervention are to provide prevention education and early identification and treatment aimed at minimizing the severity and duration of eating disorders.

Course and Outcome

The course and outcome for individuals with anorexia nervosa are highly variable. Some people fully recover after a single bout with this disorder, others exhibit a fluctuating pattern of weight gain followed by a relapse, and others experience a chronically deteriorating course of the illness over many years. In some cases, hospitalization is required to help restore weight and to manage fluid and electrolyte imbalances. The long-term consequences of intractable anorexia nervosa can be catastrophic. In the treated, nonathletic population, anorexia nervosa has a 10–18% mortality rate (Ratnasuriya et al., 1991). Of individuals admitted to university hospitals, the long-term mortality from anorexia nervosa is more than 10% (American Psychiatric Association, 1994). In these cases, death most commonly results from starvation, suicide, or electrolyte imbalance. The long-term outcome of bulimia nervosa is unknown (American Psychiatric Association, 1994).

A recent retrospective study using the EDI-2 and visual analog scales compared current and past eating disorder symptoms between former college gymnasts and controls matched for age, height, and weight (O'Connor et al., 1996). The mean EDI-2 scores for the former gymnasts were lower than normative means for every subscale. The former gymnasts were similar to the control subjects on all variables, ex-

TABLE 4-4. *Main Components of Clinical Treatment of Female Athlete Triad*

1) Decrease overall training by 10-20%
2) Increase calorie intake slowly by 10-20%
3) Aim to increase body weight by 2-3%
4) Increase dietary calcium to 1,500 mg/day
5) Prudent resistance training to boost muscle and bone strength
6) Consider treating sustained amenorrhea (6-12 months) with oral contraceptives

cept that the former gymnasts had significantly lower asceticism and body dissatisfaction scores did than the controls. Study results also indicated that symptoms of eating disorders abated after retirement from the sport. In addition, the study demonstrated that weight preoccupation was stable across the life span for controls, but it was lower before former gymnasts began training and higher for former gymnasts when they were participating in college gymnastics.

Clinical eating disorders rarely occur before puberty, but there are indications that the severity of associated mental disturbances may be greater and prognosis for recovery poorer among prepubertal individuals who develop disorders than when the disorders begin in early adolescence, between ages 13 and 18 y (American Psychiatric Association, 1994). Recovery from eating disorders also varies with the stage of development of the disorder, duration of the disorder, and previous history of counseling intervention, but early intervention tends to improve the chances for a better outcome (Szmukler & Russell, 1986).

Effective Treatment of Eating Disorders

Increased awareness of the multidimensional nature of eating disorders and education on how to screen for and treat the disorders are necessary for prevention and early identification. An awareness of risk factors for eating disorders, as well as signs and symptoms of disordered eating patterns and their health and sport performance consequences, may help detect problems early and initiate prompt treatments (Grooms, 1996). Therefore, athletes, parents, coaches, training staff, physicians, and athletic administrators need to be educated about risk factors for eating disorders, warning signs and symptoms of disordered eating and exercise practices, and adverse health and performance consequences of subclinical and clinical eating disorders, which for females include menstrual dysfunction and osteoporosis. Education also needs to be provided on methods to screen for eating disorders, the importance of and guidelines for healthy eating and exercise practices, appropriate expectations concerning body weight and body composition, and available local resources for prevention and treatment of eating disorders. In addition, coaches, trainers, and parents need to be educated on how they may influence the development of eating disorders in their athletes.

Warning Signs. Disordered eating practices are typically well-kept secrets, so it is important for everyone working with athletes to be aware of subtle warning signs that can be related to the presence of disordered eating or exercise practices. Table 4-5 summarizes the list of warning signs for anorexia nervosa and bulimia nervosa that was distributed to coaches, athletes, and athletic officials by the National Collegiate Athletic Association (Brownell & Rodin, 1992).

TABLE 4-5. *Warning Signs for Eating Disorders*

Warning Signs for Anorexia Nervosa
• Dramatic weight loss
• A preoccupation with food, calories, and weight
• Wearing baggy or layered clothing
• Relentless, excessive exercise
• Mood swings
• Avoiding food-related social activities

Warning Signs of Bulimia Nervosa
• A noticeable weight loss or gain
• Excessive concern about weight
• Bathroom visits after meals
• Depressive moods
• Strict dieting followed by eating binges
• Increased criticism of one's body

Treatment Approaches. The likelihood that athletes will receive appropriate support, education, and treatment are improved and stress on staff is reduced when athletes, trainers, coaches, and other staff members who work closely with athletes have developed a plan for use in the prevention, intervention, and treatment of eating disorders. These plans include knowing the risk factors for eating disorders, having a screening program to identify athletes who are at risk for eating disorders, being aware of triggering events or practices that can contribute to the onset of eating disorders, recognizing the warning signs and symptoms, knowing what treatment options are available in the community, and having guidelines for what steps to take if a problem is suspected or identified (Am. Diet. Assoc., 1994; Grandjean, 1991; Grooms, 1996; Leon, 1991; Johnson, 1994; Nattiv & Lynch, 1994; Van De Loo & Johnson, 1995).

Screening for Signs and Symptoms. The preparticipation physical examination, educational meetings, or workshops can be used to conduct screenings for signs and symptoms of disordered eating and other triad disorders. Screening instruments that address both the behavioral and psychological characteristics of eating disorders should be used. When assessing individuals who participate in sports or regular exercise, it is important to be aware that several screening instruments contain items on rigorous exercise that may produce spuriously high "eating-disordered" scores (Wolf & Akamatsu, 1994). For example, in a study by Wolf and Akamatus (1994) several exercisers would have exceeded the EAT cutoff of 30 if the three exercise items in the inventory had been taken into account. When athletes with disordered eating attitudes or practices are identified by a screening program, then athletes need to be approached to initiate appropriate interventions. Guidelines on how to approach these athletes and refer them to appropriate treatment have been published (Clark, 1994; 1996; Thompson & Sherman, 1993).

Team-based Development of Treatment Goals and Plans. The immediate goals of treatment are to preserve the athlete's psychological and medical well being (Nattiv & Lynch, 1994). The ideal method of treating athletes with eating disorders is a multidisciplinary team approach involving people experienced in the management of eating disorders (Johnson, 1994). The physician monitors medical status and athletic participation and often coordinates care; the dietitian or nutritionist provides appropriate nutritional guidance; and the mental health professional addresses the psychological issues. Important ancillary team members can include trainers, coaches, nurses, physician's assistants, and exercise physiologists. For young athletes who live at home, family involvement in treatment is often necessary.

Whereas individuals who have the full range of symptoms and signs of subclinical and clinical eating disorders require comprehensive treatment plans, those with only a limited array of disordered eating concerns and practices could benefit from an appropriate preventive, educational or dietary intervention. Well-designed preventive educational programs, including seminars, workshops, and individual consultations, all can help increase awareness of warning signs and symptoms as well as provide guidance for how to obtain appropriate prevention and treatment assistance for eating disorders. Specific guidelines for screening for and treating people with eating disorders and other disorders of the female athlete triad have been published (Clark, 1993; 1994; Dueck et al., 1996b; Grandjean, 1991; Johnson, 1994; Lindeman, 1994; Manore, 1996; Nattiv & Lynch, 1994; Nattiv et al., 1995; Sandri, 1993; Thompson & Sherman, 1993; Wichmann & Martin, 1993; Woscyna, 1991).

Resources for Treatment. Private organizations, sport governing bodies, and sports medicine organizations have developed educational resources for use in eating disorder prevention programs. These resources include books, articles, pamphlets, videos, and numerous sites on the Internet. The National Collegiate Athletic Association developed a three-part video series on nutrition and eating disorders and distributed it to all member institutions. The videos include guidelines that sports-related personnel can use to manage eating disorders in athletes. The American College of Sports Medicine has developed educational resources for use in programs related to The Female Athlete Triad: Disordered Eating, Amenorrhea, and Osteoporosis. Table 4-6 lists organizations that provide educational resources for use in the prevention and treatment of eating disorders for athletes.

Summary. The scope of the problems of eating disorders goes beyond the individual athlete. High levels of athletic performance provide prestige and money for athletes, parents, coaches, athletic programs,

TABLE 4-6. *Resources for Education and Support for Preventing and Treating Eating Disorders Organizations.*

Organizations:

American Anorexia/Bulimia Association, Inc. (AABA); 165 W. 46th Street, Suite 1108, New York, NY 10036; Phone: 212/278-0697; Web Site: http://members.aol.com/AmAnBu

American Dietetic Association (ADA); 216 W. Jackson Blvd., Suite 800; Chicago, IL 60606-6995; Phone: 800/877-1600; Web Site: http://www.eatright.org

Anorexia Nervosa and Related Eating Disorders, Inc., (ANRED); P.O. Box 5102, Eugene, OR 97405; Phone: 541/344-1144; Web Site: http://www.anred.com

Eating Disorders Awareness & Prevention, Inc. (EDAP); 603 Stewart Street, Suite 803; Seattle, WA 98101; Phone: 206/382-3587; Web Site: http://members.aol.com/edapinc/home.html

International Center for Sports Nutrition (ICSN); 502 S. 44th St., Suite 3012; Omaha, NE 68105-1065; Phone: 402/559-5505

National Eating Disorders Organization (NEDO); 6655 S. Yale Avenue, Tulsa, OK 74136; Phone: 918/481-4404; Web Site: http://www.laureate.com/nedo-con.html

National Association of Anorexia Nervosa and Associated Disorders (ANAD), P.O. Box 7, Highland Park, IL 60035; Phone: 847/831-3438; e-mail: anad20@aol.com

National Osteoporosis Foundation, Suite 500, 1150 17th St., NW, Washington, DC 20036-4603; Phone: 202/223-2226; Web Site: http://www.nof.org

and schools. The message to "win at all costs" encourages athletes to be willing to do anything to improve their performance and attain success in their sports (Nattiv & Lynch, 1994). To enable athletes to participate and to succeed in their sports via the healthiest and safest means possible, effective ways to help modify dysfunctional, institutionalized, sociocultural pressures that promote disordered eating and exercise practices need to be addressed. This is a daunting mission that needs to be addressed as part of future research and education efforts.

DIRECTIONS FOR FUTURE RESEARCH

The presence of the spectrum of eating disorders has been determined in most studies by the use of self-report questionnaires that typically included various forms of the EAT and EDI. Research is clearly needed to validate these instruments in athletes and to identify the conditions under which forthright responses are likely to be given. Because of their limitations, a diagnosis of clinical eating disorders cannot be based solely on responses obtained with these instruments. In future studies, the use of psychiatric interviews or other clinical measures that more specifically assess the presence of diagnostic criteria for eating disorders will help determine the actual prevalence of clinical and subclinical eating disorders (American Psychiatric Association, 1994; Leon, 1991, Sundgot-Borgen, 1993b).

Well-designed longitudinal studies are also needed to determine if the prevalence and incidence of eating disorders are higher in athletes than in nonathletes and among athletes in specific sports. The key question that needs to be addressed by these types of studies is whether or not participation in some sports causes the disturbances or if individuals with eating problems or with psychosocial problems that increase the risk of eating disorders are drawn to certain sports (Brownell, 1995).

Currently, with the exception of anorexia athletica, classifications for cases of subclinical eating disorders are not based on unique diagnostic criteria (Beals & Manore, 1994; Sundgot-Borgen, 1993b). The features of anorexia athletica as described by Sundgot-Borgen (1993b) need to be refined (Beals & Manore, 1994). Therefore, research is needed to further define and describe the unique characteristics of subclinical eating disorders such as anorexia athletica and to determine the prevalence of these disorders in the athletic population. Recommendations on how to proceed in conducting this research have been proposed (Beals & Manore, 1994).

Many young athletes are concerned about their body weight and shape, yet they do not develop eating disorders (French et al., 1994). It has been hypothesized that psychological traits associated with eating disorders, such as depression, stress reactivity, sexual and maturity concerns, autonomy, and control needs, may be less likely to be present in young athletes. As a result, sports participation could represent a protective factor for the development of eating disorders by increasing self-esteem and feelings of autonomy, control, and social support, while decreasing feelings of depression and stress (French et al., 1994). French has further speculated that environmental factors, such as sociocultural norms for extremely low body weight (typical for women in current, dominant, industrialized cultures, and particularly pronounced in certain subcultures, such as some types of athletes) and low levels of social support may be necessary secondary cofactors related to an increased risk for the development of eating disorders. Prospective research is needed to evaluate these provocative hypotheses as well as to determine the role of genetics in the development of eating disorders.

The current cultural emphasis on fitness and health has influenced the promotion of participation in regular exercise. There is a pressing need for better understanding of the association between exercise levels, body image, and disordered eating, not only because of the methodological limitations of previous research, but because of the social relevance and potential health-related consequences of this issue.

Little is known about the long-term physical and psychological effects of early intensive athletic training and the female athlete triad on the young female athlete or about the most effective means of preventing premature osteoporosis in vulnerable female athletes. Questions regarding the prevention of premature osteoporosis in these female athletes need to be addressed.

In addition to the need for further research in all the areas related to determining the development, prevalence, risk factors, consequences, and treatment of eating disorders, there is also a critical need to evaluate the effectiveness of approaches to the prevention and treatment of disordered eating and exercise practices. Additional research is needed to develop models that can accurately identify athletes who are at risk for eating disorders. Development of more effective ways for athletes, coaches, trainers, parents, and physicians to treat eating disorders and to prevent the development of eating disorders is essential to good health and success in sports.

SUMMARY

Strictly defined, clinical eating disorders include anorexia nervosa, bulimia nervosa, and eating disorders not otherwise specified. These are the extreme disorders in a spectrum of disordered eating and exercise patterns that can result in significant morbidity and even mortality. Disturbances in the perception of body shape and weight are essential characteristics of both of these eating disorders. Anorexia nervosa is further distinguished by refusal to maintain a minimally normal body weight and by the presence of amenorrhea in post menarcheal females. Bulimia nervosa is characterized by repeated episodes of binge eating, fear of inability to stop eating, and use of purging behaviors to avoid weight gain. Individuals with bulimia nervosa are able to maintain body weight at or above a minimally normal weight.

Evidence indicates that pathological eating and weight control practices and the psychological aspects of eating disorders, such as preoccupation with body shape and weight, occur among recreational exercisers and competitive athletes. Definitive information on the prevalence of eating disorders related to exercise and among athletes is not currently available because of the methodological limitations of studies estimating the prevalence of eating related problems in these groups. Disordered eating appears to be more prevalent in females than in males and in sports where low body weight is considered important to performance, e.g., distance running, rowing, or wrestling, or in appearance sports, e.g., body building, diving, dancing, gymnastics, and figure skating.

Various factors, including sociocultural, biological, psychological, exercise, and sport participation may predispose athletes to the development of disordered eating and exercise practices and subsequent adverse health and performance consequences. The term Female Athlete

Triad is used to describe the interrelationships of disordered eating, menstrual dysfunction, and osteoporosis in physically active females. This triad can lead to many psychological and physiological problems that may, at the extreme, affect every organ system and even lead to premature death. Recovery from eating disorders varies according to age of onset, duration of the disorder, extent of disturbed relationships, and previous history of counseling, but early intervention tends to improve the chances for a better outcome. In the medically treated nonathletic population, anorexia nervosa has a 10–18% mortality rate. Prevention and early detection of disordered eating and exercise practices is essential to enabling athletes to participate and succeed in their sports in the healthiest and safest way.

In societies that place a great deal of emphasis on thinness and specific ideal body images, some people will use extreme means to try to reshape their bodies. Athletes risk developing dysfunctional eating and exercise practices as they attempt to meet a rigid weight standard or lose weight because they think it will improve performance. Until society in general and sport leaders in particular eliminate the pressures that encourage these behaviors, there will be a need to recognize, treat, and prevent disordered eating and exercise practices. It is also important to continue to promote the message that regular exercise has many health-related benefits and to provide guidelines for safe and healthy exercise practices.

A global prevention and treatment plan for the Female Athlete Triad has been developed through collaborative efforts of the US Congress' Women's Health Equity Act and the American College of Sports Medicine's Ad Hoc Task Force on Women's Issues in Sports Medicine. An action plan has been developed to address strategies for future prevention and treatment of eating disorders and the associated disorders of the female athlete triad. Through such global efforts progress can be made in developing more effective approaches for early detection, prevention, and treatment of eating disorders.

Publications:

Pre-Season Meeting Handbook. Available from: National Federation of State High School Associations TARGET Program; P.O. Box 20626, Kansas City, MO 64195

Helping Athletes with Eating Disorders, by Ron A. Thompson, Ph.D. and Roberts Trattner Sherman, Ph.D. Available from: USA Gymnastics Merchandise Dept., Pan American Plaza, Suite 300, 201 S. Capitol, Indianapolis, IN 46225; Phone: 317/237-5050

Gatorade Sports Science Institute; P.O. Box 049005; Chicago, IL. 60604-9005; Phone: 312/222-7704; Web Site: http://www.gssiweb.com

Audiovisuals:

Nutrition and Eating Disorders in College Athletes Video Series. Produced by the National Collegiate Athletic Association (NCAA), Available from: Karol Video, 350 N. Pennsylvania Avenue, P.O. Box 7600, Wilkes Barre, PA 18773; Phone: 800/526-4773

Female Athlete Triad: Disordered Eating, Amenorrhea and Osteoporosis. Available through: American College of Sports Medicine: ACSM, c/o Triad, P.O. Box 1440, Indianapolis, IN 46206-1440; Phone: 317/637-9200

Smart Choices (video). Gatorade Sport Sciences Institute; P.O. Box 049005; Chicago, IL 60604-9005; Phone 312/222-7704

Sports Nutrition Fundamentals. Gatorade Sport Sciences Institute; P.O. Box 049005; Chicago, IL 60604-9005; Phone 312/222-7704

ACKNOWLEDGEMENTS

I wish to thank E. Randy Eichner, M.D.; Yvonne Satterwhite, M.D.; Suzanne Steen, D.Sc., R.D.; and Melinda Manore, Ph.D., R.D. for sharing their insights and perspectives in the development of this chapter. I would like to acknowledge Jennifer Ricketts, Ph.D., R.D.; Nicole Ayan; and Leah Brown for their assistance in the preparation of this chapter.

BIBLIOGRAPHY

American College of Sports Medicine (1997). Position Stand. The female athlete triad. *Med. Sci. Sports Exerc.* 29:1–9.

American Dietetics Association (1994). Position of the American Dietetics Association: Nutrition intervention in the treatment of anorexia nervosa, bulimia nervosa, and binge eating. *J. Am. Diet. Assoc.* 94:902–907.

American Psychiatric Association (1994). *Diagnostic and Statistical Manual of Mental Disorders-IV* (4th ed.) Washington, DC: American Psychiatric Association. pp. 539–550.

Anderson, A.E. (1990a). Diagnosis and treatment of males with eating disorders. In: A.E. Anderson (ed.) *Males with Eating Disorders*. New York: Brunners/Mazel, Publishers, pp. 133–162.

Anderson, A.E. (1995). Eating disorders in males. In: K.D. Brownell and C.G. Fairburn (eds.) *Eating Disorders and Obesity*. New York: The Guilford Press, pp.177–182.

Anderson, A.E. (1990b). A proposed mechanism underlying eating disorders and other disorders of motivated behavior. In: A.E. Anderson (ed.) *Males with Eating Disorders*. New York: Brunners/Mazel, Publishers, pp. 221–254.

Anderson, S.L., K. Zager, R.K. Hetzler, M. Nahikian-Nelms, and G. Syler (1996). Comparison of eating disorder inventory (EDI-2) scores of male bodybuilders to the male college student subgroup. *Int. J. Sports Nutr.* 3:255–262.

Ashley, C.D., J.F. Smith, J.B. Robinson, and M.T. Richardson (1996). Disordered eating in female collegiate athletes and collegiate females in an advanced program of study: a preliminary investigation. *Int. J. Sport Nutr.* 6:391–401.

Beals, K.A., and M.M. Manore (1994). The prevalence and consequences of subclinical eating disorders in female athletes. *Int. J. Sports Nutr.* 4:175–195.

Benardot, D., K. Engelbert-Fenton, K. Freeman, C. Hartsough, and S. Nelson Steen (1994). Eating disorders in athletes: the dietician's perspective. *Sports Sci. Exchange Roundtable* 5:1–8.

Benson, J.E., G.E. Allemann, G.E. Theintz, and H. Howard (1990). Eating problems and calorie intake levels in Swiss adolescent athletes. *Int. J. Sports Med.* 11:249–252.

Blumenthal, J.A., L.C. O'Toole, and J.L. Chang (1984). Is running an analogue of anorexia nervosa? An empirical study of obligatory running and anorexia nervosa. *J.A.M.A.* 252:520–523.

Bouchard, C. (1992). Genetic aspects of human obesity. In: P. Bjorntorpp and B.N. Brodoff (eds.) *Obesity.* Philadelphia: Lippincott, pp. 343–351.

Brewerton, T.D., E.J. Stellefson, N. Hibbs, E.L. Hodges, and C.E. Cochrane (1995). Comparison of eating disorder patients with and without compulsive exercising. *Int. J. Eating Disord.* 4:413–416.

Brooks-Gunn, J., M.P. Warren, and L.H. Hamilton (1987). The relation of eating problems and amenorrhea in ballet dancers. *Med. Sci. Sports Exerc.* 19:41–44.

Brownell, K.D. (1995). Eating disorders in athletes. In: K.D. Brownell and C.G. Fairburn (eds.) *Eating Disorders and Obesity.* New York: The Guilford Press, pp.191–196.

Brownell, K. D., and J. Rodin (1992). Prevalence of eating disorders in athletes. In: K.D. Brownell, J. Rodin, and J.H. Wilmore (eds.). *Eating, Body Weight and Performance in Athletes: Disorders of Modern Society.* Philadelphia: Lea & Febiger, pp. 128–145.

Brownell, K.D., S. Nelson Steen, and J.H. Wilmore (1987). Weight regulation practices in athletes: analysis of metabolic and health effects. *Med. Sci. Sports Exerc.* 19:546–555.

Bryant-Waugh, R., and B. Lask (1995). Childhood-onset eating disorders. In: K.D. Brownell and C.G. Fairburn (eds.) *Eating Disorders and Obesity.* New York: The Guilford Press, pp. 183–187.

Button, E.J., and A. Whitehouse (1981). Subclinical anorexia nervosa. *Psychol. Med.* 11:509–516.

Cann, E.E., M.C. Martin, H.K. Genant, and R.B. Jaffe (1984). Decreased spinal mineral content in amenorrheic woment. *J.A.M.A.* 251:626–629.

Clark, N. (1994). Counseling the athlete with an eating disorder: A case study. *J. Am. Diet. Assoc.* 94:656–658.

Clark, N. (1996). How to handle eating disorders among athletes. *Gatorade Sports Sci. Institute Coaches' Corner.*

Clark, N. (1993). How to help the athlete with bulimia: practical tips and a case study. *Int. J. Sports Nutr.* 3:450–460.

Crago, M., C.M. Shisslak, and L.S. Estes (1996). Eating disturbances among American minority groups: a review. *Int. J. Eating Disord.* 19:239–248.

Crisp, A., and T. Burns (1983). The clinical presentation of anorexia nervosa in males. *Int. J. Eating Disord.* 2:5–10.

Davis, C., and M. Cowles (1989). A comparison of weight and diet concerns and personality factors among female athletes and non-athletes. *J. Psychosoma. Res.* 33:527–536.

Davis, C., and J. Fox (1993). Excessive exercise and weight preoccupation in women. *Addict. Behav.* 18:201–211.

DePalma, M.T., W.M. Koszewski, J.G. Case, R.J. Barile, B.F. DePalma, and S.M. Oliaro (1993). Weight control practices of lightweight football players. *Med. Sci. Sports Exerc.* 25:694–701.De

De Souza, M.J., and D.A. Metzger (1991). Reproductive dysfunction in amenorrheic athletes and anorexic patients: a review. *Med. Sci. Sports Exerc.* 23:995–1007.

Dick, R.W. (1991). Eating disorders in NCAA athletic programs. *Athletic Training J.N.A.T.A.* 26:136–140.

Drinkwater, B.L., R. Bruemmer, and C.H. Chestnut III (1990). Menstrual history as a determinant of current bone density in young athletes. *J.A.M.A.* 263:545–548.

Drinkwater, B.L., K. Nilson, S. Ott, and C.H. Chestnut (1986). Bone mineral density after resumption of menses in amenorrheic athletes. *J.A.M.A.* 256:380–382.

Dueck, C.A., M.M. Manore, and K.S. Matt (1996a). Role of energy balance in athletic menstrual dysfunction. *Int. J. Sports Nutr.* 6:165–190.

Dueck, C.A., K.S. Matt, M.M. Manore, and J.S. Skinner (1996b). Treatment of athletic amenorrhea with a diet and training intervention program. *Int. J. Sports Nutr.* 6:24–40.

Dummer, G.M., L.W. Rosen, W.W. Heusner, P.J. Roberts, and J.E. Counsilman (1987). Pathogenic weight-control behaviors of young competitive swimmers. *Phys. Sportsmed.* 15:75–84.

Eichner, E.R. (1992). General health issues of low body weight and undereating in athletes. In: K.D. Brownell, J. Rodin, and J.H. Wilmore (eds.). *Eating, Body Weight and Performance in Athletes: Disorders of Modern Society.* Philadelphia: Lea & Febiger, pp. 191–201.

Emmons, L. (1994). Predisposing factors differentiating adolescent dieters and nondieters. *J. Am. Diet. Assoc.* 84:725–728, 731.

Epling, W.F., and W.D. Pierce (1988). Activity-based anorexia: a biobehavioral perspective. *Int. J. Eat. Disord.* 7:475–485.

Epling, W.F., and W.D. Pierce (1996). An overview of activity anorexia. In: W.F. Epling and W.D. Pierce (eds.). *Activity Anorexia: Theory, Research, and Treatment.* Mahwah, NJ:Lawrence Erlbaum Assoc., Publishers, pp. 3–12.

Epling, W.F., W.D. Pierce, and L. Stefan (1983). A theory of activity-based anorexia. *Int. J. Eat. Disord.* 3:27–46.

Evers, C.L. (1987). Dietary intake and symptoms of anorexia nervosa in female university dancers. *J. Am. Diet. Assoc.* 87:66–68.

French, S.A., C.L. Perry, G.R. Leon, and J.A. Fulkerson (1994). Food Preferences, eating patterns, and physical activity among adolescents: correlates of eating disorders symptoms. *J. Adolesc. Health* 15:286–294.

French, S.A., M. Story, B. Downes, M.C. Resnick, L.J. Harris, and R. Blum (1995). Frequent dieting among adolescents: psychosocial and health behavior correlates. *Am. J. Public Health* 85:695–701.

Friday, K.E., B.L. Drinkwater, B. Bruemmer, C. Chestnut III, and A. Chait (1993). Elevated plasma low-density lipoprotein and high-density lipoprotein cholesterol levels in amenorrheic athletes: Effects of endogenous hormone status and nutrient intake. *J. Clin Endocrin. and Metabol.* 77:1605–1609.

Frusztajer, N.T., S. Dhuper, M.P. Warren, J. Brooks-Gunn, and R.P. Fox (1990). Nutrition and the incidence of stress fractures in ballet dancers. *Am. J. Clin. Nutr.* 51:779–783.

Gadpaille, W.J., C.F. Sanborn, and W.W. Wagner (1987). Athletic amenorrhea, major affective disorders and eating disorders. *Am. J. Psychiatry* 144:939–942.

Garner, D.M. (1991). Eating Disorder Inventory-2: Professional Manual. Odessa, Florida: Psychological Assessment Resources, Inc. 1991.

Garner, D.M., and P.E. Garfinkel (1979). The eating attitudes test: an index of the symptoms of anorexia nervosa. *Psychol. Med.* 9:273–279.

Garner, D.M., M.P. Olmsted, and J. Polivy (1984). Manual of Eating Disorder Inventory (EDI). Odessa, Florida: Psychological Assessment Resources.

Garner, D.M., M.P. Olmstead, Y. Bohr, and P.E. Garfinkel (1982). The eating attitudes test: Psychometric features and clinical correlates. *Psychol. Med.* 12:871–878.

Grandjean, A.C. (1991). Eating disorders—the role of the athletic trainer. *Athletic Training, J.N.A.T.A.* 26:105–112.

Grooms, A.M. (1996). The female athlete triad. *J. Florida M.A.* 83:479–481.

Hamilton, L.H., J. Brooks-Gunn, M.P. Warren, and W.G. Hamilton (1988). The role of selectivity in the pathogenesis of eating problems in ballet dancers. *Med. Sci. Sports Exerc.* 20:560–565.

Herzog, D.B., and P.M. Copeland (1985). Eating disorders. *N. Engl. J. Med.* 313:295–303.

Hetland, M.D., J. Haarbo, and C. Christiansen (1993). Running induces menstrual disturbances but bone mass is unaffected, except in amenorrheic women. *Am J. Med.* 95:53–60.

Hickerson, J.F., T.E. Johnson, W. Lee, and R.J. Sidor (1990). Nutrition and the precontest preparations of a male bodybuilder. *J. Am. Diet. Assoc.* 90:264–267.

Holland, A.J., N. Sicotte, and J. Treasure (1988). Anorexia nervosa: Evidence for a genetic basis. *J. Psychosom. Res.* 32:561–571.

Hsu L.K.G. (1980). Outcome of anorexia nervosa: A review of the literature (1954 to 1978). *Arch. Gen. Psych.* 37:1041–1046.

Ibrahim, H., and N. Morrison (1976). Self-actualization and self-concept among athletes. *Res. Q.* 47:68–79.

Johnson, C. (1986). Initial consultation for patients with bulimia and anorexia nervosa. In: D.M. Garner and P.E. Garfinkel (eds.) *Handbook of Psychotherapy of Anorexia Nervosa and Bulimia.* New York: Guilford Press, pp. 19–33.

Johnson, M.D. (1994). Disordered eating in active and athletic women. *Clinics in Sports Med.* 13:355–369.

Joy, E., N. Clark, M.L. Ireland, J. Martire, A. Nattiv, and S. Varechok (1997b). Team Management of the Female Athlete Triad, Part 1: What to Look for, What to ask. *Phys. Sportsmed.* 25:94–96, 101–102, 104, 107–108, 110.

Joy, E., N. Clark, M.L. Ireland, J. Martire, A. Nattiv, and S. Varechok (1997a). Team Management of the Female Athlete Triad, Part 2: Optimal Treatment and Prevention Tactics. *Phys. Sportsmed.* 25:55–57, 60–61, 65–69.

Joyce, J.M., D.L. Warren, L.L. Humphries, A.J. Smith, and J.S. Coon (1990). Osteoporosis in women with eating disorders: comparison of physical parameters, exercise, and menstrual status with SPA and DPA evaluation. *J. Nucl. Med.* 31:325–331.

Kaiserauer, S.K., A.C. Snyder, M. Sleeper, and J. Zierath (1989). Nutritional, physiological, and menstrual status of distance runners. *Med. Sci. Sports Exerc.* 21:120–125.

Keizer, H.A., and A.D. Rogol (1990). Physical exercise and menstrual cycle alterations: What are the mechanisms? *Sports Med.* 10:218–235.

King, M. (1989). Eating disorders in a general practice population: Prevalence, characteristics and follow-up at 12 to 18 months. *Psychol. Med.* 14:S3–11.

Kirchner, E.M., R.D. Lewis, and P.J. O'Connor (1996). Effect of past gymnastics participation on adult bone mass. *J. Appl. Physiol.* 80:226–232.

Kirchner, E.M., R.D. Lewis, and P.J. O'Connor (1995). Bone mineral density and dietary intake of female college gymnasts. *Med. Sci. Sports Exerc.* 27:543–549.

Kleiner, S.M., T.L. Bazzarre, and M.D. Litchford (1990). Metabolic profiles, diet, and health practices of championship male and female bodybuilders. *J. Am. Diet. Assoc.* 90:962–967.

Klemchuk, H.P., C.B. Hutchinson, and R.I. Frank (1990). Body dissatisfaction and eating-related problems on the college campus: Usefulness of the Eating Disorder Inventory with a nonclinical population. *J. Counsel. Psychol.* 37:297–305.

Kurtzman, F.D., J. Yager, J. Landsverk, E. Wiesmeier, and D.C. Bodurka (1989). Eating disorders among selected female student populations at UCLA. *J. Am. Diet. Assoc.* 89:45–53.

Leon, G.R. (1991). Eating disorders in female athletes. *Sports Med.* 12:219–227.

Lindeman, A.K. (1994). Self-esteem: Its application to eating disorders and athletes. *Int. J. Sports Nutr.* 4:237–252.

Loosli, A.R., and J. Benson (1990). Nutritional intake in adolescent athletes. *Pediatr. Clin. North Am.* 37:1143–1152.
Loucks, A.B. (1990). Effects of exercise training on the menstrual cycle: existence and mechanisms. *Med. Sci. Sports Exerc.* 22:275–280.
Loucks, A.B., J. Vaitukaitis, J.L. Cameron, A.D. Rogol, G. Skrinar, M.P. Warren, J. Kendrick, and M.C. Limacher (1992). The reproductive system and exercise in women. *Med. Sci. Sports Exerc.* 24:S288–S293.
Manore, M.M. (1996). Chronic dieting in active women: What are the consequences? *Women's Health Issues* 6:332–341.
Mortenson, G.M., S.L. Hoerr, and D.M. Garner (1993). Predictors of body satisfaction in college women. *J. Am. Diet. Assoc.* 93:1037–1039.
Nattiv, A., and L. Lynch (1994). The female athlete triad: Managing an acute risk to long-term health. *Phys. Sportsmed.* 22:60–68.
Nattiv, A., R. Agostini, B. Drinkwater, and K. Yeager (1994). The female athlete triad. *Clinic in Sports Med.* 13:405–418.
Noden, M. (1994). Special report: dying to win. Sports Illustrated 81:52–60.
Nudelman, S., J.C. Rosen, and H. Leitenberg (1988). Dissimilarities in eating attitudes, body image distortion, depression, and self-esteem between high-intesnity male runners and women with bulimia nervosa. *Int. J. Eating Disord.* 7:625–634.
O'Connor, P.J., R.D. Lewis, and E.M. Kirchner (1995). Eating disorder symptoms in female college gymnasts. *Med. Sci. Sports Exerc.* 27:550–555.
O'Connor, P.J., R.D. Lewis, E.M. Kirchner, and D.B. Cook (1996). Eating disorder symptoms in former female college gymnasts: relations with body composition. *Am. J. Clin. Nutr.* 64:840–843.
Olson, M.S., H.N. Williford, L.A. Richards, J.A. Brown, and S. Pugh (1996). Self-reports on the Eating Disorder Inventory by female aerobic instructors. *Percep. & Motor Skills* 82:1051–1058.
Otis, C. (1992). Exercise-associated amenorrhea. *Clin. Sports Med.* 11:351–362.
Parry-Jones, B., and W.L. Parry-Jones (1995). History of Bulimia and Bulimia Nervosa. In: K.D. Brownell and C.G. Fairburn (eds.) *Eating Disord. Obesity.* New York: The Guilford Press, pp. 145–150.
Piran, N., P. Lerner, P.E. Garfinkel, S.H. Kennedy, and C. Brouilette (1988). Personality disorders in anorexic patients. *Int. J. Eating Disord.* 7:589–599.
Pugliese, M.T., F. Lifshitz, G. Grad, P. Fort, and M. Marks-Katz (1983). Fear of obesity. A cause of short stature and delayed puberty. *New Engl. J. Med.* 309:513–518.
Putukian, M. (1994). The female triad. *Medical Clinics of North America* 78:345–356.
Ratnasuriya, R.H., I. Eisler, G.I. Szmukler, and G.F. Russell (1991). Anorexia nervosa: Outcome and prognostic factors after 20 years. *Brit. J. Psychol.* 158:495–502.
Rencken, M.L., C.H. Chesnut III, and B.L. Drinkwater (1996). Bone density at multiple skeletal sites in amenorrheic athletes. *J.A.M.A.* 276:238–240.
Robinson, T.L., C. Snow-Harter, D.R. Taaffe, D. Gillis, J. Shaw, and R. Marcus (1995). Gymnasts exhibit higher bone mass than runners despite similar prevalence of amenorrhea and oligomenorrhea. *J. Bone Min. Res.* 10:26–35.
Rodin, J. (1993). Cultural and psychosocial determinants of weight concerns. *Ann. Intern. Med.* 119:643–645.
Rodin, J., and L. Larson (1992). Societal factors and the ideal body shape. In: K.D. Brownell, J. Rodin, and J.H. Wilmore (eds.). *Eating, Body Weight and Performance in Athletes: Disorders of Modern Society.* Philadelphia: Lea & Febiger, pp. 146–158.
Root, M.P. (1991). Persistent, disordered eating as a gender-specific, post traumatic stress response to sexual assault. *Psychotherapy* 28:96–102.
Rosen, L.W., and D.O. Hough (1988). Pathogenic weight-control behaviors of female college gymnasts. *Phys. Sportsmed.* 16:141–144.
Rosen, L.W., D.B. McKeag, D.O. Hough, and V. Curley (1986). Pathogenic weight-control behavior in female athletes. *Phys. Sportsmed.* 14:79–86.
Rucinski, A. (1989). Relationship of body image and dietary intake of competitive ice skaters. *J. Am. Diet. Assoc.* 89:98–100.
Russell, G. (1979). Bulimia nervosa: An ominous variant of anorexia nervosa. *Psych. Med.* 9:429–448.
Sandri, S.C. (1993). On dancers and diet. *Int. J. Sports Nutr.* 3:334–342.
Serdula, M.K., M.E. Collins, D.F. Williamson, R.F. Anda, E. Pamuk, and T.E. Byers (1993). Weight control practices of U.S. adolescents and adults. *Ann. Intern. Med.* 119:667–671.
Silverman, J.A. (1995). History of anorexia nervosa. In: K.D. Brownell and C.G. Fairburn (eds.) *Eating Disorders and Obesity.* New York: The Guilford Press, pp. 141–144.
Silverstone, P.H. (1992). Is chronic low self-esteem the cause of eating disorders? *Med. Hypotheses* 39:311–315.
Slemenda, C.W., and C.C. Johnson (1993). High intensity activities in young women: Site specific bone mass effects among female figure skaters. *Bone Miner.* 20:125–132.

Snow-Harter, C.M. (1994). Bone health and prevention of osteoporosis in active and athletic women. *Clinics in Sports Med.* 13:389–404.
Steen, S.N., and K.D. Brownell (1990). Patterns of weight loss and regain in wrestlers: Has the tradition changed? *Med. Sci. Sports Exerc.* 22:762–768.
Steen, S.N., and J.H. Wilmore (1987). Weight regulation practices in athletes: Analysis of metabolic and health effects. *Med. Sci. Sports Exerc.* 19:546–56.
Stephenson, J.N. (1991). Medical consequences and complications of anorexia nervosa and bulimia nervosa in female athletes. *Athletic Training, J.N.A.T.A.* 26:130–135.
Story, M., S.A. French, D. Neumakar-Sztainer, B. Downes, M.D. Resnick, and R.W. Blum (1997). Psychosocial and behavioral correlates of dieting and purging in Native American adolescents. *Pediatr.* 99:e8 (Electronic Article).
Stoutjesdyk, D., and R. Jevne (1993). Eating disorders among high performance athletes. *J. Youth Adolesc.* 22:271–282.
Sundgot-Borgen, J. (1994a). Eating disorders in female athletes. *Sports Med.* 17:176–188.
Sundgot-Borgen, J. (1993a). Nutrient intake of female elite athletes suffering from eating disorders. *Int. J. Sport Nutr.* 3:431–442.
Sundgot-Borgen, J. (1993b). Prevalence of eating disorders in elite female athletes. *Int. J. Sport Nutr.* 3:29–40.
Sundgot-Borgen, J. (1994b). Risk and trigger factors for the development of eating disorders in female elite athletes. *Med. Sci. Sports Exerc.* 26:414–419.
Sundgot-Borgen, J., and J. Corbin (1987). Eating disorders among female athletes. *Phys. Sportsmed.* 15:89–95.
Szmukler, G., and G. Russell (1985). Outcome and prognosis of anorexia nervosa. In: K.D. Brownell, J. Rodin, and J.H. Wilmore (eds.). *Handbook of Eating Disorders: Physiology, Psychology and Treatment of Obesity, Anorexia, and Bulimia.* New York:Basic Books, pp. 283–300.
Sykora, C., C.M. Grilo, D.E. Wilfley, and K.D. Brownell (1993). Eating, weight, and dieting disturbances in male and female lightweight and heavyweight rowers. *Int. J. Eating Disord.* 14:203–211.
Thompson, R.A., and R.T. Sherman (1993). *Helping Athletes with Eating Disorders.* Champaign, Il: Human Kinetics, pp.97–170.
Thornton, J.S. (1990). Feast or famine: Eating disorders in athletes. *Phys. Sportsmed.* 18:116–122.
Tipton, C.M, and R.A. Oppliger (1984). The Iowa wrestling study: Lessons for physicians. *Iowa Med.* 74:381–385.
Van De Loo, D.A., and M.D. Johnson (1995). The young female athlete. *Clinics in Sports Med.* 14:687–707.
Walberg, J.L., and C.S. Johnston (1991). Menstrual function and eating behavior in female recreational weight lifters and competitive body builders. *Med. Sci. Sports Exerc.* 23:30–36.
Warren, B.J., A.L. Stanton, and D.L. Blessing (1990). Disordered eating patterns in competitive female athletes. *Int. J. Eating Disord.* 9:565–569.
Webster, S., R. Rutt, and A. Weltman (1990). Physiological effects of a weight loss regimen practiced by college wrestlers. *Med. Sci. Sports Exerc.* 22:229–234.
Weight, L.M., and T.D. Noakes (1987). Is running an analog of anorexia?: A survey of the incidence of eating disorders in female distance runners. *Med. Sci. Sports Exerc.* 19:213–217.
Wichmann, S., and D.R. Martin (1993). Eating disorders in athletes. *Phys. Sportsmed.* 21:126–135.
Wilmore, J.H. (1991). Eating and weight disorders in the female athlete. *Int. J. Sport Nutr.* 1:104–117.
Wilmore, J.H., K.C. Wambsgans, M. Brenner, C.E. Broeder, I. Paijmans, J.A. Volpe, and K.M. Wilmore (1992). Is there energy conservation in amenorrheic compared with eumenorrheic distance runners? *J. Appl. Physiol.* 72:15–22.
Wolf, E.M., and T.J. Akamatsu (1994). Exercise involvement and eating-disordered characteristics in college students. *Eating Disorders: The Journal of Treatment and Prevention* 2:308–318.
Woscyna, G. (1991). Nutritional aspects of eating disorders: Nutrition education and counseling as a component of treatment. *Athletic Training, J.N.A.T.A* 26:141–147.
Yates, A. (1992). Biologic consideration in the etiology of eating disorders. *Pediat. Ann.* 21:739–744.
Yates, A. (1989). Current perspectives on the eating disorders: I. History, psychological, and biological aspects. *J. Am. Acad. Child Adolesc. Psychiatry* 6:813–828.
Yates, A., K. Leehey, and C.M. Shisslak (1983). Running—An analogue of anorexia? *N. Engl. J. Med.* 308:251–255.
Yates, A., C.M. Shisslak, J. Allender, M Crago, and K. Leehey (1992). Comparing obligatory to nonobligatory runners. *Psychomatics.* 33:180–189.
Yates, A., C. Shisslak, M. Crago, and J. Allender (1994). Overcommitment to sport: Is there a relationship to the eating disorders? *Clin. J. Sport Med.* 4:39–46.
Yeager, K.K., R. Agostini, A. Nattiv, and B. Drinkwater (1993). The female athlete triad: Disordered eating, amenorrhea, osteoporosis. *Med. Sci. Sports Exer.* 25:775–777.

190   *PERSPECTIVES IN EXERCISE SCIENCE*

DISCUSSION

STEEN: Please describe some of the strategies used to treat eating disorders in athletes.

HOUTKOOPER: There needs to be a person other than the coach who intercedes to initiate treatment. In part, this is because coaches are not trained in this area and in part because some coaches believe that some of the practices, i.e., having a very low body weight and being amenorrheic, are normal indicators of adequate training. As a result, some coaches won't allow athletes to gain weight and regain their menses because the coaches think that will decrease the performance of the athletes. Ideally, a physician or psychologist who has a great deal of authority and experience in this area is probably one of the most powerful people to initiate and coordinate treatment. Certainly, psychological counseling is very critical in effective recovery. Also, I think nutritionists need to be a key part of this team. It is also important that athletic trainers and administrators in schools be aware of these problems because effective approaches to prevent or treat eating disorders will require modifying the culture of high-risk sports. All of one's efforts in trying to get an athlete to change behavior will not be effective without support of family, trainers, sport judges, health professionals, coaches, and school athletic administrators. Early education starting in grade school regarding what is desirable body fat or body weight is a first step. Also, we need to provide education for effective coping strategies to deal with the psychological issues that contribute to disordered eating and weight-control problems. We should also take a proactive approach and talk about how we can help people learn to eat healthfully to manage their weight. We also need to modify sport culture so that judges and coaches accept a different image of what is a desirable weight or physique in a sport. That's a daunting challenge.

SATTERWHITE: From a physician's standpoint, I find quite frustrating the fact that the best way to identify eating disorders in athletes is through clinical interviews, and I certainly hope someone will eventually be able to develop a screening technique that is reliable and valid for athletes. Annually we physicians administer preparticipation physicals, but there is simply not enough time to screen or identify athletes with possible eating disorders. Also, you mentioned that there is an equal tendency toward eating disorders in both male and female lightweight rowers, and I think it would be helpful to design tracking studies for females and males in other weight-category sports such as USA wrestling, USA boxing, and USA weight lifting. These are sports in which females are only now becoming involved, and so there may be an opportunity even at the high-school level to evaluate girls just entering the sport and then track them to determine their risk of developing eating disorders over a period of several years. Lastly, as for categories, it would be interesting to look at sports that are considered annual sports, as opposed to seasonal sports. Athletes such as cheerleaders participate year-long in competition, not just nationally or regionally, but amongst themselves to determine who will perform certain roles on the team. Other sports characterized by annual preparation and competition include body building and weight lifting, especially if the athletes use the periodization cycle that was developed by Medvedev. Such training is very intense, and every time the athlete enters the weight room, the athlete has the mentality of entering a competition, and body weight must be adjusted up or down throughout the year. It would be interesting to compare groups that compete year-round versus seasonally and determine the prevalence of eating disorders.

Finally, I think people with eating disorders not only have a preoccupation with "thinness," but a fear of "fatness." Some of the people with eating disorders are exposed via the press to a perceived epidemic of fatness, and they fear that fatness may be "communicable." Thus, they tenaciously hold on to their beliefs of maintaining or decreasing weight because the press emphasizes just how fat everyone is becoming.

HOUTKOOPER: There is another issue that is related. Even though exercise is healthy and good for people, it's just like a nutrient, i.e., a certain amount is really desirable and essential, but beyond a certain amount, there are some negative consequences to excess nutrient intake or excessive exercise. At the American College of Sports Medicine meeting this year, there were concerns expressed regarding the negative message about excess exercise consequences for young women. Excessive exercise can lead to demineralized bones. That is really an extreme, affecting a small percentage of female athletes. But the message that gets picked up in the popular press is that exercise can really create health problems. That's not the message we want to send out to young women. We know there are healthy ranges of physical activity.

MAUGHAN: One area you did not cover in depth is the relationship between body composition, eating habits, and performance. In sports such as distance running there may be a very clear improvement in performance if one reduces body fat to levels that are far lower than those that we would say are consistent with good health. These athletes are also often obsessive, but I don't think one can be an Olympic champion without being obsessive and without being concerned about eating. There must be a danger that we are classifying these people as having disorders when they are doing what is necessary to achieve success in a given sport. Reducing body weight in men and women to extremely low levels in some sports will improve performance.

HOUTKOOPER: That's an important point. It appears that in sports where restricting weight and restricting body fat are important for performance, some people maintain low body weight, perform well, and remain fairly healthy. I think we need to study those successful athletes who get their body weight down really low but don't have the negative metabolic or health consequences that can be associated with having a low body weight.

MAUGHAN: My concern about identifying athletes as suffering from disordered eating is that the criteria are not individualized to allow for some of the behaviors of the elite athlete. If weight is maintained, even at extremely low levels of body fat, then intake must be sufficient to match expenditure. The difficulties arise when intake is restricted. This will limit the training load, and performance will then suffer. If such athletes then gain weight, their performance will be impaired.

HOUTKOOPER: Maybe their short-term performance is fine, but what are the long-term health or medical consequences for them? Maybe for some of these women, there are none because they are eating well. If they are making the best food choices possible and doing other things to control their stress, and they don't have psychological distress and a sense of being out of control or being controlled by their condition, having a low body weight or fat level may be fine. I have been doing a development program for about 7 y with USA Track and Field elite female athletes, and we measure their body composition using multiple component models. Most of these athletes are lean, i.e., 9% to 10% body fat, and yet they have bone mineral density that is about 112 -135% of their age and ethnic match ed controls. Most of them eat pretty well. So I don't worry about them, even though their body fat is really low because they don't seem to have negative health consequences.

COYLE: Ron, you mentioned that you assumed that the athletes really know what's best and that they look at us and say, "You don't understand that you have to be 10% body fat to be a top distance runner." I don't agree. I think the athletes are often ill informed. I work with the women's athletic program at the University of Texas, and we formed a performance team to address these issues. It became difficult to do because these eating disorders, of course, are very sensitive issues, and they can't be discussed in committee. However, we found a lot of these athletes were misinformed. In particular, runners were trying to be much too lean; we gave them food supplements, and their performance improved. However, group dynamics are exceptionally complex. The volleyball team at Texas is a good example. Our women's volleyball team had a great coach; he discouraged disordered eating, and the team was first and second in the national championships. Then from one year to the next, athletes on the team changed the dynamics because they thought, "Well, to really compete, we have to be leaner than is realistic." And within one year in the same group of athletes, eating disorders on the team were relatively common because some athletes had the mistaken impression that they had to become much leaner to be the starters. The coach thought their performance was deteriorating but had a hard time convincing some athletes of that. What I'm saying is that we have to convince the athletes that what they hear from one another isn't always correct. We have to use valid performance measures to counteract ignorance. And then we must rely upon some of the athletes who are resistant to all this misinformation to educate the others.

HOUTKOOPER: That's another important point. The University of Texas, Austin, has one of the premiere programs in the country for dealing with eating disorders. Also, related to this performance question, there is a group at Arizona State University (Manore and Dueck) who have tried to address this issue in female runners. In their first case study, the runner was amenorrheic. They decreased her training by one day per week and had her drink a commercial liquid meal (Gator-Pro®) as a daily supplement in addition to what she was eating. She was able to regain her menstrual cycle and improve her performance. This study supports the energy-drain theory. Getting the right level of energy intake can ameliorate metabolic problems and improve performance. Trying this approach is difficult because there is a widely held belief among some female and male athletes, coaches and trainers that leaner is always better. A female athlete credo is "Get thin and win."

PASSE: You mentioned that the EAT or the EDI were not all that successful at predicting the DSM-IV eating disorder categories. Could you comment on whether you believe that those clinical descriptions are the gold standards that ought to be operative here? Should we be using less stringent criteria?

HOUTKOOPER: The American Psychiatric Association has set those criteria. They are arbitrary but are the current "gold standard." Sundot-Borgen is attempting to expand the criteria to include the category of anorexia athletica. We don't know what the psychological or performance implications are for athletes diagnosed with eating disorders using current criteria.

PASSE: Are eating disorders prevalent in athletes in other cultures that have lower incidence rates of eating disorders than in the West? In other words, is participation in sport an independent risk factor in the development of eating disorders?

HOUTKOOPER: Research indicates that sport participation is not an independent risk factor except in certain sports where appearance is critical or where a low body weight is perceived to improve performance, or in sports with weight categories. There seems to be a little higher prevalence of eating disorders among those specific athletic groups. But among other athletes, definitely, there does not appear to be any greater prevalence of eating disorders.

MCCAY: Is there a role of pharmacotherapy in treating eating disorders? My reason for this question is that many psychological disorders have a neurochemical basis.

HOUTKOOPER: The pharmacotherapy used most often is antidepressants, but behavioral approaches are usually the first line of therapy.

CLARKSON: My question involves the role of weight cycling at an early age in the development of obesity. I work with classical ballet dancers who start dieting at about 10 years old, which I understand is about the age that the general population of young girls is starting to diet. These girls would be considered of normal weight, but a bit heavy for ballet. Those who diet get quite thin, go through the weight cycling, end up gaining more weight than they might have, and drop out of ballet. These girls don't appear on any of the surveys determining the incidence of eating disorders. They drop out of the sport because they end up not being able to control their weight. Several of these girls that I have kept in contact with over the years are now obese. Did these girls have some predisposition towards obesity that the weight cycling triggered? Have you any information on the possible role of weight cycling at an early age and its negative consequences in later life?

HOUTKOOPER: No, I don't.

DESPRES: The NIH has had a consensus conference on weight cycling. There's no evidence that it makes individuals prone to become more obese. In this case you might be dealing with girls who were more prone to eventually become obese.

CLARKSON: But the NIH conference did not discuss kids who began weight cycling at an early age.

DESPRES: The issue is far from being resolved. My bias would be that they are more prone to becoming obese, and they adjust their intake accordingly.

JOHNSEN: We have 225,000 high-school coaches in Nebraska who work with 6 million student athletes, and one problem that we experience is the denial by the parents that the student athlete has a weight-control problem; our hands are tied in how much further we can take this. What would your suggestions be? If coaches perceive a problem, society will not allow them to deal with it because of the legal and educational systems.

HOUTKOOPER: That is a challenge at all fronts with any kind of behavior for kids. Surveys indicate that an athlete typically gets advice and information on eating and weight control from other athletes, someone in their family, or the media. Education programs that have a family component can offer some basic suggestions to families about desirable levels of body weight or body fat and about healthy eating patterns and weight control approaches. We need some creative approaches to education that will engage parents. Maybe the approach might be to try to find some parents who are willing to be role models and to help provide education. Peer-to-peer education sometimes is very effective.

BAR-OR: I have a comment and a question. The comment is regarding thermoregulation in anorexia nervosa. Clinicians are familiar with the low tolerance to cold (and, sometimes, heat) of these patients. There is one preliminary report (Davies & Fohlin, *J. Physiol.* (London) 268:8P-9P, 1977) suggesting that during prolonged exercise, the ambient temperature range in which female patients can maintain constant core temperature is narrower than normal. Bearing in mind that young athletes with anorexia are often exposed to heat stress, more research should be conducted in this field.

My question is regarding sports retirees. Is there any information about prevalence, incidence and prognosis of eating disorders among these people?

HOUTKOOPER: There isn't a great deal of information published in that area. There was one study dealing with retired collegiate female gymnasts done at the University of Georgia (O'Connor et al.). They compared the gymnasts to a control group matched for age, height, and weight, and found that there was excellent recovery in these female gymnasts. In fact, the gymnasts actually had a greater body satisfaction than the comparison group, were at a normal weight, and did not have any negative medical consequences.

EICHNER: In gymnasts, too, it may be not the female athlete triad, but the female athlete diad. There are about 10 studies of female gymnasts, albeit cross-sectional, and in none is there any decrease in bone density. So, it seems that the impact loading of the sport keeps the bones strong despite a high prevalence of disordered eating and menstrual problems.

ARAGON-VARGAS: You have mentioned that early intervention is very important. What is the message we're actually trying to convey to the young athletes? You had this illustration about eating disorders being like canoeing in a river away from a waterfall. Are we trying to tell these young athletes: "Don't get into the canoe at all," or are we trying to find a place where they need to jump off the canoe? We certainly encourage them to restrict their fat intake. What should the message be for them? I think that's a very practical issue that we need to explore so we can be effective once we have determined that a problem exists.

HOUTKOOPER: We're telling athletes they need to get in the canoe, that it's important to exercise and participate in sports. What we're also trying to do is help athletes know the boundaries when they are crossing over to unhealthy and detrimental eating, weight control and exercise practices.

SPRIET: The mortality data you show for people who are diagnosed with eating disorders is very alarming. One point that you made is that if they're involved in a program in which they receive dietary counseling, then the mortality rate goes down. My question is, what experimental data led you to conclude this, and how significantly do the mortality rates decrease?

HOUTKOOPER: The mortality data that I presented were for the nonathletic population because we don't know what it is in the athletic population. The actual clinical studies that have been done have shown that psychological counseling was the most effective intervention and that nutrition counseling was also helpful. Psychological counseling has been the most effective because it's treating underlying psychological causes for eating disorders. Eating disorders really are psychological disorders that end up manifesting themselves in symptoms of pathological exercise practices, eating behavior, and weight control practices.

SPRIET: How strong are the data?

HOUTKOOPER: Not very. The data were collected by people who do intervention studies in which they examined athletes who had frank eating disorders and developed major problems versus athletes who recovered from the disorder. So these are self-reported survey data. I don't think there has ever been any kind of randomized prospective trial testing different approaches to treating or preventing eating disorders. We really need to do research to determine strategies for effective prevention and treatment of eating disorders.

M. WILLIAMS: Recently, the state of Wisconsin initiated a weight-control program for high-school wrestlers, and it seems to have been fairly successful. I wonder if you think a similar type of program could be developed for other young athletes in sports such as gymnastics and distance running?

HOUTKOOPER: In gymnastics, a program is being developed for the national team to educate coaches, athletes, and judges about healthier criteria for physique in that sport. I'm not aware of any other sport in which that's happening. These might be good models for people to emulate in other sports.

5

Changing Body Weight and Composition in Athletes

JANET WALBERG-RANKIN, PH.D.

INTRODUCTION

A wrestler runs while wearing a rubber suit to make the desired weight class; a bodybuilder sets an alarm to wake every 2 h to eat since she has heard that frequent consumption of small meals is critical to weight loss (Steen, 1991); and a cheerleader is devastated when she is removed from the squad because she exceeded the body weight standards. These are examples of athletes caught up in their concerns about body weight.

Many nonathletes believe that athletes don't need to worry about their body weights. The assumption seems to be that athletes' high energy expenditures allow effortless weight management. Numerous studies show that this is not true for many athletes. This is illustrated in the question posed by Parr et al.(1984) to almost 3000 high school and collegiate athletes in various sports. When asked for their primary nutrition concerns, the most common answer was "body weight."

Athletes have many motives for weight change, some of which can be predicted by the natures of their sports. Some are focused on reducing body weight, whereas others are more concerned about body fat. While long distance runners might want to reduce total weight to reduce the energy cost of running, volleyball players and basketball players may want to reduce body fat to improve power-to-body weight ratios for a better jump. Gymnasts, dancers, figure skaters, and body builders are concerned about aesthetic appearance because judges expect very low body fat in these athletes. Other athletes, such as wrestlers and weight lifters, lose weight rapidly over a short time, often using dehydration to achieve a lower competitive weight class. Wrestlers hope to quickly regain the lost body weight prior to a match and face an opponent who may have less muscle mass and power. Overlying these performance motives are the social expectations for a lean physique for men and, especially, for women. This review will present the weight loss practices of athletes and the possible consequences of weight reduction and will recommend strategies for developing body weight goals and managing weight. This review will purposely avoid discussion of true eating disorders in athletes and will focus on typical and unusual but not necessarily pathogenic weight loss practices.

WEIGHT LOSS PRACTICES OF ATHLETES

Sufficient evidence is available on the weight control practices of athletes in the sports that will be discussed in the following sections. Data will be presented to illustrate the concern about weight as well as the dietary practices of these athletes. Use of drugs or supplements for weight control will not be included because that topic is covered elsewhere in this volume.

It is important to note that almost all data on food consumption of athletes relies on self-report, typically using a food record. These records are tedious for individuals to complete and may, by themselves, alter food choices. Underreporting of food consumption in diet records is common for any study population. For example, significant training of 263 individuals on appropriate procedures for keeping food records still resulted in substantial inaccuracies, when compared to the measured intake required to maintain their weights (Mertz et al., 1991). Eighty-nine percent of these individuals either under- or overestimated actual energy intake by more than 413 kJ/d (100 kcal/d). The average underestimate was 2890 kJ/d (700 kcal/d) less than maintenance energy requirement.

Accuracy of reporting may be even worse for some subgroups. Obese individuals who claimed inability to lose weight underreported their food intake by an average of 47%, compared to 19% underestimation by obese subjects who did not claim dieting resistance (Lightman et al., 1992). Edwards et al.(1993) found that the energy intake of nine female runners over 7 d was 32% lower than the energy expenditure measured using doubly labeled water. Since body weight did not change over this period, it suggests underreporting of food consumption. There was a negative correlation between body weight and energy intake and with body weight and body image. This suggests that underreporting may be more of a problem in heavier athletes, who may be less comfortable with their bodies. In summary, most individuals tend to underreport food intake, and those with special concerns about their body weights may be more likely to grossly underestimate their food consumption. This has implications for the nutritional intake data collected from athletes; all the self-report dietary data presented in this review should be interpreted with caution.

Runners

Female long distance runners, in particular, have been reported to apparently subsist on low energy intakes in spite of long-distance workouts. For example, the female runners studied by Myerson et al. (1991) ran an average of 83 km/wk but consumed insignificantly more—826 kJ/d (200 kcal/d)—than the comparison group of sedentary women. Resting metabolic rate, when expressed per unit body weight was not different between the eumenorrheic runners and the sedentary controls. Thus, one would expect that the additional expenditure of their running would increase the total energy needs of the runners substantially, relative to sedentary women. Although the energy intake from 3-d food records was less than the estimated energy expenditure using heart rate monitors for both controls and female distance runners studied by Beidleman et al. (1995), the discrepancy between reported intake and expenditure was greater for runners (−4131 kJ/d), compared to controls (−1652 kJ/d).

Some runners admit to purposely restricting food consumption in order to lose weight. Armstrong et al. (1990) found that of the 930 female runners who responded to a questionnaire at a road race, 69% of the women reported they had changed their food choices over the last 5 y to either a "moderate" or "great" extent. When asked why they had changed their dietary selections, 63% answered "to lose weight." Nutter (1991) presented the dietary intakes of female athletes in a variety of sports as well as the incidence of dieting for weight loss. Four of the six cross-country runners in the study claimed they were dieting during their season; five of these runners were dieting after the competitive season was completed. It is interesting, however, that querying a group of nonathletes at the same university showed that 18 of the 24 were dieting during the recording period. Thus, dieting is common in females and may be even more prevalent in female runners.

Although this concern about low body weight is most prevalent in females, individual male runners may also be extremely concerned about weight loss. Yates et al. (1983) first described several case studies of "obligatory" male runners whose obsession with running was motivated by a desire for leanness. Kiernan et al. (1992) found that weekly running distance was associated with degree of concern about eating and body weight, as measured by the Eating Attitudes Test (EAT), in a group of 2459 male runners who responded to a survey placed in a national running magazine. A greater proportion of runners who ran more than 72 km/wk had elevated EAT scores than did those who ran lesser distances. Interestingly, distance running was not associated with the EAT score for female runners completing the survey.

Swimmers

The concern about body weight in swimmers was shown in a survey done on highly competitive adolescent swimmers at a swim camp (Dummer et al., 1987). Almost 40% of the female swimmers claimed that they worried about weight often or almost always; only about 14% of the male swimmers answered similarly. Sixty percent of the girls who were classified as normal weight for height and 18% of those classified as underweight were trying to lose weight. When asked for their motives for weight loss, 80.5% of the swimmers reported that they wanted to look better. The males were more frequently motivated by the possibility of performance improvement. The researchers attempted to determine the source of pressures for body weight in these athletes. The most common source of a message that they were overweight was parents (53.7%), whereas their coaches had told only 25.8% of the athletes that they should lose weight.

Since swimmers are typically fatter than distance runners in spite of prolonged workouts, there is a common misconception that exercise in water preserves body fat stores and makes fat loss more difficult. Several studies argue against this perception. Flynn et al. (1990) had runners, swimmers, and triathletes perform 45 min of swimming or running at 75% of their aerobic capacities. Although the energy expended during recovery from the exercise bouts was similar, the indirect calorimetry measurements showed that more fat was oxidized after the swim than after the run. Barr and Costill (1992) confirmed that a strenuous swim-training season did not change body weight but reduced body fat in male collegiate swimmers. The swimmers had increased their energy intakes during the increased swim volume period, but those intakes were below requirements, causing utilization of body fat stores. Thus, the evidence does not support a unique fat-preserving effect of swimming.

Dancers and Gymnasts

Dancers and gymnasts do anaerobically-biased workouts that are strenuous but do not utilize as much overall energy as do sports that incorporate more aerobic activity. Thus, by restricting energy intake, dancers and gymnasts often attempt to create a negative energy balance. Benson et al. (1985) analyzed diet records from over 90 adolescent elite ballet dancers. Although the average energy intake was reasonable— 7802 kJ/d (1890 kcal/d), about 29% recorded less than 6192 kJ/d (1500 kcal/d), and 11% ate less than 4954 kJ/d (1200 kcal/d) during the measurement period. The 25 adult professional ballet dancers studied by Calabrese et al. (1983) reported consuming an average of only 5606 kJ/d (1358 kcal/d). Twenty-four of the 25 said they consumed less than 85% of the RDA for folate and iron. Most were also consuming low amounts of vitamins B12, A, and D, and calcium.

Twenty-six collegiate female gymnasts given a food frequency questionnaire to assess their diet (Kirchner et al., 1995) reported consuming an average of only 5701 kJ/d (1381 kcal/d). This was significantly less than the 7203 kJ/d (1745 kcal/d) determined from the diet records of a control group matched by body weight.

Rowers

Heavyweight rowers do not have any body weight restrictions, whereas lightweight rowers have a maximal average weight for the boat as well as a maximal individual body weight requirement. Some lightweight rowers use food restriction (McCargar et al., 1993), whereas others may practice acute dehydration (Burge et al., 1993) to achieve the body weight required for competition. The rowers who restrict energy to lose weight may begin dieting about 1 mo before competition begins (McCargar et al., 1993). Although the seven female rowers in that study who were classified as weight cyclers (they had lost more than 5 kg four times in the previous 5 y) lost 4.2 kg between preseason and peak season, dietary records indicated only a minimal change (about 949 kJ less daily energy intake) in their energy intake during that period. This modest negative energy balance may have been effective if chronically maintained over many months; alternatively, it is possible that their scheduled dietary recording periods did not match the times of more severe energy restriction. Almost all the weight lost was regained by 6–8 wk after the last competition.

Rowers surveyed by Sykoro et al. (1993) used more severe methods to lose weight—13% of the women used vomiting; 67% of the lightweight rowers used fasting as a weight control method. Gender differences were also uncovered; male rowers (lightweight and heavyweight combined) tended to lose weight more times during the season (5.4 versus 0.4 times) and used fasting more often than did women (57% versus 25%).

Bodybuilders

Bodybuilding is a unique sport; the participants desire great muscle tissue mass concurrent with extremely low body fat. They are judged not only on muscle size and symmetry but also on how well defined or "cut" their muscles are at competition time. They eat very different diets during times when they are trying to increase muscle mass ("bulking") than when they are preparing for a competition ("cutting").

The "cutting" phase may involve months of dietary restriction to reduce body fat. For example, 55% of the male and 75% of the female bodybuilders studied by Kleiner et al. (1990) began dieting 2-4 mo before a competition. Thus, they are an interesting group in which to study the effects of chronic energy restriction. Comparison of energy intake during the "cutting" phase compared to the "bulking" phase for several studies shows a 40–50% lower energy intake during the weight-loss period (Walberg-Rankin, 1995). Two case studies of male bodybuilders preparing for competitions have published detailed dietary information (Hickson et al., 1990; Steen, 1991). Each of these individuals ate a progressively more energy-restricted diet during the period before competition. For example, the subject studied by Steen (1991) dropped his energy intake from 17,309 kJ/d (4193 kcal/d) during the bulking phase to

12,466 kJ/d (3020 kcal/d) 3 mo before and 7992 kJ/d (1936 kcal/d) during the week before the contest. Interpretation of these cases is clouded by admission of use of anabolic steroids by both bodybuilders; these drugs may influence dietary intake.

We included 103 women involved in weight training in a survey of their feelings about their body weights and eating habits (Walberg & Johnston, 1991). The weight trainers scored higher on the "Drive for Thinness" subscale of the Eating Disorder Inventory, were more obsessed with food, were more likely to use laxatives for weight control, and were more terrified of becoming fat than were inactive women. This was particularly pronounced among the subset of 12 women who had competed in bodybuilding competitions. Sixty-seven percent of these women claimed that they were terrified of becoming fat.

To get more specific information about the dietary habits and weight loss patterns of competitive bodybuilders, we followed a group of six female bodybuilders while they were preparing for competitions (Walberg-Rankin et al., 1993). Diet and body weight records were kept 1 mo before, 1 wk before, 2 d before, immediately after, and 3 wk after the competitions. The women lost an average of 2.7 kg over the month before competition, with a range of 0.4–6.4 kg. This was accomplished with moderate, chronic restriction in energy intake. Even the woman who lost 6.4 kg never reported less than 5779 kJ/d (1400 kcal/d). This rate of weight loss, approximately 0.7 kg/wk, was within the recommended range.

The composition of the weight reduction diets consumed by the women in our study was more restrictive than were their energy intakes; average dietary fat was kept as low as 6.4% during the 2 d before competition. The common perception among bodybuilders is that weight loss cannot be accomplished unless dietary fat is kept extremely low (Steen, 1991). This is misinformation because the energy content rather than the fat content of a diet determines weight change.

The food choices of body builders during the "cutting" phase tend to be limited and repetitive. Sandoval and Heyward (1991) found that the average number of different foods dropped over 30% during preparation for competition. Many bodybuilders avoid red meat and dairy products during the "cutting" phase. The impact of these repetitive diets will be discussed later with regard to micronutrient deficiencies.

Not surprisingly, the remarkable dietary control the bodybuilders display while preparing for competition disappears after the competition. The male body builder followed by Steen (1991) consumed 22,126 kJ (5360 kcal) the day after the competition, with 45% of those calories as fat. The reported energy intake of the six bodybuilders we studied increased by 80%, and the total grams of dietary fat increased by a factor of ten (Walberg-Rankin et al., 1993). Weight gain was rapid after the contest, with an average weight gain of almost 1 kg over the immediate days after competition and almost 4 kg within 3 wk.

In summary, bodybuilders begin losing weight months prior to their competitions by restricting energy intake and drastically reducing dietary fat. They are a unique group in their rigorous commitment to dietary modification for weight loss over a long period.

Wrestlers

Many wrestlers lose weight repeatedly and rapidly during each season to achieve a particular weight class. Their goal is to drop weight temporarily while maintaining muscle tissue and, therefore, muscle strength and power. Forty-one percent of the collegiate wrestlers at a major tournament reported they lost between 5 and 9 kg each week of the season (Brownell et al., 1987). Weight loss is typically accomplished over several days by energy and fluid restriction, sweating, and increased exercise. However, extreme methods of weight reduction, including vomiting and the use of rubber suits during exercise, have been reported.

We asked six collegiate and ten high-school wrestlers to keep food records just before and after four matches over their season (Pesce et al., 1996). The average weight loss diet reported by the wrestlers on the day before the match was moderately low in average energy—7319 kJ/d (1773 kcal/d) and 4140 kJ/d (1003 kcal/d) for high school and college, respectively. However, average energy intakes on the day of the match prior to weigh-in were drastically reduced to 2336 kJ (566 kcal) and 120 kJ (29 kcal) for the high school and college athletes. Clearly, most of the college athletes fasted prior to the weighin.

One study compared the weight loss methods of 125 high school wrestlers to their parents' perceptions of their weight loss practices (Weissinger et al., 1991). Seventy percent of the wrestlers worried about their weight "often" or "almost always." The proportion of the wrestlers "always" using one or more particular techniques for weight loss was as follows: 77% exercised, 30% spit, 28% drank less fluid, 15% used sauna or steam rooms, and 11% exercised in rubber suits. Fifteen percent used vomiting either "always" or "occasionally". Many used modest energy restriction methods such as skipping a daily meal (29%) or cutting out snacks (69%), but a full 13% "always" used fasting and 38% used it "occasionally" to make weight.

Parents underestimated the amount of weight their sons were losing. The wrestlers indicated that they lost an average of 5.3 kg, whereas the parents thought they lost only 3.5 kg. Some parents didn't even realize their sons lost weight; only 64% of parents reported that their sons lost weight while 81% of their sons said they did. Many of the wrestlers felt there was too much pressure for weight loss. Forty-two percent believed that wrestlers should compete at their normal weights with less emphasis on weight loss.

WEIGHT GAIN PRACTICES

Little has been written about the methods used by athletes to gain weight. Wolf et al. (1979) asked 137 Big-Ten college coaches from a variety of sports if they prescribed diets to decrease or increase body weight of their athletes. Sixteen percent of the male and female coaches were involved in developing plans to have their athletes gain weight, less than the 26% and 39% of male and female coaches who prescribed weight loss. This study did not inquire about the actual weight change plans that the coaches recommended.

Baer et al. (1994) focused on the recommendations given by 135 high school football coaches to athletes who desired a gain in lean tissue. Ninety-eight percent of them claimed that they had advised their athletes on weight gain. All of them believed that weight training and 97% thought diet had important roles to play in gaining lean mass. Only 10% answered that protein was important to weight gain, but 30% recommended protein powders as valuable.

Jacobson and Aldana (1992) asked more than 800 collegiate athletes about their nutritional practices and beliefs. Of the male athletes who reported taking protein and vitamin supplements, 49% and 27%, respectively, believed that these supplements would aid their weight gain. Football and baseball had the highest proportions of athletes who believed these nutrients had value for weight gain.

Many bodybuilders focus on protein intake as a critical dietary component to accelerate weight gain. A review of reported average protein intakes (1.7–2.8 g/kg) for male bodybuilders indicates that this nutrient typically accounts for 19–26% of the energy intake (Walberg-Rankin, 1995), significantly above the RDA of 0.8 g/kg for adult males. Even though their diets are typically rich in protein, it is not unusual for them to also consume protein supplements. Evaluation of the nutritional supplements marketed to bodybuilders indicated that the most frequently promoted benefit was muscle growth; about 60% of the products claimed this effect (Philen et al., 1992). Protein powder and other weight gain formulas were consumed by 59% and 26% of the bodybuilders competing in a sample of 309 competitors in state competitions (Brill & Keane, 1994). When asked to list the reasons that they took dietary supplements, about 53% answered that the supplements aided weight gain.

JUSTIFICATION FOR BODY WEIGHT AND
FAT LOSS IN ATHLETES

Coaches have been known to administer penalties to those athletes who don't conform to rigid body weight or fat requirements. Is it true that a lower body weight and lower body fat are advantageous to physical performance? Several correlational studies have shown that body weight and body fat are negatively related to performance in events such as the long jump, running sprints, and the mile run. For example, performances of 61 military recruits in the long jump and 75-yd dash were negatively correlated with body weight (−0.13 and −0.22, respectively) and even more closely with body fat (−0.61 and −0.52, respectively) (Riendeau et al., 1958). These subjects did not do any endurance tests, but Katch et al. (1973) evaluated the association of body fat to performance of a 12-min run in 36 college women. They found a similar negative correlation, −0.55, between body fat and performance but no relationship between body weight and distance covered. So, individuals with a leaner body composition tend to do better than fatter individuals for many events.

Not surprisingly, swimming performance is less associated with body weight or fat because the additional fat does not necessarily increase energy cost and may actually reduce it by improving buoyancy. Stager and Cordain (1984) compared the best swim times for 100 yd of 284 female swimmers age 12–17 y. The performance time was unrelated to percent body fat and only moderately predicted by lean body mass (r = −0.26).

It is important to note that even for the running or jumping events there is not a perfect correlation between performance and body fat or weight. Correlation is likely to be very high when comparing individuals with widely varying body weights and compositions but will be lower when comparing similar subjects. In other words, body fat is likely to be strongly correlated with performance of an endurance run if the range of body fat is 3%–30%. However, confining the sample to elite male athletes whose body fat range may be only 3–8% will show less association between performance and body fat. Many factors other than body weight and composition are involved in predicting performance at the elite level. There are clearly some individuals on every team having body fat at the higher end of the spectrum who perform better than the leanest athletes. In addition, the data defining an association between performance and body fat are from cross-sectional studies. Studies have not determined whether or not performance of the fatter runners, for example, improved when they lost body fat and weight.

NEGATIVE CONSEQUENCES TO WEIGHT LOSS IN ATHLETES

Dehydration Effects on Physiology

Horswill (1991) reviewed the effects of dehydration on health and performance of high-intensity exercise. Physiological changes occur even with small fluid deficits; decreases in plasma volume, stroke volume, and blood pressure, along with increases in heart rate, can occur with only a 2% reduction in body weight via dehydration. Thus, organs such as the kidney and muscles will receive less blood flow in a dehydrated state. The ability to sweat may also be compromised, causing problems with thermoregulation. Finally, copious sweat loss will result in depletion of body electrolytes, which may precipitate muscle cramping and fatigue. The severity of these changes rises as the magnitude of dehydration increases. Most of these changes are temporary and will be alleviated with fluid ingestion. However, dehydration of greater than 5% of body weight may increase susceptibility to heat exhaustion as physical effort continues in this state (Horswill, 1991).

Menstrual and Endocrine Disturbances

Female athletes have a high incidence of menstrual dysfunction, as defined as oligomenorrhea or amenorrhea. Because weight loss without exercise is known to influence the reproductive cycle, the "energy drain" hypothesis and metabolic changes that occur during negative energy balance have been suggested as explanations for menstrual changes in some athletes (DeSouza & Metzger, 1991). Kapen et al. (1981) presented a case report of a woman who lost 20 lb via dieting and developed secondary amenorrhea. Further hormonal analysis at 20-min intervals over the day showed a pattern of blood concentrations of luteinizing hormone (LH) similar to that seen at puberty. Once she had regained 75% of the weight lost, her 24-h LH pattern returned to that of an adult. Bullen et al.(1985) reported that women who lost weight (0.45 kg/wk) concurrent with a progressive increase in running distance were more likely to have changes in their cycles than were women who maintained their body weights during training. For example, 75% of the weight-loss group but only 33% of the weight-maintenance group lost their midcycle LH surges by the end of the two-menstrual-cycle training period. Seventy-five percent of the women who lost weight had delayed menstrual periods, compared to only 11% of those who did not lose weight.

Some studies comparing energy intake of women with menstrual abnormalities to those with eumenorrhea reported a lower energy intake in the former athletes. For example, Kaiserauer et al. (1989) found that amenorrheic runners reported consuming an average of 6530 kJ/d (1582 kcal/d), significantly below the 10,279 kJ/d (2490 kcal/d) of regularly menstruating women running a similar amount. Of course, there is a possibility of differential underreporting on diet records by members of these two groups.

Bonen et al.(1983) had women run on a treadmill for 60 min in a state of energy balance and after a 24-h fast. They found that plasma concentrations of hormones such as growth hormone and cortisol were higher during exercise when the women had been fasted. Some hormones, such as cortisol and beta-endorphin, cause negative feedback to the hypothalamus and can reduce the production of gonadotropin-releasing hormone (De Souza & Metzger, 1991). Thus, a link between reduced energy intake and menstrual change may be alterations in hormone levels during negative energy balance that may influence cyclicity.

We examined this hypothesis in female weight trainers because we had previously noted a higher incidence of menstrual irregularity in this population, along with a high degree of concern about food consumption and body fat (Walberg & Johnston, 1991). We had five eumenorrheic experienced resistance trainers do a controlled resistance bout while they were in energy balance and then when they were energy restricted to 2064 kJ/d (500 kcal/d) for 2 d (Walberg-Rankin et al., 1992). All tests were done during the luteal phase of the women's cycles on d 18 and 20. Blood was withdrawn before, immediately after, and up to 30 min after the bout. Analysis of serum beta-endorphin and estradiol indicated that concentrations of both hormones increased as a result of resistance exercise in energy balance. The increases for both hormones were greater when the women were in negative energy balance. This suggests that the acute changes in some anti-reproductive hormones that occur as a result of exercise may be more robust when women are losing weight. An increase in these hormones would be expected to reduce LH pulsatility and thus disrupt the normal pattern of reproductive hormones.

Williams et al.(1995) systematically studied the effects of acute energy restriction (60% of maintenance energy requirement) and/or dramatic increases in exercise on 24-h LH pulsatility in four eumenorrheic runners. Only energy restriction concurrent with increased exercise caused a change in LH pattern, a reduction in LH pulse frequency. Increased exercise alone had no effect on LH pattern. This is strong evidence for the important role of negative energy balance rather than of exercise alone in precipitating menstrual disturbance in female athletes.

There may also be hormonal effects of weight reduction in male athletes. One study evaluated blood concentrations of a variety of hormones in 19 male wrestlers at the peak of their competitive season and again two months after the end of the season (Straus et al., 1985). Serum concentration of testosterone and prolactin were significantly lower during the season than after the season and were correlated with body weight and fat. A later follow up to this study was performed on a single wrestler over two seasons (Strauss et al., 1993). As the collegiate wrestler's body fat fell to 4% during the season, serum testosterone, LH, thyroxine, estradiol, and prolactin concentrations fell to low levels, as did the subject's reported sexual activity. There was a high correlation between reductions in body weight and fat with all measured hormone concentrations and with sexual activity. The wrestler competed at a higher weight class the next year, requiring less weight loss during this season. Testosterone as well as reported sexual activity remained at pre season levels during this second season.

In summary, efforts to lose weight with energy restriction are likely to reduce reproductive hormone levels in both male and female athletes. This may be expressed as menstrual disorders in women and reduced hormone concentrations and sexual interest in men. The reproductive dysfunction is probably explained by changes in the hypothalamic-pituitary axis, possibly via increases in anti-reproductive hormones that occur as a result of negative energy balance alone or concurrent with exercise. Increases in energy intake and weight are likely to stimulate the return to normal hormone levels and menstrual patterns.

A potentially negative effect of prolonged periods of menstrual disruption, reduced bone mineralization, may not be totally reversible. Drinkwater et al. (1990) assessed the bone mineral density of female athletes along with their present and past menstrual patterns. There was a linear relationship between bone mineral and incidence of menstrual disturbance when patterns in the past and at present were combined. This suggests that there may be residual effects of menstrual dysfunction on bone strength in women.

Reduced Lean Body Mass

Those who treat obesity with energy restriction know that loss of lean body mass is likely if a substantial loss of body weight occurs. For example, Yang and Van Itallie (1976) calculated that the weight lost over 10 d of a 3302 kJ/d (800 kcal/d) mixed diet was about 60% fat and 40% lean mass. Using the nitrogen balance technique, these researchers estimated that most of the lean mass loss in the obese subjects was water, 37%, but that body protein contributed 3.4% of the total weight loss over the 10 d.

Amino acids such as alanine are good substrates for liver gluconeogenesis to provide glucose to the body when carbohydrate intake and stores are low. The source of these amino acids is not entirely clear but could at least partly come from breakdown of muscle enzymes or contractile proteins. Russell et al. (1984) observed significant muscle fiber atrophy and necrosis in obese women who consumed 1674.4 kJ (400 kcal)/d for 2 wk.

Short-term net losses of body protein were evident in athletes undergoing resistance training during 7 d of a hypoenergy diet (73.3 kJ/kg) containing the RDA for protein (Walberg et al., 1988). However, because the body adapts over time to energy restriction by reducing the breakdown of amino acids, these athletes were nearly in nitrogen balance on the seventh day of the study. Thus, repeated dieting for 3–4 d may be more detrimental to the maintenance of lean body mass than is sustained, moderate energy restriction.

Reduction in total lean body mass has been noted for bodybuilders who are chronically reducing their energy intakes in preparation for a contest. Hydrodensitometry assessment of the male subject studied by Hickson et al.(1990) for the month prior to the competition showed that 2.3 kg of the 7.1 kg total weight loss was fat-free mass (in spite of admitted anabolic steroid use). Heyward et al. (1989) studied 9 male and 12 female bodybuilders before competition (6–17 wk prior to and just before competition). The average lean body mass fell by 1.3 kg over the measurement period, with 75% of the bodybuilders losing lean tissue during this dieting phase. Those bodybuilders from this group who lost the most lean mass consumed the fewest calories. Thus, the belief that a high protein diet and substantial resistance training can prevent lean tissue loss is erroneous.

Lean body mass loss has been observed in wrestlers during their season. Park et al. (1990) noted a reduction (3 kg) in fat-free mass over the scholastic wrestling season. Melby et al. (1990) also measured an average 4.5 kg reduction in fat-free mass in collegiate wrestlers during their season, but their average lean mass rose to preseason values by 5 6 wk after the wrestling season. High school wrestlers studied over their season as well as 3.5 months after the season showed less gain in arm muscle area and peak power over their season than did recreationally active controls (Roemmich & Sinning, 1996). However, these variables rebounded to or were higher than pre-season levels at the post-season assessment.

Parents are often concerned that the growth of athletes involved in "making weight" will be permanently impaired. Theintz et al. (1989, 1993) addressed this issue by examining the growth patterns of 12–13 year old elite female gymnasts (a sports group known to frequently consume low energy diets) and trained swimmers. The gymnasts had been training for approximately 5 y, whereas the swimmers had begun training about 3 y prior to the study. Examination of the athletes showed that the gymnasts were lighter than swimmers but that their growth was appropriate based on parental heights and growth history. These athletes were followed for a mean of 2.35 y to determine if the continued training affected growth. A stunting of leg-length growth and an attenuation of the increase in bone age was noted in gymnasts relative to swimmers. Predicted height based on bone age did not change over the measurement period for swimmers but declined for gymnasts. The authors concluded that intensive gymnastics training might stunt growth such that final height does not reach genetic potential. Because this study did not assess diet, it is not clear if these negative effects on growth were due to excessive exercise or to a poor diet of the gymnasts. However, it suggests that further research should be done to clarify the effects of weight loss on growth in adolescent athletes.

These studies illustrate that it is unlikely that a reduction in lean body mass can be prevented when there is substantial total weight loss. However, the lean tissue will likely be regained when energy intake and body weight rise.

Metabolic Rate

The literature regarding obesity treatment illustrates that a reduction in basal metabolic rate is expected with energy restriction. For example, our laboratory observed an 8% drop in resting metabolic rate (RMR) within 1 wk and about a 20% reduction after 4 wk on an average energy intake of 2188 kJ/d (530 kcal/d) in obese women (Mathieson et al., 1986). The reduction in (RMR) may be partially explained by the reduction in lean body mass mentioned above. However, because the drop in metabolic rate is typically greater than could be explained by lean body mass change, other factors, including changes in thyroid hormone concentrations, have been implicated (Mathieson et al., 1986).

The effect of energy restriction on (RMR) and changes in thyroid hormones in athletes has not been thoroughly studied. Only McCargar et al.(1993) measured thyroid hormones as well as RMR in athletes losing weight. The RMR and T3 of lightweight female rowers assessed before, during, and after their season followed a similar pattern in that there was a significant decrease in both factors during peak season with a rebound at the post-season measurement. This coincided with a 4.2 kg reduction in body weight during the season and a 4.0 kg regain after the season. Other experimenters have examined thyroid hormone changes but not RMR during weight loss in wrestlers. Strauss et al. (1985) reported that, along with a reduction in body weight and fat, serum thyroxine concentration tended to decrease in a group of 18 collegiate wrestlers during their competitive season (7.9 ng/dL) compared to 5 mo after the season (9.1 ng/dL). A subsequent case study of one wrestler whose hormone concentrations were measured many times over his competitive season showed a reduction in thyroxine that correlated significantly with weight loss (r = 0.69) and body-fat loss (r = 0.77) (Straus et al., 1993). McCargar and Crawford (1992) assessed wrestlers about 6 wk prior to their first competition, near the end of the season, and 5 mo after the season. Serum T3 fell over time, with the pre-season concentration significantly higher than that during the offseason.

Weight cycling, repeated cycles of weight loss and gain, has been a focus of research in the obesity literature. It has been suggested that weight gain after a period of energy restriction is likely to replace more fat than lean tissue—ultimately causing a reduction in resting energy needs. Repeated cycles of weight loss followed by gain may make future weight loss efforts more difficult due to a reduction in total lean body mass and thus metabolic rate. Data to support this theory came mainly from cross-sectional studies using obese subjects categorized as "weight cyclers" and "non-weight cyclers". It was tempting to ascribe the observed lower basal metabolic rate in the weight cyclers to a response to repeated dieting and gain. However, an alternative theory is that the "weight cyclers" may have started with a lower inherited metabolic rate, and this contributes to their repeated efforts to lose weight. Most of the more recent longitudinal studies have not found that weight cycling has a permanent effect on basal metabolic rate. For example, Jebb et al. (1991) had 11 obese women lose weight for three periods of 2 wk each, separated by 4 wk of ad libitum feeding. RMR returned to baseline during each of the ad libitum periods and was not different from baseline at the end of the three cycles.

Another hypothesis was that weight cycling in wrestlers precipitated a higher body fat and lower metabolic rate over time. Early work by Steen et al. (1988) divided high school wrestlers into weight cyclers and noncyclers based on their self-reported weight loss history. Measurement of resting metabolic rate indicated that the cyclers had 14% lower resting energy expenditures, in spite of similar body weights and compositions. As in the obesity research area, longitudinal studies did not support the weight-cycling hypothesis. Melby et al. (1990) measured resting metabolic rates in wrestlers over a season when they were repeatedly losing and gaining weight. Although RMR was reduced during the season while the wrestlers were actively losing weight, there was no difference in RMR after the season ended, compared to that prior to the competition period. This laboratory continued to evaluate these wrestlers over a second wrestling season (Schmidt et al., 1993) and compared them to a group of noncycling wrestlers. No difference in RMR was observed between the groups. In addition, both wrestling groups had higher RMR than did noncycling, nonwrestling controls. These data suggest that the brief weight loss and gain cycles in wrestlers do not have a permanent effect on metabolic efficiency. Some of the discrepancies in the results of studies may relate to contradictory effects of different weight loss methods on RMR, i.e., dehydration tends to increase RMR, whereas energy restriction reduces RMR.

It is still possible bodybuilders and other athletes who undergo longer periods of energy restriction may experience a change in lean body mass and, therefore, RMR. Unfortunately, there has not been a systematic analysis of the effect of chronic dieting on RMR in athletes such as bodybuilders.

Immune Function

Immune function is sensitive to reductions in energy intake. For example, severe protein-energy malnutrition impairs most immune system functions and increases susceptibility to infection (Chandra, 1991). Treatment of obesity with very-low-energy diets has been shown to decrease mitogen-stimulated lymphocyte proliferation (Field et al., 1991). It is unclear in many of these studies whether the low energy or the lower vitamin and mineral intake is responsible for the immune deficits.

Nieman et al. (1996) reported a detrimental effect of more moderate energy restriction and weight loss in obese women with maintenance of micronutrient intake. A loss of 9.9 kg over 12 wk in 13 obese women who used energy restriction caused significant impairments in several markers of immune function. For example, total counts of leukocytes, neutrophils, monocytes, and natural killer cells decreased for the obese but did not change for the normal-weight control subjects over the 12 wk. Phagocytosis, B-cell counts and T-cell counts were not changed by weight loss. Because micronutrient intake was not significantly depressed during the weight loss period, the experimenters ascribed the immune system changes to weight loss rather than to poor nutrient intake.

One study has shown that energy restriction in athletes depresses cell-mediated immunity (Kono et al., 1988). Nine female swimmers were asked to consume a 5366 kJ/d (1300 kcal/d) diet over 2 wk. Coinciding with a 2-kg reduction in body weight, an approximate 10% reduction in phagocytic response of monocytes to zymosan and sheep erythrocytes containing IgG was observed. On the other hand, no significant changes were observed for lymphocyte production of IgG, IgA, or IgM after weight loss. These changes suggest that energy restriction may reduce the athletes' cell-mediated defense against some microorganisms and potentially result in more illnesses. It is important to point out that the swimmers' phagocytic responses were still slightly greater than those for controls after weight loss. No data are currently available to support or refute the hypothesis of increased illness in athletes who consume insufficient energy.

Both the latter two studies illustrate that moderate dietary restriction resulting in weight loss of less than 1 kg/wk was associated with depression of the immune system. It is possible that the more restricted diets used by some athletes may have more severe effects on immunity.

Vitamin and Mineral Status

Inadequate intake of micronutrients is more likely as the energy content and the variety of foods consumed is reduced. We found that diet records completed by female bodybuilders showed that the frequency of dietary intakes less than 67% of the RDA for vitamins and minerals increased as competition approached. The vitamins for which consumption was most often inadequate in prior to the bodybuilding competitions were vitamins A, B12, C, and folate. Reported mineral intake was even less optimal than that for vitamins. Minerals most likely to be found in suboptimal amounts in the diet records were, in order: zinc, calcium, copper, and magnesium. The calcium intake was particularly problematic because the intake of calcium was substantially less than the RDA for all measurement periods during the month prior to competition for all women. (Walberg-Rankin et al., 1993). Other research groups have also reported poor micronutrient intake, especially calcium, of female bodybuilders during preparation for competition (Heyward et al., 1989, Kleiner et al., 1990, Lamar-Hildebrand et al., 1989, Sandoval et al., 1989). Most of these studies, as well as ours, reported that these low intakes disappeared during the postcompetition diet when energy intake and the variety of foods chosen increased. Thus, the low vitamin and mineral intakes are due partly to reduced energy intake and partly to avoidance of certain foods (e.g., milk and red meat).

Not surprisingly, the average in-season wrestler's food intake is inadequate for numerous micronutrients. Steen and McKinney (1986) analyzed the diets of wrestlers during their wrestling season. The 4-d records included the 2 d before a match, the day of the match, and the day after the match. Thirty percent of the 42 college wrestlers consumed a diet with less than 67% of the RDA for vitamin C; the respective proportions for other micronutrients were: 48% vitamin A, 81% B6, 31% thiamin, 27% iron, 64% magnesium, 52% zinc. It should be noted that these percentages might be even worse if only the weight loss days were computed (i.e., these data also include the day after the match, which is likely to be high in energy intake).

It is emphasized again that food records are known to have limitations and may not accurately portray the dietary intake of an individual. In addition, low nutrient intakes do not guarantee biochemical and functional impairment because the true nutrient requirement of some individuals is well below the RDA. Thus, it is important to confirm biochemical nutrient status in athletes involved in weight loss. In one of the few studies to actually test biochemical nutrient status in athletes, Horswill et al. (1990b) found over the competitive season in wrestlers a reduction in pre-albumin and retinol-binding protein, which are plasma proteins used as indicators of protein status. They also observed a decrease in the ratio of essential to total amino acids. The relative changes in body fat were correlated with the changes in pre-albumin and retinol-binding protein.

Folgelholm et al. (1993) examined micronutrient intake and biochemical status in male judo competitors and wrestlers who either lost weight rapidly using energy restriction along with dehydration over 2.4 d or reduced weight more gradually with energy restriction alone over 3 wk. Micronutrient intake was less than 100% of the Nordic recommendations for thiamin, riboflavin, magnesium, iron, and zinc during the rapid procedure; only zinc was slightly below recommended levels during the gradual procedure. Interestingly, evaluation of blood biochemistry revealed that B6 and magnesium status deteriorated during the gradual but not the rapid weight loss procedure. Unfortunately, the authors did not report the B6 intake during the gradual weight loss, but the magnesium intake was not significantly different during the gradual weight loss procedure, compared to baseline intake. Thus, at least the deterioration of magnesium status was not secondary to reduced intake of that nutrient during energy restriction; negative energy balance and weight loss themselves had a negative effect on nutrient status. Biochemical indicators of thiamin (erythrocyte-TKAC), riboflavin (erythrocyte-GRAC), iron (serum ferritin), potassium (serum potassium), and zinc (serum zinc) were not influenced by either weight loss regimen.

In summary, changes in diet designed for weight loss typically cause a reduction in consumption of a variety of micronutrients. A limited amount of research suggests that weight loss impairs biochemical status of some nutrients. Additional research on biochemical indicators of nutritional status would be valuable to predict potential functional problems associated with weight loss in athletes.

Mood

Several negative effects on psychological status have been confirmed in chronically dieting athletes. Lightweight football players claimed that their weight control efforts caused interference with their thought and extracurricular activities "often" or "always" (Depalma et al., 1993). The bodybuilder studied by Steen (1990) over 6 mo reported feeling "angry, hostile and irritable" during the dieting period before his competition. Moods of eight other bodybuilders were assessed three times over 12 wk of dieting for a competition (Newton et al., 1993). The vigor scale of the Profile of Mood States (POMS) questionnaire showed significant reductions, and depression, as measured by the Beck Depression Inventory, became significantly elevated as the duration of dieting progressed.

Horswill et al. (1990a) used the POMS to examine psychological effects of short-term dieting in wrestlers. Scores for confusion, depression, anger, fatigue, and tension were significantly increased, whereas vigor dropped after 4 d of energy restriction. On average, when they had been dieting the athletes also had a higher personal assessment of effort (Rating of Perceived Exertion (RPE)) after a high-intensity, intermittent arm crank test. Even 27 h of fasting caused significant increases in the POMS scores for fatigue in male marathon runners (Nieman et al., 1987). Also, the RPE of the runners was higher throughout a run to exhaustion at 70% of $\dot{V}O_2$max. Thus, dieting for weight loss is likely to cause deterioration of mood and increase perceived difficulty of an exercise session.

Performance

The effect of weight loss on physical performance is inconsistent among studies. It is difficult to compare the effects of weight loss on performance because different weight loss methods (dehydration, energy restriction, or both), lengths of weight loss (ranging from hours to months), and performance tests were used. This discussion will emphasize those studies that involved energy restriction with only a brief discussion of dehydration because that has been fully reviewed elsewhere (see Fogelholm, 1994, Horswill, 1991).

Dehydration and Exercise Performance. Dehydration is known to impair aerobic exercise performance. For example, $\dot{V}O_2$max decreased by 3%, and time to complete a 10,000-m run increased 6.7% when diuretics were used to reduce body weights of competitive runners (Armstrong et al., 1985). The decrement in performance of the endurance run was correlated with the reductions in body weight of the subjects. This is a classic illustration of the detrimental effect of dehydration on aerobic performance.

The reported effects of dehydration on anaerobic exercise performance are mixed. Viitasalo et al. (1987) reported a 7.8% reduction in isometric strength in athletes dehydrated via sauna but a significant increase in mechanical power tested using the vertical jump after diuretic use. Jacobs (1980) found no effect of dehydration via sauna on a 30-s Wingate test in college wrestlers.

Energy Restriction Alone or with Dehydration. *Aerobic Performance.* Short-term energy restriction with dehydration has either been observed to have no effect (Houston et al.,1981) or a detrimental effect

(Webster et al.,1990) on $\dot{V}O_2$max. However, some animal research has actually reported an ergogenic benefit of energy restriction on aerobic endurance. Rats fasted for 24 h ran longer before exhaustion than did fed rats (Dohm et al., 1983). A suggested mechanism for this enhancement of performance was the Randle effect; the increase in fat utilization may slow body depletion of carbohydrate and thus delay exhaustion.

Several studies have examined whether or not there is a similar ergogenic effect of fasting in humans. It appears that humans react differently than rats because both cycling and running endurance are impaired with short-term fasting. Loy et al. (1986) had competitive cyclists fast for 24 h and ride at either 86% or 79% of $\dot{V}O_2$max until exhaustion. Although some of the metabolic effects of the brief fast, e.g., maintenance of initial muscle glycogen and increased plasma fatty acid levels, suggest improved metabolic state for endurance exercise, fatigue occurred more rapidly when the athletes were fasted. Fatigue appeared to coincide with depleted bodily carbohydrate reserves; hypoglycemia and muscle glycogen depletion were observed when the athletes could not maintain power outputs equivalent to 65% $\dot{V}O_2$max.

Similar results were seen by Nieman et al. (1987) in their study of 27-h-fasted marathon runners. Time to exhaustion at 70% $\dot{V}O_2$max was reduced by almost 45% in the fasting condition. The fast in this study tended to reduce initial muscle glycogen by 17%, but this was not statistically significant. Although the fasting enhanced fat utilization, this did not translate to lower muscle glycogen utilization during the run. The metabolic cause for fatigue was unclear because none of the metabolites or hormone changes correlated with fatigue. The authors concluded that there was no clear metabolic explanation for the reduction in endurance performance with fasting; it was likely a result of a combination of metabolic and psychological factors (e.g., increased perception of fatigue).

Anaerobic Performance. Several studies have reported significant reductions in muscle strength after short-term energy restriction. A study from our laboratory examined the effect of 10 d of energy restriction on peak torque in a five-repetition isokinetic test for elbow flexion and knee extension. The hypoenergy diet resulted in 3.3 kg of weight loss and approximately an 8% reduction in peak torque for both biceps brachii and quadriceps muscles (Walberg-Rankin et al. 1994). Houston et al. (1981) also used an isokinetic device to test muscle force development following weight loss in athletes. They observed a significant reduction in peak quadriceps torque produced at the slowest speed, 30°/s, within 48 h of a weight-loss period in wrestlers. The quadriceps strength remained depressed during 48 additional hours of weight loss.

Webster et al. (1990) observed a reduction in upper body (chest press and latissimus pull) but not lower body strength as measured with a hydraulic resistance machine after 36 h of self-imposed dehydration and energy restriction (average 4458 kJ/d (1080 kcal/d), with no food for the 12 h immediately prior to the testing). A reduction in maximal leg isometric force production was evident in athletes who lost weight with a combination of diet restriction and diuretic (Viitasalo et al., 1987). These studies show that acute weight loss via energy restriction alone or with dehydration can reduce maximal muscle force development in athletes.

Muscle endurance was also compromised in male weight trainers who lost 3.8 kg over 7 d of a formulated, hypoenergy diet (Walberg-Rankin et al., 1988). Quadriceps endurance, as measured by the fall in force development during 10 repeated isometric contractions, was significantly lower in a group who consumed a 50% carbohydrate diet with 74.3 kJ/kg (18 kcal). Biceps brachii isometric endurance was unaffected by this diet (Figure 5-1).

Another study in our laboratory measured a significant increase in biceps endurance after 10 d of energy restriction in resistance trainers

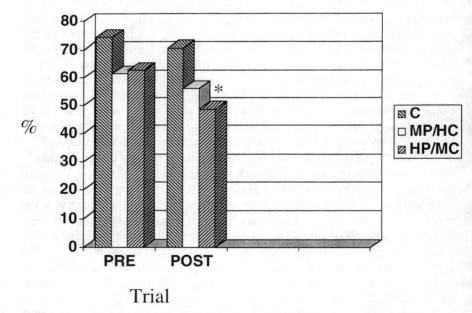

FIGURE 5-1. *Quadriceps endurance ratio before and after energy restriction in resistance trainers. Values are means ± SEM. Ratio is calculated by dividing the total area under the torque curve for the last two of ten contractions by that from the first two contractions. C = control; MP/HC moderate protein with high carbohydrate; HP/MC = high protein with moderate carbohydrate.*

(Walberg-Rankin et al., 1994). However, because peak torque was reduced in these athletes, there may have been a confounding effect on endurance ratio, i.e., the initial force for the first of the repeated contractions was lower after energy restriction and thus easier to maintain.

Two studies that assessed vertical jump ability after energy restriction reported increases in muscle power (Fogelholm et al., 1993, Viitasalo et al.. 1987). In the first study, subjects who lost weight over 3 wk with modest energy restriction were able to jump higher when loaded with 50% of their body weight during the vertical jump test than they did before weight loss. The fact that the athletes had lost 5% of their body weight over this time contributed to their ability to jump higher. It is important to note that the athletes in this study were given a 5-h "refeeding" period between the weight loss and the performance test. Thus, some short-term changes concurrent with energy restriction could have been overcome during the recovery period.

Some of the studies have incorporated a Wingate-type test of 30–60 s in length. Two studies using Wingate tests of 30 or 40 s (McMurray et al., 1991, Webster et al., 1990) in wrestlers during weight loss showed reductions in total work done. Two studies using tests of approximately 1 min (Fogelholm et al., 1993, Houston et al., 1981) detected no effect of weight loss on performance.

An intermittent-intensity arm crank test was developed by Hickner et al. (1991) to improve the specificity of tests designed to mimic a wrestling match. The original test involved alternating bouts of 15 s of maximal-effort isokinetic cranking and 30 s of low-intensity cranking for a total of eight cycles. Consumption of a liquid diet of 102.8 kJ/kg (24.9 kcal/kg) for 3 d caused a significant reduction in the total work done during the high-intensity intervals. Use of an identical test by Horswill et al.(1990a) also showed a lower total sprint work done by wrestlers who had lost 6.3% body weight over 4 d of an energy restricted diet. In both of these studies the wrestlers used dehydration as well as energy restriction to reduce their body weights. Our laboratory had collegiate wrestlers lose weight using only energy restriction for 3 d. We used a modification of the test developed by Hickner et al. (1991) (eight bouts of 15 s of maximal-effort cranking against a resistance of 0.04 kg/kg body weight followed by 20 s unloaded cranking)and found a 7.6% reduction in total work done by the wrestlers during the high-intensity segments of the test in the negative energy balance state (unpublished, Figure 5-2)

Mechanisms explaining performance impairment during energy restriction might include reduction in energy stores (e.g., glycogen or phosphocreatine), changes in enzyme activity, modification of the function of the sarcoplasmic reticulum, or structural alterations in the mus-

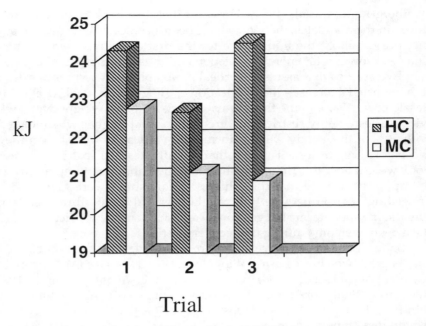

FIGURE 5-2. *Total work done by wrestlers during the high-intensity intervals of the performance test performed before (Trial 1) and after (Trial 2) weight loss and after a 5-h refeeding period (Trial 3). The performance during Trial 2 for both groups was significantly less than that during Trial 1. The interaction between Trials and Groups was not significant (P = 0.10). HC = high-carbohydrate refeeding diet; MC = moderate carbohydrate refeeding diet.*

cle. Few studies on energy-restricted athletes have evaluated these factors. Research examining impairments of muscle function in obese individuals during weight loss is useful for discussion of possible effects in athletes because more sophisticated analyses of muscle function and biochemistry have been performed in studies of obese individuals. For example, the potential mechanisms for the reduction in maximal electrically-stimulated force production after 2 wk of a 1651 kJ/d (400 kcal/d) diet in energy-restricted obese individuals (Russel et al., 1983) included reductions in the activities of various enzymes involved in ATP generation and disturbances in electrolytes and other minerals. Intracellular sodium and potassium were decreased, while calcium concentration was elevated. Thus, change in calcium transfer between the sarcoplasmic reticulum and the cytosol may have influenced force generation capacity. Structural changes, such as reductions in the number and size of type-II muscle fibers, loose and collapsed basement membranes, and less distinct Z bands, were also present in muscle biopsies from the energy-restricted patients (Russel et al., 1984).

Similar histochemical measurements have not been done on muscles from athletes undergoing energy restriction to see if these changes might coincide with performance decrements. Only Houston et al. (1981) took muscle biopsies from the athletes before and after weight loss. Their analyses of the fuel stores in muscle biopsies from the wrestlers who lost weight over 4 d showed that muscle glycogen, but not concentrations of phosphocreatine or ATP, were significantly reduced at the same time that the peak quadriceps torque was impaired. However, reduced muscle glycogen is unlikely to be the limiting factor for performance of just five maximal muscle contractions. Other factors that may have played a part in muscle force generation were not measured.

In summary, short-term weight loss using energy restriction is likely to cause decrements in maximal muscle strength and power tests, impairments for tests of maximal effort of 30–40 s, no effect for tests lasting approximately 1 min, and decrements when maximal efforts of 15–20 s are repeated with short recovery (20–30 s) between efforts. This suggests that anaerobic events that rely primarily on phosphocreatine for fuel are more likely to be impaired by energy restriction than are those depending more on anaerobic glycolysis. Effects of longer-term energy restriction on physical performance in athletes have not been well studied.

DETERMINING BODY WEIGHT GOALS

Decisions on appropriate body weight and fat for athletes should be made based on body composition, not just on height and weight data. This avoids the situation in which a heavy but lean individual is told to achieve some arbitrary weight. It is critical to use personnel experienced in the body composition assessment technique to obtain reliable readings. Standardized technique and equations for skinfold measurement have been published (Lohman et al., 1988). A body fat goal can be developed for the athlete based on the body composition assessment, realistic expectations (i.e., rate of weight loss should not be greater than 0.5-1 kg/wk), and ranges of optimal body fat for the sport. Body fat ranges have been suggested, but they are based more on common sense and averages for elite athletes than on specific performance data. In general, the goal of female athletes should not be less than 12–14% body fat and that of males not less than 5–7% body fat (American College of Sports Medicine, 1996). The higher end of the body fat spectrum for athletes tends to be about 15% for males and 18% for females. An equation that can be used to calculate a body weight goal once current body composition and goal body composition have been established is presented in Table 5-1.

TABLE 5-1. *Calculation of body-weight goal when considering body composition in a program of weight loss.*

1. Analyze body composition to estimate current percent body fat and percent lean mass.
2. Estimate the percent body fat and percent lean mass that are appropriate for the sport, for optimal health; ensure also that a reasonable rate of weight loss will accomplish these goals.
3. Divide the current lean body mass (kg) by the desired percent of lean body mass (expressed as a decimal fraction). Multiply this quotient by 100 to obtain the desired body weight. *(These calculations assume that all of the lost weight will be fat tissue.)*

Leaders in the sport of wrestling have tried to limit inappropriate weight standards and weight loss practices. The American College of Sports Medicine (1996) has produced a revised position stand on this topic to discourage unhealthy weight loss in wrestlers. One state, Wisconsin, has extended the efforts to make wrestling a safer sport by initiating the Wrestler Minimum Weight Project (WMWP) in 1989 (Oppliger et al., 1995a). This project, initiated by the Wisconsin Interscholastic Athletic Association, recommended some guidelines on minimum weight and maximum weight loss as well as a nutrition education program. Specifically, the organization used 7% as the minimum body fat and no more than 3 lb of weight lost per week as the requirements for wrestling eligibility. This required implementation of consistent and valid body composition procedures among teams. A training program for testers using the skinfold technique and an equation validated on wrestlers was developed. The certified testers analyze the body composition of all high school wrestlers in the state before the first competition and send this information to the state office in order to allow the wrestler to compete during the season. This information determines the minimum weight class for each wrestler.

Nutrition education was recognized as a critical part of this project. The Wisconsin Interscholastic Athletic Association solicited the input from the Wisconsin Dietetic Association and the Wisconsin Department of Public Instruction to develop a nutrition education module that could be presented by dietitians trained in the program. Oppliger et al. (1995b) reviewed the changes in weight-loss practices in the sport after two years of the new rules. The average for most weight lost, weekly weight cycled, and the longest fast were significantly reduced in a sample of high school wrestlers following the implementation of the new rules. It is interesting that although more than 60% of coaches were initially opposed to the program, over 95% were supportive of the program several years after it was in place (Opplinger et al., 1995a). This program illustrates that rule changes along with education can reduce the practice of extreme weight loss in athletes.

RECOMMENDATIONS FOR WEIGHT LOSS

Nutrition

Dehydration for weight loss cannot be recommended due to previously mentioned potential adverse effects on health as well as performance. In addition, the use of drug-assisted dehydration is banned by the NCAA and International Olympic Committee. Even use of heat exposure for dehydration is banned by some sport governing bodies (e.g., National Federation of High School Associations and NCAA wrestling championships) (Horswill, 1991).

Energy restriction, if modest, can be recommended to reduce body weight and fat. Ideally, moderate energy reduction should occur prior to the start of the season so that performance impairments during negative energy balance do not occur during competition. Typically, the maximum rate of weight loss recommended is 0.5–1.0 kg/wk. This translates into energy restriction of 2064–4128 kJ/d (500–1000 kcal/d) or a more modest restriction along with an increase in energy expenditure via added activity. Quicker weight loss than this is likely to result in some or all of the negative consequences discussed in this chapter.

Several studies have demonstrated the value of a high-carbohydrate weight-loss diet in athletes. The wrestlers studied by Horswill et al. (1990a) and by McMurray et al. (1991) could maintain high-power performance on a high-carbohydrate, hypoenergy diet of 66% and 70%, respectively; performance was impaired in the same athletes when they consumed 41% or 55% carbohydrate, respectively. Horswill et al. (1990a) speculated that the differences in performance with different diets was associated with an effect on body acid load. During energy restriction, especially when carbohydrate is low, ketone bodies that increase hydrogen ion concentration are produced. The body may be less able to handle the additional acid load when lactate accumulates during anaerobic exercise. Horswill et al. (1990a) observed that resting base excess was significantly lower after weight loss on the lower, compared to the higher, carbohydrate diet. A practical suggestion would be to recommend athletes consume at least 60–70% of their energy as carbohydrate while dieting.

Protein requirements increase during negative energy balance. This is particularly true during the initial week of weight loss because some of the ingested amino acids will be oxidized and/or converted to glucose due to reduced carbohydrate stores. We found that although ingestion of a hypoenergy diet with the RDA for protein (0.8 g/kg) resulted in a substantially negative nitrogen balance, consumption of twice that amount of protein during weight loss maintained net body nitrogen

(Walberg-Rankin et al., 1988). Another study found that resistance trainers consuming 1.2 g/kg protein were in nitrogen balance during energy restriction (Walberg-Rankin et al., 1994). This suggests that protein intake during weight reduction should be at least 1.2 g/kg to preserve body nitrogen. A list of practical suggestions for diet modifications for weight reduction is provided in Table 5-2.

Exercise

Aerobic exercise of long duration has typically been recommended for weight reduction of obese individuals and athletes to increase both energy expenditure and fat utilization. Thus, assuming the athlete has the time, additional aerobic activity can help to create the negative energy balance. Body builders, for example, typically add aerobic activity to their workouts as the competition approaches to accelerate body fat loss. Of course, additional exercise in an athlete who is already very active may increase the risk of overuse injuries.

A provocative Canadian cross-sectional survey suggests that the optimal exercise prescription for weight loss may be different from that typically prescribed (Tremblay et al., 1990). The investigators found that those individuals reporting higher intensity exercise had less body fat than those claiming they did moderate intensity activity. Later this group did a longitudinal study of the value of high intensity exercise for body fat loss. Tremblay et al. (1994) compared the effects of constant intensity cycling at 60% heart rate reserve (HRR) [60% HRR = resting heart + 0.6 (maximal HR-resting HR)], eventually progressing to 75% HRR, four times per week over 20 wk, to a cycling regime that included high-intensity interval training in normal-weight untrained males. Although neither program significantly altered body weight, the interval-trained group tended to have a greater reduction in body fat, as assessed by sum of six skinfold measurements. The total estimated energy cost of the interval training program was less than that of the constant intensity program. Thus, the decrease in body fat in relation to energy cost of the exercise program was significantly greater for the interval-trained group.

TABLE 5-2. *Practical tips for losing body weight.*

---

1. Reduce energy intake by about 2064 kJ/d (500 kcal/d).
   - Reduce the sizes of portions.
   - Increase the intake of fiber to 25-35 g/d.
   - Substitute lower- for higher-energy snacks.
   - Increase consumption of fruits and vegetables.
2. Consume 60-70% of energy as carbohydrate.
3. Consume 1.4-2.0 g protein per kilogram body weight daily.
4. Consider using a regular multivitamin/mineral supplement.
5. Participate regularly in aerobic exercise.

An interesting additional piece of evidence for the value of the interval training program for body fat reduction was the greater increase in activity of the muscle enzyme, hydroxyacyl-coenzyme A dehydrogenase, for the interval training group relative to the group who did constant-intensity activity. This suggests a greater capacity to oxidize fatty acids in the interval-trained group than in the constant-intensity group. Additional work needs to be done examining the potential benefits of interval and high-intensity exercise for weight loss.

NUTRITIONAL RECOMMENDATIONS FOR RECOVERY FROM BODY WEIGHT LOSS

Generally, athletes who "make weight" to prepare for a competitive weight division (e.g., wrestlers or weight lifters) have a specified interval between the weigh-in and the competition during which there is an opportunity to address dehydration, fuel depletion, and negative energy balance. This depends on the sport and the circumstances of the competition, with the period varying from 1-24 h. The exception is horse racing, where jockeys are required to weigh-in after their rides. In wrestling, the recovery period may be as brief as 1 h or as long as 24 h, depending on the match and the weight class. Houston et al. (1981) tested the muscle strength of wrestlers after 3 d of weight loss and again after 3 h of ad libitum food and fluid consumption. Because quadriceps strength as well as muscle glycogen remained depressed, 3 h was not enough time to recover from the negative effects of weight loss. However, there was no measurement or control over diet during this period. It is possible that they did not choose an optimal diet for quick recovery.

Another study refutes the belief that a short rehydration period will allow athletes to fully replace body water and any performance deficits. Burge et al. (1993) had lightweight rowers reduce body weight by an average of 5.4% within 24 h, using fluid and food restriction as well as exercise while wearing waterproof clothing. All athletes were given 1.5 L of water over a 2-h rehydration period. Both plasma volume and muscle glycogen concentration were reduced following the water ingestion, compared to values prior to the weight loss. Assessment of rowing performance using a rowing protocol designed to simulate a 2000-m race demonstrated that performance was significantly impaired after the recovery period relative to that before weight loss. Unfortunately, diet was not measured, so it is unclear how much of these changes were due to dehydration versus food restriction. Also, superior recovery may have been possible if food as well as fluid had been provided during the recovery period.

It is possible that a longer time is required for recovery after severe, acute weight loss. Fogelholm et al. (1993) allowed wrestlers and judo athletes to consume food and fluids ad libitum for 5 h after either a rapid 2.4-d or a gradual 3-wk weight-loss period and before a battery of performance tests. None of the high-power performance tests showed impairment of the athletes' abilities following weight loss. However, because performance was not tested without the refeeding period, it is not known if there was an effect of weight loss without the recovery feedings.

The 17-h recovery period offered to the wrestlers studied by Tarnopolsky et al. (1996) appears to be adequate to replace muscle glycogen. Wrestlers in this study who lost 5% of their body weights using energy and fluid restriction had a 54% reduction in muscle glycogen content. However, wrestlers who were allowed to refeed for 17 h following the weight loss had normal muscle glycogen concentrations.

We found that the performance of collegiate wrestlers after 72 h of a hypoenergy formula diet (74.3 kJ/kg) was depressed by 7.6% (Walberg Rankin et al., 1996). For 5 h following the 72-h low energy diet, half of the wrestlers were provided with a formulated refeeding diet of 86.7 kJ/kg (21 kcal/kg) with 75% carbohydrate, and the others consumed a 47% carbohydrate diet. For example, at controlled intervals over the 5-h refeeding period, a 70-kg subject received a total of 275 g of carbohydrate if in the high-carbohydrate group or 173 g of carbohydrate if in the moderate-carbohydrate group. Work done during the arm crank test was 99.1% and 91.5% of the baseline performance in the high and moderate carbohydrate groups, respectively (P = 0.1 for the interaction between groups across time) (Figure 5-2). This study, together with the previously mentioned experiments, suggests that carbohydrate is important to performance, not only for the weight loss diet but also for the recovery diet. It remains to be seen if the composition of the diet is critical when recovery time is longer than 5 h.

We were curious about the actual diet consumed by wrestlers after their weigh-ins. Six collegiate and ten high-school wrestlers were asked to keep records of food consumed between their weigh ins and the matches (Pesce et al., 1996). Not surprisingly, they tended to consume a large amount of energy, approximately 7018 kJ (1700 kcal), to attempt to recover for their match. The average recovery diet was relatively high in carbohydrate, with 60% and 66% of the energy coming from carbohydrate for high-school and collegiate athletes, respectively (Figure 5-3). However, there was significant intra- and inter-individual variation in composition and energy content of the recovery diet; high-school wrestlers consumed 35–100% carbohydrate diets, whereas collegiate wrestlers ate 28–87% of their energy as carbohydrate during the recovery period. Thus, these wrestlers could use more guidance on food choices during recovery after the weigh-in.

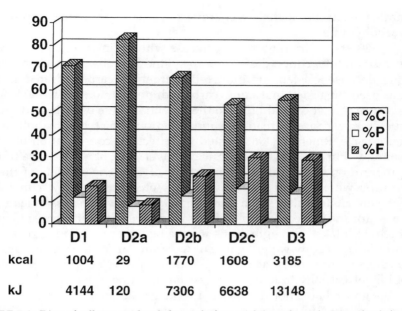

	D1	D2a	D2b	D2c	D3
kcal	1004	29	1770	1608	3185
kJ	4144	120	7306	6638	13148

FIGURE 5-3. *Diets of college wrestlers before and after weigh-in and match. D1 = day before match, D2a = portion of day of match before weigh-in; D2b = portion of day of match between weigh-in and match, D2c = portion of day of match after the match. D3 = day after the match.*

NUTRITIONAL RECOMMENDATIONS FOR WEIGHT GAIN

The most important nutritional factor to allow muscle growth is consumption of adequate energy. Because protein synthesis is a costly metabolic process, failure to consume adequate energy will depress lean tissue gain. Several studies have shown that simply increasing energy intake in resistance trainers can increase lean body mass. For example, Harberson (1988) added a 2229 kJ (540 kcal) liquid supplement (a sports meal replacement beverage) to the ad libitum diet of nine males involved in a resistance-training program. These athletes had greater increases in their average lean body mass and decreases in their percent fat as compared to individuals doing the same resistance program without any supplement. Gater et al. (1992) also observed a greater increase in lean body mass of novice male resistance trainers who consumed a 1486–2229 kJ/d (360–540 kcal/d) liquid meal supplement as compared to those who were not given a supplement. Interpretation of these studies is clouded because food records indicated that the macronutrient intake of the supplement group was different from that of the control group. More research would need to be done to separate the effect of increased energy from that of differences in protein or carbohydrate.

Resistance training must coincide with an increase in energy consumption to partition the energy to synthesis of lean rather than fat tissue. Because resistance training relies largely on carbohydrate for fuel, it has been suggested that a high carbohydrate diet may be valuable for resistance trainers. In addition to the potential value of carbohydrate as a fuel, it may cause a greater insulin secretion, which has anabolic effects on muscle. Rinehart (1988) tested the effects of consumption of a 65%, compared to a 40%, carbohydrate diet over 9 wk of a resistance training program on body composition change of 12 novices. Diets of the two groups were similar in energy and were provided by a metabolic kitchen. He found positive nitrogen balance and increases in lean body mass for the subjects, but no effects attributable to differences in carbohydrate intake. Strength gains for the bench press and leg press were correlated to body weight gain but were similar for the diet groups. The authors pointed out that although this study does not prove the value of a higher carbohydrate diet for resistance trainers, the higher carbohydrate group had a nonsignificant 1.08 kg greater increase in their fat-free mass, relative to the lower carbohydrate group. They suggested that a longer study or one with more subjects might have detected a difference in lean tissue accretion.

Several studies have investigated the potential value of protein intake at greater than the RDA in resistance trainers. Tarnopolsky et al. (1992) fed resistance-trained and inexperienced men three different diets varying in protein (0.086, 1.4, or 2.4 g/kg). Nitrogen balance tests conducted during the last 3 d of each feeding period indicated that although the lowest protein intake was adequate for the sedentary subjects, the resistance trainers were in negative nitrogen balance on that protein intake. The 1.4 g/kg protein intake resulted in nitrogen balance and high rates of whole-body protein synthesis. Increasing the protein intake to 2.4 g/kg conferred no additional benefit for protein retention or synthesis.

Protein requirements may be affected by training status of the individual. Lemon et al. (1992) had novices begin a vigorous 6 d/wk resistance training program and added daily supplements of either carbohydrate or protein at 1.5 g/kg. The total protein intake averaged 334% of RDA for the protein-supplemented and 124% of RDA for the carbohydrate-supplemented group. Nitrogen balance, assessed for 3 d after 3.5 wk on the diet, was negative (−3.4 g/d) for the carbohydrate-supplemented but positive (+8.9 g/d) for the protein-supplemented group. Thus, the higher protein intake was advantageous relative to the lower protein group with regard to total body nitrogen. However, this did not translate to differences in muscle strength or change in body mass between dietary groups.

In summary, the critical nutritional factor for weight gain is energy. Those desiring to gain lean tissue should increase their energy intakes by up to 2064 kJ/d (500 kcal/d). Although more research is required to identify the optimal protein intake for maximal body protein retention, a number of studies suggest that protein intake should be greater than the RDA, possibly 1.4–2.0 g/kg. Longer-term studies are necessary to determine if the greater nitrogen retention that accompanies higher protein diets allows greater muscle mass and strength gains in resistance trainers. Practical diet and exercise suggestions for weight gain are provided in Table 5-3.

SUMMARY

Because body composition is correlated with performance of many athletic events, some athletes would like to lose body fat or increase lean mass. Decisions on body weight change for athletes should be determined with the help of an appropriate professional (e.g., sports nutritionist, team physician, athletic trainer) and should be based on flexible guidelines that allow for individual differences. A body weight goal should be based on body composition data and should include the objective of optimizing physical performance without compromising the health of the athlete. Athletes who lose weight faster than the recommended 0.5–1.0 kg/wk (~1–2 lb/wk) may experience loss of lean tissue, reduction in metabolic rate, impairment of certain immune functions, and depression of reproductive hormones and mood. Micronutrient intake and biochemical status may deteriorate. Aerobic exercise performance is almost certainly impaired during significant weight loss, whether achieved through dehydration or energy restriction. Muscle strength and endurance as well as repeated high-intensity interval exer-

---

TABLE 5-3. *Practical tips for gaining body weight.*

1. Increase energy intake by about 2064 kJ/d (500 kcal/d).
   - Increase the frequency of daily meals.
   - Increase the sizes of meal portions.
   - Substitute higher- for lower-energy snacks.
   - Consider liquid "sports meals" as supplements.
2. Consume less than 30% of daily energy as fat.
3. Consume 1.4-2.0 g protein per kilogram body weight daily.
4. Participate in a regular resistance training program.

---

cise performance may also be reduced during negative energy balance. Thus, athletes whose performance is likely to improve with weight loss should make these efforts during the off season. Experience of the Wisconsin Minimum Weight Project for wrestlers shows that intervention by sport governing bodies can decrease excessive in-season weight loss among athletes.

Total energy intake is the most important dietary factor for weight loss or gain. A reduction or addition of approximately 2064 kJ/d (500 kcal/d) is a guideline for realistic and safe weight change. Adequate carbohydrate in the diet (60–70% of energy) is also of importance during weight loss, and dietary protein (1.4–2.0 g/kg) may be of value for optimal gain of lean tissue.

DIRECTIONS FOR FUTURE RESEARCH

Review of the research regarding weight loss in athletes shows that most of the research has focused on effects of general energy restriction on physical performance. It would be of value to increase study of the composition of the hypoenergy diet (e.g., macronutrients and vitamins) to determine if a particular diet composition results in superior performance or improved health consequences, e.g., improved biochemical status of micronutrients and enhanced immune function. Most of these studies employ laboratory-based performance tests that may not be specific to athletic events; more field studies would be of value. In addition, analysis of biochemical and histochemical changes in muscle might provide insight into the mechanisms for change in physical performance with weight loss. The limited data on the effects of energy restriction on immune function in athletes are provocative but need to be further developed to assess the consequences of frequent illness or infection and to determine whether or not manipulation of dietary quality can influence these consequences. Additional practical research concerning the best dietary and resistance-training strategies for lean tissue gain would be valuable. Efforts should be made to tease out the effects of particular added macronutrients from that of additional energy. The data provided by studies as described above will allow the professional to make more specific recommendations to athletes who would profit from body weight change.

BIBLIOGRAPHY

American College of Sports Medicine (1996). Position stand on weight loss in wrestlers. *Med. Sci. Sports Exerc.* 28:ix–xii.
Armstrong, J.E., E.L. Lange, and D.E. Stem (1990). Reported dietary practices and concerns of adult male and female recreational exercisers. *J.N.E.* 22:220–225.

Armstrong, L.E. D.L. Costill, and W.J. Fink (1985). Influence of diuretic-induced dehydration on competitive running performance. *Med. Sci. Sports Exerc.* 17:456–461.

Baer, J.T., D.J. Dean, and T. Lambrinides (1994). How high school football coaches recommend their players gain lean body mass. *J. Str. Cond. Res.* 8:72–75.

Barr, S.I., and D.L. Costill (1992). Effect of increased training volume on nutrient intake of male collegiate swimmers. *Int. J. Sports Med.* 13:47–51.

Beidleman, B.A., J.L. Puhl, and M.J. De Souza (1995). Energy balance in female distance runners. *Am. J. Clin. Nutr.* 61:303–311.

Benson, J., D.M. Gillien, K. Bourdet, and A.R. Loosli (1985). Inadequate nutrition and chronic calorie restriction in adolescent ballerinas. *Phys. Sportsmed.* 13(10):79–90.

Bonen, A., F.J. Haynes, W. Watson-Wright, M.M. Sopper, G.N. Pierce, M.P. Low, and T. E. Graham (1983). Effects of menstrual cycle on metabolic responses to exercise. *J.Appl. Physiol.* 55:1506–1513.

Brill, J.B., and M.W. Keane (1994). Supplementation patterns of competitive male and female bodybuilders. *Int. J. Sport Nutr.* 4:398–412.

Brownell, K.D., S. Nelson Steen, and J.H. Wilmore (1987). Weight regulation practices in athletes: analysis of metabolic and health effects. *Med. Sci. Sports Exerc.* 19:546–556.

Bullen, B.A., G.S. Skrinar, I.Z. Beitins, G. von Mering, B.A. Turnbull, and J.W. McArthur (1985). Induction of menstrual disorders by strenuous exercise in untrained women. *N.Eng.J. Med.* 312:1349–1353.

Burge, C.M., M.F. Carey, and W.R. Payne (1993). Rowing performance, fluid balance, and metabolic function following dehydration and rehydration. *Med. Sci. Sports Exerc.* 25:1358–1364.

Calabrese, L.H., D.T. Kirkendall, M. Floyd, S.Rapoport, G.W. Williams, G.G. Weiker, and J.A.Bergfeld (1983). Menstrual abnormalities, nutritional patterns and body composition in female classical dancers. *Phys. Sportsmed.* 11(2):86–98.

Chandra, R.K (1991). Nutrition and Immunity: lessons from the past and new insights into the future. *Am. J. Clin. Nutr.* 53:1087–1101.

Depalma, M.T., W.M. Koszewski, J.G. Case, R.J. Barile, B.F. Depalma, and S.M. Oliaro (1993). Weight control practices of lightweight football players. *Med. Sci. Sports Exerc.* 25:694–701.

DeSouza, M.J., and D.A. Metzger (1991). Reproductive dysfunction in amenorrheic athletes and anorexic patients: a review. *Med. Sci. Sports Exerc.* 23:995–1007.

Dohm, G.L, E.B. Tapscott, H.A. Barakat, and G.J. Kasparek (1983). Influence of fasting on glycogen depletion in rats during exercise. *J. Appl. Physiol.* 55:830–833.

Drinkwater, B.L., B.Bruemner, and C.H. Chesnut (1990). Menstrual history as a determinant of current bone density in young athletes. *J. Am. Med. Assoc.* 263:545–548.

Dummer G.M., L.W. Rosen, W.W. Heusner, P.J. Roberts, and J.E. Counsilman (1987). Pathogenic weight-control behaviors of young competitive swimmers. *Phys. Sportsmed.* 15(5):75–84.

Edwards, J.E., A.K. Lindeman, A.E. Mikesky, and J.M. Stager (1993). Energy balance in highly trained female endurance runners. *Med. Sci. Sports Exerc.* 25:1398–1404.

Field, C.J., R. Gougeon, and E.B. Marliss (1991). Changes in circulating leukocytes and mitogen responses during very-low-energy all-protein reducing diets. *Am. J. Clin. Nutr.* 54:123–129.

Flynn, M.G., D.L. Costill, J.P. Kirwan, J.B. Mitchell, J.A. Houmard, W.J. Dink, J.D. Beltz, and L.J. D'Acquisto (1990). Fat storage in athletes: Metabolic and hormonal responses to swimming and running. *Int. J. Sports Med.* 11:433–440.

Fogelholm, G.M (1994). Effects of bodyweight reduction on sports performance. *Sports Med.* 18:249–267.

Folgelholm, G. M., R. Koskinen, J.Laakso, T. Rankinen, and I. Ruokonen (1993). Gradual and rapid weight loss: effects on nutrition and performance in male athletes. *Med. Sci. Sports Exerc.* 25:371–377.

Gater, D.R., D.A. Gater, J.M. Urige, and J.C. Bunt (1992). Impact of nutritional supplements and resistance training on body compsoition, strength and insulin-like growth factor-1. *J. Appl. Sports Sci. Res.* 6:66–76.

Haberson, D.A (1988). Weight gain and body composition of weight lifters: Effects of high-calorie supplementation v. anabolic steroids. In: *Muscle Development: Nutritional Alternatives to Anabolic Steroids.* Columbus, OH: Ross Laboratories.

Heyward, V.H., W.M. Sandoval, and B.C. Colville (1989). Anthropometric, body composition, and nutritional profiles of bodybuilders during training. *J.Appl. Sports Sci. Res.* 3:22–29.

Hickner, R.C., C.A. Horswill, J.M. Welker, J.Scott, J.N.Roemmich, and D.L. Costill (1991). Test development for the study of physical performance in wrestlers following weight loss. *Int. J. Sports Med.* 12:557–562.

Hickson, J.F., T.E. Honson, W.Lee, and R.J. Sigor (1990). Nutrition and the precontest preparations of a male bodybuilder. *J. Am. Diet. Assoc.*90:264–267.

Horswill, C.A (1991). Does rapid weight loss by dehydration adversely affect high-power performance? *Gatorade Sports Sci. Exch.* 3(30).

Horswill C.A., R.C. Hickner, J.R. Scott, D.L. Costill, and D. Gould (1990a). Weight loss, dietary carbohydrate modifications, and high intensity physical performance. *Med. Sci. Sports Exerc.* 22:470–477.

Horswill, C.A., S.H. Park, and J.N. Roemmich (1990b). Changes in protein nutritional status of adolescent wrestlers. *Med. Sci. Sports Exerc.* 22:599–604, 1990.

Houston, M.E., D.A. Marrin, H.J. Green, and J.A. Thompson (1981). The effect of rapid weight loss on physiological functions in wrestlers. *Phys. Sportsmed.* 9(11):73–78.

Jacobs, I (1980). The effects of thermal dehydration on performance of the Wingate anaerobic test. *Int. J. Sports Med.* 1:21–24.

Jacobson, B.H., and S.G. Aldana (1992). Current nutrition practice and knowledge of varsity athletes. *J.Appl. Sports Sci. Res.* 6:232–238.

Jebb, S.A., G.R. Goldberg, W.A. Coward, P. R. Murgatroyd, and A.M. Prentice (1991). Effects of weight cycling caused by intermittent dieting on metabolic rate and body composition in obese women. *Int. J. Obes.* 15:367–374.

Kaiserauer, S., A.C. Snyder, M. Sleeper, and J. Zierath (1989). Nutritional, physiological, and menstrual status of distance runners. *Med. Sci. Sports Exerc.* 21:120–125.

Kapan, S., E. Sternthal, and L. Braverman (1981). A "pubertal" 24–hour luteinizing hormone (LH) secretory pattern following weight loss in the absence of anorexia nervosa. *Psychosom. Med.* 43:177–182.

Katch, F.I., W.D. McArdle, R. Czula, and G.S. Pechar (1973). Maximal oxygen uptake, endurance running performance, and body composition in college women. *Res. Q.* 44:301.`

Kiernan, M., J. Rodin, and K.D. Brownell (1992). Relation of level of exercise, age, and weight-cycling history to weight and eating concerns in male and female runners. *Health Psychol.* 11:418–421.

Kirchner, E.M., R.D. Lewis, and P.J. Conner (1995). Bone mineral density and dietary intake of female college gymnasts. *Med. Sci. Sports Exerc.* 27:543–549.

Kleiner, S.M. R.L Bazzarre, and M.D. Litchford (1990). Metabolic profiles, diet, and health practices of championship male and female bodybuilders. *J.Am. Diet. Assoc.* 90:962–967.

Kono, I., H. Kitao, M. Matsuda, S.Haga, H. Fukushima, and H. Kashiwagi (1988). Weight reduction in athletes may adversely affect the phagocytic function of monocytes. *Phys. Sportsmed.* 16:56–65.

Lamar-Hildebrand, N, L. Saldanha, and J. Endres (1989). Dietary and exercise practices of college-aged female bodybuilders. *J. Am. Diet. Assoc.* 89:1308–1310.

Lemon, P., M.A. Tarnopolsky, J.D. MacDougall, and S.A. Atkinson (1992). Protein requirements and muscle mass/strength changes during intensive training in novice bodybuilders. *J. Appl. Physiol.* 73:767–775.

Lightman, S.W., K.Pisarska, E. R. Berman, M.Pestone, H. Dowling, E. Offenbacher, H.Weisel, S. Heshka, D.E. Matthews, and S. B. Heymsfield (1992). Discrepancy between self-reported and actual caloric intake and exercise in obese subjects. *N. Eng. J. Med.* 327:1893–1898.

Lohman, T.G., A.F. Roche, and R. Martolell, eds. *Anthropometric Standardization Reference Manual* Human Kinetics, Champaign IL 1988.

Loy, S.F., R.K. Conlee, W.W. Winder, A.G. Nelson, D.A. Arnall, and A.G. Fisher (1986). Effects of 24–hour fast on cycling endurance time at two different intensities. *J. Appl. Physiol.* 61:654–659.

Mathieson, R.A., J.L. Walberg, F.C. Gwazdauskas, D.E. Hinkel, and J.M. Gregg (1986). The effect of varying carbohydrate content of a very-low-caloric diet on resting metabolic rate and thyroid hormones. *Metabolism* 35:394–398.

McCargar, L.J., and S.M. Crawford (1992). Anthropomentric changes with weight cycling in wrestlers. *Med. Sci. Sports Exerc.* 24:1270–1275.

McCargar, L.J., D.Simmons, N.Craton, J.E. Taunton, and C.L. Brimingham (1993). Physiological effects of weight cycling in female lightweight rowers. *Can. J. Appl. Physiol.* 18:291–303.

McMurray, R.G., C.R. Proctor, and W.L. Wilson (1991). Effect of caloric deficit and dietary manipulation on aerobic and anaerobic exercise. *Int. J. Sports Med.* 12:167–172.

Melby, C.L., W.D. Schmidt, and D. Corrigan (1990). Resting metabolic rate in weight-cycling collegiate wrestlers compared with physically active, noncycling control subject. *Am. J. Clin. Nutr.* 52:409–414.

Mertz, W., J.C. Tsue, J.T. Judd, S. Reiser, J.Hallfrisch, E.R. Morris, P.D. Steele, and E. Lashley (1991). What are people really eating? The relation between energy intake derived from estimated diet records and intake determined to maintain body weight. *Am. J. Clin. Nutr.* 54:291–295.

Myerson, M., B. Gutin, M.P. Warren, M.T. May, I. Contento, M.Lee, F.X. Pi-Sunyer, R.N. Pierson, and J. Brooks-Gunn (1991). Resting metabolic rate and energy balance in amenorrheic and eumenorrheic runners. *Med. Sci. Sports Exerc.* 23:15–22.

Newton, L.E., G.Hunter, M.Bammon, and R. Roney (1993). Changes in psychological state and self-reported diet during various phases of training in competitive bodybuilders. *J. Strength Cond. Res.* 7:153–158.

Nieman, D.C. K.A. Carlson, M.E. Brandstater, R.T. Naegele, and J.W. Blankenship (1987). Running endurance in 27–h-fasted humans. *J. Appl. Physiol.* 63:2502–2509.

Nieman, D.C., S.L. Nehlsen-Cannarells, D.A. Henson, D.E. Butterworth, O.R. Fagoago, B.J. Warren, and M.S. Rainwater.(1996). Immune response to obesity and moderate weight loss. *Int. J. Obesity Res.* 20:353–360.

Nutter, J. (1991). Seasonal changes in female athletes' diets. *Int. J. Sport Nutr.* 1:395–407.

Oppliger, R.A., R.D. Harms, D.E. Herrmann, C.M. Streich, and R.R. Clark (1995a). The Wisconsin wrestling minimum weight project: a model for weight control among high school wrestlers. *Med. Sci. Sports Exerc.* 27:1220–1224.

Oppliger, R.A. , G.L Landry, W.W. Foster, and A.C. Lambrecht (1995b). Wisconsin minimum weight rule curtails weightcutting practices of high school wrestlers. *Med. Sci. Sports Exerc.* S12.

Park, S.H., J.N. Roemmich, and C.A. Horswill (1990). A season of wrestling and weight loss by adolescent wrestlers: effect on anaerobic arm power. *J. Appl. Sport Sci. Res.* 4:1–4.

Parr, R.B., M.A. Porter, and S.C. Hodgson (1984). Nutrition knowledge and practice of coaches, trainers, and athletes. *Phys. Sportsmed.* 12:127–138.

Pesce, T., J. Walberg-Rankin, E. Thomas, D. Sebolt, and J.Wojcik (1996). Nutritional intake and status of high school and college wrestlers prior to and after competition. *Med. Sci. Sports Exerc.* 28:S91.

Philen, R.M., D.I. Ortiz, S.B. Auerbach, and H. Falk (1992). Survey of advertising for nutritional supplements in health and bodybuilding magazines. *J.A.M.A.* 268:1008–1011.

Riendeau, R.P., B.E. Welch, C.E. Crisp et al. (1958). Relationships of body fat to motor fitness scores. *Res. Q.* 29:200, 1958.

Rinehardt, K.F (1988). Effects of diet on muscle strength gains during resistive training. In: *Muscle Development: Nutritional Alternatives to Anabolic Steroids.* Columbus, OH: Ross Laboratories, pp. 79–82.

Roemmich, J.N., and W.E. Sinning (1995). Sport-seasonal changes in body composition, growth, power and strength of adolescent wrestlers. *Int. J. Sports Med.* 17:92–99.

Russell, D. L.A. Leiter, J. Whitwell, E.B. Marliss, and K.N. Jeejeebhoy (1983). Skeletal muscle function during hypocaloric diets and fasting: a comparison with standard nutritional assessment parameters. *Am. J. Clin. Nutr.* 37:133–138.

Russell, D.M., P.M. Walker, L.A. Leiter, A.A. Sima, W.K.Tanner, D.A. Mickle, J. Whitwell, E.B. Marliss, and K. N. Jeejeebhoy (1984). Metabolic and structural changes in skeletal muscle during hypocaloric dieting. *Am. J. Clin. Nutr.* 39:503–513.

Sandoval, W.M., and V.H. Heyward (1991). Food selection patterns of bodybuilders. *Int. J. Sport Nutr.* 1:61–68.

Sandoval, W.M., V.H. Heyward, and T.M. Lyons (1989). Comparison of body composition, exercise and nutritional profiles of female and male bodybuilders at competition. *J. Sports Med. Phys. Fit.* 29:63–70.

Schmidt, W.D., D. Corrigan, and C. L. Melby (1993). Two seasons of weight cycling does not lower resting metabolic rate in college wrestlers. *Med. Sci. Sports Exerc.* 25:613–619.

Stager, J.M., and L. Cordain (1984). Relationship of body composition to swimming performance in female swimmers. *J. Swim. Res.* 1:21.

Steen, S.N (1991). Precontest strategies of a male bodybuilder. *Int. J. Sport Nutr.* 1:69–78.

Steen, S.N., and S. McKinney (1986). Nutrition assessment of college wrestlers. *Phys. Sportsmed.* 14(11):100–116.

Steen, S.N., R.A. Oppliger, and K.D. Brownell (1988). Metabolic effects of repeated weight loss and regain in adolescent wrestlers. *J. Am. Med. Assoc.* 260:47–50.

Strauss, R.H., R.R. Lanese, and W.B. Malarkey (1993). Decreased testosterone and libido with severe weight loss. *Phys. Sports Med.* 21(12):64–71.

Strauss, R.H., R.R. Lanese, and W.B. Malarkey (1985). Weight loss in amateur wrestlers and its effect on serum testosterone levels. *J.Am. Med. Assoc.* 245:3337–3338.

Sykoro, C., C.M. Grilo, D.E. Wilfley, and K.D. Brownell (1993). Eating, weight, and dieting disturbances in male and female lightweight and heavyweight rowers. *Int. J. Eat. Dis.* 14:203–211.

Tarnopolsky, M.A., S.A. Atkinson, J.D. MacDougall, A.Chesley, S.Phillips, and P.F. Schwarcz (1992). Evaluation of protein requirements for trained strength athletes. *J. Appl. Physiol.* 73:1986–1995.

Tarnopolsky, M.A., N. Cipriano, C. Woodcroft, W.J. Pulkkinen, D.C. Robinson, J.M. Henderson, and J.D. MacDougall (1996). Effects of rapid weight loss and wrestling on muscle glycogen concentration. *Clin. J. Sport Med.* 6:78–84.

Theintz, G.E., H. Howald, Y. Allemann, and P.C. Sizonenko (1989). Growth and pubertal development of young female gymnasts and swimmers: a correlation with parental data. *Int. J. Sports Med.* 10:87–91.

Theintz, G.E., H. Howald, U. Weiss, and P.C. Sizonenko (1993). Evidence for a reduction of growth potential in adolescent female gymnasts. *J. Pediatr.* 122:306–313.

Tremblay, A., J.P. Depres, C. Leblanc, C.L. Craig, B. Ferris, T. Stephens, and C. Bouchard (1990). Effect of intensity of physical activity on body fatness and fat distribution. *Am. J. Clin. Nutr.* 51:153–157.

Tremblay, A., J.Simoneay, and C. Bouchard (1994). Impact of exercise intensity of body fatness and skeletal muscle metabolism. *Metabolism* 43:814–818.

Viitasalo, J.R., H. Kyrolainen, C. Bosco, and M. Alen (1987). Effects of rapid weight reduction on force production and vertical jumping height. *Int. J. Sports Med.* 8:281–185.

Walberg, J.L., and C.S. Johnston (1991). Menstrual function and eating behaviour in female recreational weight lifters and competitive bodybuilders. *Med. Sci. Sports Exerc.* 23:30–36.

Walberg-Rankin, J. (1995). A review of nutritional practices and needs of bodybuilders. *J.Strength Cond. Res.* 9:116–124.

Walberg, J.L., M.K. Leidy, D.J. Sturgill, D.E. Hinkle, S.J. Ritchey et al. (1988). Macronutrient content of a

BODY WEIGHT AND COMPOSITION/ATHLETES **235**

hyopenergy diet affects nitrogen retention and muscle function in weight lifters. *Int. J. Sports Med.* 9:261–266.

Walberg-Rankin, J., C.E. Edmonds, and R.C. Gwazdauskas (1993). Detailed analysis of the diets and bodyweights of six female bodybuilders before and after competition. *Int. J. Sport Nutr.* 3:87–102.

Walberg-Rankin, J. W.D. Franke, and F. C. Gwazdauskas (1992). Responses of beta-endorphin and estradiol to resistance exercise in females during energy balance and energy restriction. *Int. J. Sports Med.* 13:5421–547.

Walberg-Rankin, J., C.E. Hawkins, D.S. Fild, and D.R. Sebolt (1994). The effect of oral arginine during energy restriction in male weight trainers. *J. Strength Cond. Res.* 8:170–177, 1994.

Walberg Rankin, J., J.V. Ocel, and L.L. Craft (1996). Effect of weight loss and refeeding diet composition on anaerobic performance in wrestlers. *Med. Sci. Sports Exerc.* 28:1292–1299.

Webster, S., R.Rutt, and A. Weltman (1990). Physiological effects of a weight loss regimen practiced by college wrestlers. *Med. Sci. Sports Exerc.* 22:229–234.

Weissinger, E., R.J. Housh, G.O. Johnson, and S.A. Evans (1991). Weight loss behavior in high school wrestling: wrestler and parent perceptions. *Pediat. Ex. Sci.* 3:64–73.

Williams, N.I., J.C. Young, J.W. McArthur, B.Bullen, G.S. Skrinar, and B.Turnbull (1995). Strenuous exercise with caloric restriction: effect on luteinizing hormone secretion. *Med. Sci. Sports Exerc.* 27:1390–1398.

Wolf, E.M.B., J.C. Wirth, and T.G. Lohman (1979). Nutritional practices of coaches in the Big Ten. *Phys. Sportsmed.* 7(2):113–124.

Yang, M., and T.B. Van Itallie (1976). Composition of weight lost during short-term weight reduction. *J. Clin. Investig.* 58:722–730.

Yates, A., K. Leehey, and C.M. Shisslack (1983). Running—an analogue of anorexia? *N.Engl. J. Med.* 308:251, 1983.

DISCUSSION

COYLE: When athletes, especially endurance athletes, train intensely while experiencing a negative balance of fat and carbohydrate energy, they have tremendous difficulty with training. With a negative carbohydrate balance, their moods are bad, which may be linked to the etiology of some eating disorders. Athletes who are training intensely and trying to recover receive all sorts of signals telling them to eat and especially to eat carbohydrate because something is wrong. It seems that as an athlete tries to repeatedly ignore these signals, it is very psychologically difficult and possibly depressing. Does this observation have any scientific validity? Should athletes on a low energy diet try to maximize their carbohydrate intake and maintain adequate protein intake?

WALBERG-RANKIN: Craig Horswill did a study using wrestlers, and he contrasted two weight-loss diets over a 4–d period. One contained about 42% and the other about 66% carbohydrate with the same energy content. They administered the Profile of Mood States questionnaire. They found that, in general, the weight reduction made them feel worse with less vigor, more fatigue, but that mood was even worse if they had the low-carbohydrate diet compared to the higher-carbohydrate diet. This fits in with your theory that carbohydrate is critical for mood during weight loss. So, from a performance standpoint and a mood standpoint, I would recommend that at least 60% of the energy in the diet come from carbohydrate. Secondly, most of the weight-control efforts, if possible, should take place during the off-season to minimize the mood and performance impairments during competition. We know that doesn't always happen, but we can at least give some education and assistance to encourage athletes to reduce weight during the off-season.

HORSWILL: There are a couple of other reasons why we always recommend high carbohydrate diets for these athletes who are losing weight. First, the carbohydrate may help stimulate secretion of insulin, which helps prevent the breakdown of the body proteins and may minimize the loss of lean body mass. Second, a high carbohydrate diet versus no food or a high fat diet may help maintain insulin responsiveness and management of the glucose coming into the body when the athlete refeeds after the weigh-in.

COYLE: If this theory is correct, it agrees with some of the concepts that Chris Melby introduced; that is, the body is telling the athlete to maintain carbohydrate stores; it's not responding to changes in body fat. Is that a fair conclusion?

MELBY: That ties in with the glycogenostatic theory. There really is not very much evidence that this is operative in humans. There is some evidence that decreasing glycogen stores causes subsequent increases in carbohydrate intake, but this is not easy to study in humans. In work in mice by J.P. Flatt, there is some evidence for the glycogenostatic theory, that carbohydrate deprivation or depletion on one day will lead to greater carbohydrate intake the next day.

DAVIS: I also have a possible explanation for alterations in fatigue and mood that occur with dieting and/or low carbohydrate intake. It certainly could relate to the strong relationship between the increase in plasma free-fatty acids that occurs in these situations and an increase in plasma free tryptophan that would likely increase brain serotonin. Elevated serotonin has been associated with increased fatigue and negative mood alterations. Although there are no specific studies on this as yet, there is a sound theoretical argument that prolonged elevations in free-fatty acids and the associated increase in free tryptophan could elevate brain serotonin; that may cause people to feel bad.

BURKE: I agree that there is an impression in the swimming community that something is different about swimming in terms of weight control. Swimmers, despite very high energy expenditure from their prolonged workouts, tend to have higher body fat levels than other endurance athletes. Coaches typically feel that unless over-fat swimmers undertake some dry-land training (cycling or running), they can't successfully lose body fat. You reviewed the literature for us and found that the scientific evidence fails to support differences in energy considerations between swimming and other modes of exercise. Do you have any other ideas to explain the frustration of over-fat swimmers and their coaches?

WALBERG-RANKIN: It's an excellent question that has received little attention in the literature. Flynn et al. did a study in which they had subjects perform a controlled swim or run at 75% of $\dot{V}O_2$max for 45 min. They found higher fat utilization after the swim than the run. So, this does not support the idea that weight control is more difficult in swimmers. However, we need to listen to the individuals involved in the sports and the coaches. Maybe we just haven't set up these studies correctly and haven't asked the right questions. Are there any insights that you have based on your involvement with swimmers?

BURKE: After running or cycling, we typically see a period of appetite suppression that may help to control total energy intake, but this doesn't seem to happen in swimming. When I prepare menus for swimmers, I notice they get out of the pool with hearty appetites. Swimmers may find it more difficult to achieve an energy deficit through reduced food intake. There may also be a selection process involved. In other words, people who are naturally selected to be good swimmers and who continue swimming for many years may be genetically predisposed to have higher body-fat levels. If they were programmed to have lower body-fat levels, they might have been runners instead.

I have a question that deals with the weight-making sports. You presented some evidence to suggest that the techniques that the athletes in these sports use to lose body weight have detrimental effects on performance. Of course, these athletes don't need to perform optimally, but rather to perform better than their opponents. What evidence is there that "making weight" is actually a bad thing to do from a performance standpoint? If you are a wrestler or a lightweight rower, or weight lifter, is it better to compete in a lower weight division? Will you be more successful if you do that, or should you compete against a heavier and stronger opponent?

WALBERG-RANKIN: I did avoid recommending dehydration, even though it is very common in certain sports. First of all, the Olympic Committee and NCAA already ban drug-induced dehydration; some high-school federations ban even thermal dehydration. It's probably true that short-term, modest dehydration is not necessarily detrimental to health. But, I am concerned that athletes overdo this such that their health and performance are compromised. (*Editor's note: In the autumn of 1997, acute dehydration was implicated in the deaths of three university wrestlers.*)

HORSWILL: We studied wrestlers at the NCAA tournament, measuring their weight gain during the period between when they weighed in and when they stepped on the mat to compete. We made the assumption that rapid weight gain in this interval indicated weight loss that occurred prior to making weight. We could not find any relationship between the amount of weight they regained and their success in the tournament or their success in the first match, for which we knew the weight difference between the opponents. We saw neither negative effects nor advantages of weight loss for collegiate wrestlers. There are a couple of papers in review for publication in *Med. Sci. Sports Exerc.* showing that at the high-school level, wrestlers might be more successful if they've regained more weight after the weigh-in. If collegiate or high-school wrestlers have 20 h between the weigh-in and competition, they may be pretty well recovered. Tarnopolsky et al. showed that muscle glycogen levels increase by about 50% during these 20 h in college-level wrestlers.

LAMB: Craig, what is your opinion about whether it is good to lose weight to compete in a lower weight class or not so good?

HORSWILL: It may be not that these guys are getting an advantage by losing weight, but they're avoiding a disadvantage. I think when wrestlers cut weight quickly, wrestlers can retain power and strength performance, despite losing endurance. Within the scoring system of the sport, a wrestler can win before the time of the match expires, that is, winning by a fall, or a boxer can win with a knockout; therefore, there can be an advantage to gaining power per kilogram of body mass by losing weight. With the longer recovery periods now in wrestling at the international, national and even at some of the high-school levels, there is even more motivation to drop down to lower weight classes. If you're the wrestler who is not dropping down in weight, you could be competing at a serious disadvantage.

C. WILLIAMS: Is it preferable to prescribe dietary carbohydrate as g/kg body weight because it is independent of the size of the daily energy intake?

WALBERG-RANKIN: I worry about using a recommendation for an absolute amount of carbohydrate, especially when I'm comparing the genders. It's very difficult for many women who are consuming lower amounts of energy to consume the 7–10 g carbohydrate/kg that has been recommended by many authorities. I agree that it could be useful to have some realistic recommendations for total as well as relative carbohydrate intake.

C. WILLIAMS: Our nutritional surveys show that endurance athletes actually consume about 4–5 g of carbohydrate/kg body weight. For rapid recovery, a carbohydrate intake of 9–10 g/kg body weight is effective.

Also, I wonder if the difference in body fat between swimmers and runners is linked to sustained thermoregulation. We know that the major protection against cold is a behavioral response to leave the cold environment and then eat. In swimming, perhaps there is a subliminal signal which says, "You're in a threatening environment, and you have to do two things: 1) get out and 2) eat." Perhaps installing a vending machine at poolside and supplying a set of tokens to the swimmers on two occasions could test this hypothesis. On one occasion, you lower the temperature of the water and monitor how much they spend on the vending machine; on another occasion, you raise the pool temperature to a non-threatening level, and again you monitor how much is spent at the vending machine.

WALBERG-RANKIN: The study by Flynn et al. was very controlled without any food consumption. It's possible that appetite and, therefore food intake, may be affected differently by swimming than running. Perhaps swimmers maintain their core temperatures during a workout, whereas runners and cyclists get an increase in body temperature that causes a reduction in appetite.

BURKE: Kern presented a paper at ACSM in which she described a "pilot study" of the Zone diet. She had 32 women follow the Zone dietary restrictions, which halved their energy intake for 12 wk. At the end of this period, they had sustained an average weight loss of about 10 lb. Unfortunately, a key criticism of the study is that there was no control group. We don't know if a similarly hypocaloric diet, but with a different macronutrient ratio, could achieve similar results. The other finding was that fat loss appeared to account for the total amount of weight lost. Of course, this sounds terribly attractive. However, body composition changes were measured by skinfold assessment. We know this is not a reliable and sensitive technique for monitoring changes in lean-body mass, so the study also suffers from the problem of measurement error with an important outcome variable. Clearly, more studies need to be undertaken with more careful design before the Zone diet can be assessed.

WALBERG-RANKIN: We need a comparison group to determine the value of this particular diet.

NADEL: There's an important point about dehydration that I wish to make. When wrestlers, for example, exercise in the heat to shed weight, they also lose electrolytes, particularly sodium. But when they restore the fluid lost, they generally do so with water. If they don't replace the sodium lost, then they will have a low-body sodium content that will have important implications. Takamata and colleagues published a study in 1994 in which sodium intake was restricted for 24 h after thermal dehydration in which 10% of body sodium was lost. When these subjects were allowed to rehydrate without sodium restoration, their plasma volumes remained reduced by about 5%, and their body-water content remained reduced as well. So, certain body fluid and composition derangements occur without appropriate restoration of the lost sodium, and these can impair subsequent performance.

WALBERG-RANKIN: I think the whole issue of recovery following weight loss achieved by energy and/or fluid restriction is an interesting one. We need to do more research and have some specific recommendations for athletes.

FIATARONE: It has been recommended that athletes need 2 g protein/kg body weight on a daily basis. Some of us are concerned about over-protein nutrition causing chronic renal failure, and although the RDA for protein is 0.8 g/kg/d, most people eat 1.2 g/kg/d or even more in the typical American diet. The RDA may be a little bit low because the actual need of athletes is probably closer to 1 g/kg/d to be in nitrogen balance. In fact, if you start somebody on a resistance training program, the anabolic stimulus of the resistance training causes one to be in a more positive nitrogen balance. For example, when we give older men and women protein at 0.8 g/kg/d, they are in negative nitrogen balance, but when they begin resistance training, they go into balance at the same 0.8 g/kg/d. If you give them a diet of 1.6 g protein/kg/d during resistance training, they will be in very positive nitrogen balance, but this does not improve the accretion of muscle mass or muscle performance or any other variable we have measured. Consumption of 2 g/kg/day is a very large amount of protein that may be excessive over the long term, especially given aging-related decrements in glomerular filtration rate.

WALBERG-RANKIN: Optimal protein intake for athletes has been a controversial area. The recommendation of 1.4 g/kg came partly from the Tarnopolsky et al. paper in which they did nitrogen balance and labeled leucine studies to look at whole body protein synthesis. Another study by Lemon et al. had novice weight trainers consume their regular diet plus a supplement at 1.5 g/kg of either carbohydrate or protein. They found that the group that consumed the carbohydrate supplement with a protein intake of about 0.9 g/kg was in negative nitrogen balance. The group that consumed the protein supplement was in positive nitrogen balance. Regression analysis to determine the protein intake required for balance indicated 1.4 g protein/kg as the recommended intake. Many athletes consume 2.8 g or more of protein per kilogram body weight. I'm not aware of any studies showing that consuming 2 g protein/kg/d is a health risk.

HARGREAVES: I wonder if there is some value in considering the maintenance of body weight, particularly in athletes who are undertaking a large volume of training. The guidelines or nutritional practices that they adopt to simply maintain an appropriate level of lean body mass may be quite different from those for athletes who expend less energy. In such cases the whole notion of a percent of total energy from carbohydrate may become problematic when the required total energy intake is very high. This may be part of the reason for the popularity of diets that have a higher percentage of fat and a perceived lower percentage of total energy from carbohydrates. During acute recovery, the percent of total energy from carbohydrate seems to be less important than the absolute amount of carbohydrate.

WALBERG-RANKIN: Tour de France cyclists, for example, have an incredible energy expenditure, approximately 7,000 to 8,000 kcal/d. It becomes very difficult to consume that much food, especially when you are spending most of your day exercising. My understanding is that many of these cyclists consume liquid supplements—carbohydrate supplements or sports meal supplements—that are easily digested, and they eat very frequently to get enough energy. The best recommendation I have for athletes needing a large amount of energy to match expenditure is that they eat regularly throughout the day. It may be less important to have the carbohydrate as high as 60–70% because the absolute grams of carbohydrate are so high.

DESPRES: Leptin is closely correlated with the level of total body fat, but other studies have shown that plasma leptin concentration are poorly correlated with the level of visceral fat. Thus, leptin may be the signal sent to the brain providing information about energy balance and whether there is enough energy stored for adequate reproductive function. It probably plays a greater role in reproductive function than in the etiology of obesity.

6

BODY COMPOSITION AND WEIGHT CONTROL IN OLDER ADULTS

MARIA A. FIATARONE-SINGH, M.D.

INTRODUCTION

Aging is accompanied by a series of changes in body composition and weight with direct relevance to the maintenance of health and quality of life in older adults. Aging is typically associated with a gradual increase in weight throughout mid-life, followed by stabilization or even a decline in late life. The increase in body mass is predominantly due to the accretion of adiposity, beginning as early as the fourth decade, paralleling the age-related declines in energy expenditure and physical activity (Pate et al., 1995). Even in those whose weight remains stable throughout adult life, there is a radical shift in the composition of that weight, such that increases in fat mass are matched by decreases in lean tissue (bone and muscle) beginning in mid-life and continuing into extreme old age. Thus the problems of weight control associated with young old age are predominantly those related to excess body weight and body fat, whereas those of late old age become increasingly entwined with losses of weight and shifts in body composition, especially the atrophy of skeletal muscle and bone. At both upper and lower ends of the spectrum, body mass is associated with excess mortality, and a similar relationship is emerging between extremes in body mass and disability (Andres, 1985; Harris et al., 1989).

The reasons for the alterations in body weight and composition with aging are complex, and many factors are still unknown. A model that incorporates many of the issues that must be considered is presented in Figure 6-1. The genetic predisposition to preservation of lean and accumulation of fat tissue is certainly important, but equally so are psychosocial factors, physical activity levels, nutritional intake, and the burden of diseases. Energy expenditure in physical activity is modifiable and therefore of great importance in the goal of realizing ideal body weight and composition with respect to optimal health and well-being in the older adult.

In this chapter, therefore, the major studies documenting the role of physical activity and exercise in weight control and body composition in

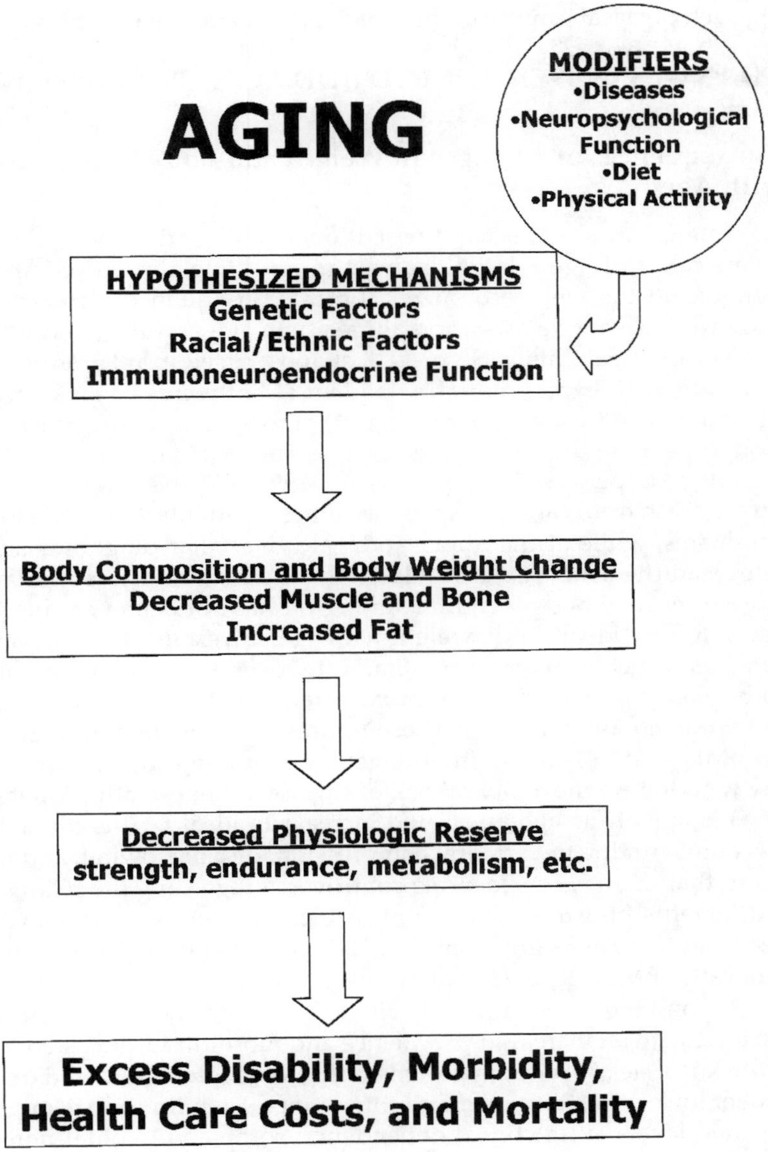

AGING

MODIFIERS
- Diseases
- Neuropsychological Function
- Diet
- Physical Activity

HYPOTHESIZED MECHANISMS
Genetic Factors
Racial/Ethnic Factors
Immunoneuroendocrine Function

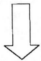

Body Composition and Body Weight Change
Decreased Muscle and Bone
Increased Fat

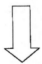

Decreased Physiologic Reserve
strength, endurance, metabolism, etc.

Excess Disability, Morbidity, Health Care Costs, and Mortality

FIGURE 6-1. *Conceptual model of factors associated with changes in weight and body composition in aging.*

the elderly will be summarized, and practical suggestions for implementing such physical activity in this unique population will be provided.

CHANGES IN WEIGHT AND BODY COMPOSITION WITH AGE

Consequences of Changes in Weight and Body Composition with Age

Interest by scientists and practitioners in the etiology and potential reversibility of age-related changes in body weight and composition stems from the well-recognized clinical consequences of extremes of body weight, muscle mass, and adiposity in older adults (Andres, 1985). Body weight exhibits a "J" or "U" shaped curve in relation to overall mortality, with excess mortality evident at both ends of the curve. This pattern is seen in several large cohorts across a broad age spectrum, although generally not inclusive of those above 85 years of age (Blair et al., 1993; Casper, 1995; Higgins et al., 1993). At the lower end of this curve, death from cancer, respiratory illness, and infectious diseases predominates, while at the upper end, cardiovascular diagnoses and diabetes lead the list of diseases related to excess mortality as compared to those of normal body weight. Although it has not been possible to precisely define "ideal" body weight with age, lowest mortality in actuarial data bases such as the Metropolitan Life Insurance population falls at a body mass index (BMI) of approximately 26–27 kg/m^2 for older men and women (Andres, 1985). These figures are considerably higher than the BMIs of 19–21 kg/m^2 in younger women found by Willett to correlate with lowest mortality or risk of cardiovascular death (Willett et al., 1995). Some of the age-associated increase in ideal BMI is explained by loss of height due to vertebral compression, disc narrowing, and kyphosis, so that there is considerable controversy regarding the relative risks and benefits of a modest amount of increase with age. However, it is clear that there are significant health risks imposed by the development of obesity (BMI $\geq$ 30 kg/m^2) at all ages.

Beyond the excess mortality cited above, obesity in the elderly is associated with an increased prevalence and morbidity from osteoarthritis of the knee, sleep apnea, hypertension, glucose intolerance and diabetes, stroke, low self-esteem, exercise intolerance, mobility impairment, and elevated levels of functional dependency, compared to older non-obese populations (Colditz et al., 1995; Harris et al., 1987, 1989; Manson et al., 1990, 1991,1992; Montgomery et al., 1988). Thus, a wide spectrum of physical, functional, and psychosocial problems in the elderly may be prevented or treated more effectively if optimal body weight was attained and maintained throughout adult life.

Although the problems of excess body weight predominate in the young old, with increasing age, and often in combination with a high burden of chronic disease, weight loss, anorexia, and undernutrition begin to surface as well. Lower than optimal body weight has been associated with excess all-cause mortality, depression, pressure ulcers, hip fracture, immune dysfunction, and increased susceptibility to infectious diseases, prolonged recovery from acute illnesses and hospitalizations, exacerbation of chronic diseases such as COPD, CHF, and chronic renal insufficiency, as well as functional impairment in the elderly (Farmer et al., 1989; Fiatarone & Evans, 1990, 1993; Losonczy et al., 1995; Morley, 1986; Morley & Kraenzle, 1994; Rumpel et al., 1993). The etiology of weight loss in frail elders appears multifactorial and may include age-related changes in neurotransmitters and humoral factors controlling hunger and satiety, functional dependency in nutrition-related activities of daily living (shopping, cooking, eating), excessive use of medications, depression and isolation, financial stresses, poor dentition, alcoholism, low energy requirements associated with extreme sedentariness and muscle atrophy, and catabolism associated with acute illnesses and certain chronic conditions such as CHF and rheumatoid arthritis(Chapman & Nelson, 1994; Fischer & Johnson, 1990; Morley & Kraenzle, 1994; Pamuk et al., 1993; Prentice et al., 1989).

Regardless of the degree to which fat mass is accumulating, concomitant losses of lean tissue (muscle and bone) pose significant health risks to the elderly. The decrease in bone mass and bone density that occurs with aging is associated with an increased risk for osteopenic fractures, primarily of the vertebrae, wrist, hip, and pelvis (Cummings et al., 1985). However, in addition to low bone density, factors related to muscle mass, including muscle strength and balance, are also important predictors of the risk of injurious falls resulting in fracture in this population (Nevitt et al., 1989). The losses of lean body mass and muscle strength are also associated with impairment of maximal aerobic capacity (Fleg & Lakatta, 1988), glucose intolerance (Pratley et al., 1995), lower resting metabolic rate (Tzankoff & Norris, 1978), immune dysfunction (Morley et al., 1995), slower gait velocity (Fiatarone et al., 1994), and functional dependency (Wagnar et al., 1992) in older adults. Age-related losses of alpha motor neurons may explain some of this muscle atrophy, but additional factors include disuse or sedentariness, catabolic illnesses, medications such as glucocorticoids and thyroid hormone, and protein or energy undernutrition in some cases (Fiatarone & Evans, 1993). Unfortunately, attempts to address the health problems of excess body fat and weight through energy restriction alone are often at odds with the goal of maintaining or increasing lean body mass in the elderly and may exacerbate age-related losses of muscle and bone.

Changes in Body Fat and Fat Distribution Patterns

Total Body Fat. Total body fat mass as well as percent body fat increases in middle and early old age, although the exact onset and magnitude of these changes is influenced by the measurement techniques available and selection bias of the population under study. Although there is a dearth of information available on the oldest old and little longitudinal data to compare to cross-sectional trends, studies from Welsh (Burr & Phillips, 1984) and French (Delarue et al., 1994) populations suggest that body fat decreases after 75 y of age; the investigators used skinfold thicknesses to estimate fat. Data from the National Health and Nutrition Evaluation Surveys (NHANES) (Hubert et al., 1993) also indicate a leveling off of subcutaneous adipose tissue after age 55. Because these studies contain no data on visceral fat stores, it is impossible to interpret changes in skinfold thickness as representative of total body fat. Data from NHANES III, which will include data on the oldest old as well as bioelectric impedance analysis, should provide some insight into these questions. Other smaller studies, such as those by Ellis (1990) and Rico et al. (1993) using isotope dilution and total body nitrogen or DXA to estimate total body fat, confirm the cross-sectional trends observed with simpler anthropometric techniques in the larger surveys. However, in the absence of longitudinal data, these apparent decreases in body fat in the oldest old may simply reflect better survival of the leaner subjects.

Percent Body Fat. Percent body fat may increase due to increases in total body fat or decreases in lean body mass or both, and may better reflect the overall metabolic balance than absolute amounts of adipose tissue. When expressed as a percentage of body weight, Going et al. (1994) reported a linear increase in percent fat between ages 40 and 81 y of about 2.2% per decade in men and 3.6% per decade in women assessed by hydrodensitometry. In a longitudinal study by Flynn et al. (1989) using serial total body potassium measurements in adults aged 28-60, similar linear increases in percent body fat of 3% per decade in men and 5.2% per decade in women were reported over an 18 y period.

Like obesity, increased body fat is linked to morbid outcomes such as glucose intolerance, diabetes, cardiovascular disease, hypercholesterolemia, and hypertension (Folsom et al., 1993; Shephard, 1994). However, because of the general lack of availability of reliable methods to estimate body fat in population studies, it has not been possible to establish "normal" or "ideal" body fat percentages for healthy aging, disease prevention, or lowest mortality, as has been done with BMI.

Regional Fat Distribution. Apart from changes in total fat mass, regional redistribution of adipose tissue with aging to truncal vs. limb, abdominal vs. lower body, and visceral vs. subcutaneous sites has been described in numerous studies using either anthropometric, computerized imaging or dual energy xray absorptiometry (DXA) techniques (Chien et al., 1975; Ley et al., 1992; Puig et al., 1990; Shimokata et al., 1988). Using image analysis of computerized tomography (CT) scans of the thigh, we have seen large amounts of intramuscular fat deposits in elderly nursing home residents (Fiatarone et al., 1990), in contrast to the primarily subcutaneous fat deposits in healthy young individuals reported in other studies (Borkan et al., 1983) (see Figure 6-2). A similar increase with age in visceral vs. subcutaneous fat distribution in the abdominal region has been described in several cross-sectional studies also using CT analysis (Borkan & Norris, 1977; Enzi et al., 1986).

Circumference measurements of the waist and hip have been used in longitudinal studies and demonstrate increases in abdominal girth and waist-to-hip ratio (WHR) with aging (Shimokata et al., 1988; Stevens et al., 1991). Importantly, increased waist circumference as well as WHR have prognostic implications, as they are associated with an elevated risk of glucose intolerance, diabetes, hyperlipidemia, hypertension, and cardiovascular disease in middle and old age (Kissebah & Krakower,

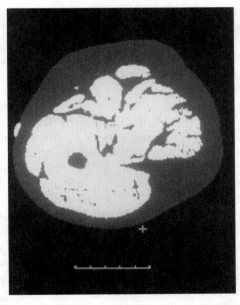

FIGURE 6-2. *Computerized tomography scan of the mid-thigh in an 89-y-old female resident of a nursing home.* The large amount of subcutaneous and intra-muscular fat is notable. In this population approximately 35% of the cross-sectional area of the mid-thigh is muscle tissue, as compared to 90% in young adults using similar imaging techniques. Data from Fiatarone and Evans, 1993.

1994; Krotkiewski et al., 1983; Ohlson et al., 1984). Thus, in addition to attempts to modify total body fat, there has been interest in the effects of physical activity and diet on modification of fat distribution patterns and on central adiposity in particular.

Changes in Lean Body Mass

Losses of lean body mass are described in numerous cross-sectional and longitudinal studies and are associated with diminished muscle and bone strength, lower basal metabolic rate and energy requirements, decreased aerobic capacity, and many clinical sequelae including osteoporosis, frailty and functional dependency, disorders of gait and balance, osteoporotic fracture, and insulin resistance (Evans, 1995; Evans & Campbell, 1993; Frontera et al., 1991; Roberts et al., 1993). Estimates of the onset and magnitude of these losses vary according to the techniques used to measure each compartment and the characteristics of the population under study, but atrophy of skeletal muscle has been described in subjects as young as 30 y of age (Imamura et al., 1983); such losses may accelerate after menopause and in extreme old age. Although lean body mass includes water, organs, skeletal muscle, bone, and connective tissue, the muscle compartment appears to undergo the greatest losses with aging (approximately 40% by age 70), relative to non-muscle lean tissue (Steen, 1988), and to have the greatest functional consequences.

Muscle Mass. Total body muscle mass is difficult to measure accurately in human studies, but estimates using urinary creatinine excretion as an index of this compartment indicate dramatic losses of nearly 50% between the ages of 20 and 90 in men from the Baltimore Longitudinal Study on Aging (Tzankoff & Norris, 1978). Investigators using total body potassium analyses have described average losses of 3–6% per decade in adult men and women, with considerable variability among individuals, however (Flynn et al., 1989). This would translate to approximately 3 kg reductions in FFM per decade between 30 and 70 y of age (Going et al., 1994)

These total body changes are mirrored by the results of regional assessments using computerized tomography scans or muscle biopsies, which show decreases in cross-sectional area of whole muscle groups or individual fibers beginning as early as the fourth decade of life (Larsson, 1983; Larsson et al., 1978, 1989; Lexell et al., 1983; Orlander et al., 1978). There appears to be a selective atrophy of Type II or fast-twitch fibers with aging, which may reflect the relative under-recruitment of these fibers as high force and/or high velocity movements become relatively infrequent in older sedentary adults (Larsson, 1983).

Bone Mass. Like muscle, bone loss is described in numerous cross-sectional and longitudinal studies beginning in middle age, with an exaggerated rate of decline at menopause in women and a fairly linear decline in men (Mazess, 1982; Orwoll et al., 1996; Prior et al., 1996; Richelson et al., 1984; Riggs et al., 1981, 1986). In general, men start with a greater bone mass than women and lose bone at a slightly slower rate, thus delaying or avoiding the bone-density threshold below which fracture risk increases markedly. However, it is clear that many factors influence the losses of bone observed, including genetics, race, nutritional intake, hormonal milieu, and physical activity levels, among others (Pocock et al., 1989).

PHYSICAL ACTIVITY, WEIGHT, AND BODY COMPOSITION IN OLDER ADULTS

Epidemiological Studies of Normal Aging

Can exercise prevent the increase in body weight and fat mass so commonly observed with aging? Many cross-sectional studies suggest a role for physical activity as a modifier of the "age-related" changes in weight and body composition described above. Some investigators have even suggested that a major portion of these changes may be due to disuse or to an "exercise deficiency syndrome"(Bortz, 1982, 1989), whereas others have described an energy imbalance with aging such that the decline in energy expenditure in physical activity is even greater than the declines in energy intake, leading to an energy surfeit that must be stored as fat (Roberts et al., 1992, 1994). For example, Meredith et al. (1987) found that percent body fat was very closely related to number of hours of training per week in runners aged 20–60, whereas age explained none of the variance in fat mass in this active group of men.

In part because an accurate epidemiololgic assessment of habitual physical activity levels over many years is difficult if not impossible to achieve, the estimates of the relative contribution of physical activity to body composition changes over time vary widely in population-based studies. In general, however, individuals who classify themselves as more active have lower body weight, BMI, percent body fat, and WHR than do sedentary age-matched individuals. For example, Romieu et al. (1988) reported that in a subset of women aged 34–59 from the Nurses' Health Study, current physical activity measured by the Harvard Alumni Activity Survey was inversely related to BMI ($r = -0.31$, $P < 0.0002$). Similarly, a survey of 25,624 women aged 20-54 y from Norway indicated that BMI was lower (24.5 kg/m^2 vs. 25.5 kg/m^2) in those who reported the highest levels of leisure time activity compared to the sedentary women (Thune et al., 1997). Importantly, among women who were consistently active over 3–5 y and who were in the lowest tertile of

BMI (<22.8 kg/m^2), the relative risk of incident breast cancer was reduced by 77%. DiPietro et al. (1993) analyzed the Behavioral Risk Factor Surveillance System Survey of 1989, a telephone sampling of 18,682 free-living adults in the US who reported that they were trying to lose weight, and found that obesity (BMI ≥30 kg/m^2) increased significantly with decreasing levels of activity (Figure 6-3). These associations strengthened with older age groups (up to age 54 y) and more intensive activities, although walking was significantly associated with leanness and was by far the most prevalent activity reported.

Regional fat distribution is related to habitual activity levels. Seidell et al. (1991) reported that in middle-aged men from six European Countries (The European Fat Distribution Study) a "sports activity index" remained a significant independent predictor of WHR and waist-to-thigh ratio after adjusting for educational level, BMI, and smoking status ($P < 0.003$ and 0.0001, respectively). Other investigators, have found that aerobic fitness levels, as surrogates for habitual activity patterns, are also inversely correlated with obesity or central adiposity (Barakat et al., 1988; Blair et al., 1989a).

Interpretation of the cross-sectional investigations cited above is obviously limited by the possibilities that differential survival will influence body composition values of older age groups, that obesity itself may preclude physical activity (i.e., obesity causes inactivity rather than the converse), and that genetic factors that influence body weight and composition may also influence activity levels.

Longitudinal studies are better suited to address the potential usefulness of exercise as a means to influence body composition in older adults, and in general the available longitudinal data are in agreement with the cross-sectional findings above. One of the larger series is a Finnish study of 4528 hypertensive men and women aged 25–59 y who were followed for 5 y to identify factors related to changes in body weight (Tuomilehto et al., 1985). There was a trend for BMI to increase more ($+0.38$ kg/m^2) in those whose leisure-time physical activity had decreased during follow-up, compared to those whose activity level had increased ($+0.07$ kg/m^2). In men, approximately 6% of the variance in BMI change was accounted for by six independent predictors: age, smoking, physical activity at work, leisure time physical activity, advice to diet, and change in intake of saturated fats. In women, less than 5% of the variance could be attributed to independent effects of smoking, blood pressure follow-up visits, study area, number of working hours and physical activity at work, and change in saturated fat intake. Thus, although exercise played a role in modifying body weight in this population, it appeared to exert relatively minor effects compared to cross-sectional data. It should be noted that the strength of associations in

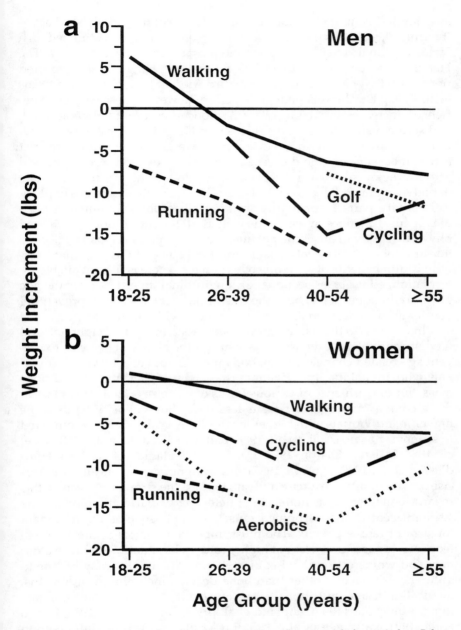

FIGURE 6-3. *The association between selected activities and mean weight by age and sex Behavioral Risk Factor Surveillance System, 1989.* Graphs based on multiple linear regression modeling, adjusting for age, race, height, education, smoking and caloric restriction. The weight increment is mean weight between those reporting the activity and those reporting no activity. Data from DiPietro et al., 1993.

such studies is limited by the accuracy of the estimate of physical activity utilized, and thus the true effect may have been underestimated. In a 3y longitudinal study of 500 premenopausal women aged 42–50 y (The Healthy Women Study), there was no overall change in self-reported physical activity level using the Harvard Alumni Questionnaire (Owens et al., 1992). During this same time period, however, these women experienced increases in weight (2.2 kg), blood pressure, total cholesterol, and serum insulin levels and decreases in HDL cholesterol. Physical activity appeared to play an important role here, as women who were least active at baseline or who decreased their energy expenditure in physical activity the most between assessments exhibited the greatest increases in body weight and decreases in HDL. Thus, voluntary changes in physical activity pattern (primarily walking or aerobics) attenuated perimenopausal changes in weight as well as HDL. The ability of increased physical activity to offset the potent effect of the perimenopausal decline in estradiol on HDL levels is significant evidence of the potential long-term health benefits of such lifestyle changes. There is little available information, either cross-sectional or longitudinal, in adults over the age of 75, so that questions about the role of physical activity in preventing obesity in the oldest old cannot be answered without further study.

In contrast to the relatively consistent data on body weight, fat, and fat distribution and exercise, consensus on the ability of exercise to prevent age-related changes in lean body mass is not yet achieved. Individuals who are habitually active may start with higher muscle and bone mass, but the influence of various forms of exercise on the rate of loss in these compartments over time is less clear. Bone density tends to be higher in individuals with higher levels of physical activity as compared to sedentary peers (Aloia et al., 1988; Bailey & McCulloch, 1990; Block et al., 1986; Dalen & Olsson, 1974; Dalsky, 1989; Hamdy et al., 1994; Huddleston et al., 1980; Santora, 1987), and weight bearing endurance exercise or weight lifting exercise appears to exert the strongest effects in this regard. Bone density is higher in athletes, particularly at regional bone sites adjacent to hypertrophied muscle groups, such as the dominant forearm of tennis players. The most important clinical sequelae of osteopenia, hip fracture, occur at higher rates in habitually sedentary older men and women (Coupland et al., 1993). However, this may be due to differences in factors other than bone density, including health status, medication usage, nutritional state, muscle and fat mass, and risk factors for injurious falls (Coupland et al., 1993; Farmer et al., 1989; Grisso et al., 1991; Lauritzen et al., 1993; Ray et al., 1987). Some intervention studies have shown that either aerobic or resistance exercise can attenuate age-related losses or even lead to increases in bone density in middle-aged and older women (Aloia et al. 1978; Dalsky et al., 1988; Kohrt et al., 1995; Krolner et al., 1983; Lohman et al., 1995; Nelson et al., 1991, 1994; Notelovitz et al., 1991; Pruitt et al., 1992). Negative results from other studies may be related to inadequate dose or intensity of the exercise intervention, imprecision in bone density measurement techniques used, or differences in populations studied (Heikkinen et al., 1991; McCartney et al., 1995; Nichols et al., 1995; Smidt et al., 1992). More information on the dose-response effect and long-term benefits and sustainability of the bone density changes are needed, but at this time exercise appears to be an important modifiable risk factor for both the prevention and treatment of osteoporosis. It should be remembered that since hypocaloric dieting typically results in losses of fat free mass, including muscle and bone, the adverse consequences of dieting or weight cycling without exercise for the postmenopausal woman with respect to preservation of bone mass may be significant (Atkinson et al., 1994). Obese women are relatively protected from hip fracture compared to thin women (Farmer et al., 1989), probably due to a combination of increased estradiol levels, higher bone density, and increased fat and muscle padding over the greater trochanter.

Due to the relative difficulty in accurately estimating muscle mass in population studies, the ability of habitual activity to modify age-related changes in this compartment is much more controversial. Although it has been speculated that there is attenuation of age-related losses of muscle in physically active individuals, review of the available data demonstrates little or no effect of exercise on this parameter (Forbes, 1992). Most studies suggest that aerobic activities such as walking have at most a modest effect on lean mass retention, and rates of loss in longitudinal follow-up have not differed by physical activity level. The greater lean body mass sometimes seen in active adults may be due to a combination of genetic factors, higher socio-economic status, lower burden of disease, and better nutritional status, all factors that are associated with higher levels of physical activity and that may serve to minimize losses of lean tissue with age (DiPietro, 1995).

In summary, it is likely that modification of body fat accretion and distribution via generalized increases in physical activities such as walking occurs by changes in energy balance over many years, whereas preservation of lean tissue (particularly skeletal muscle) requires more specific adaptations to high resistance activities (such as weight lifting) that are rarely reported in epidemiological studies because they are practiced by so few individuals.

Body Composition of Master Athletes

Studies of master athletes are useful as a means to begin to separate biological aging from disuse and disease, although such elite individuals are a small, unrepresentative group who are likely to differ genetically as well as in their lifestyle choices from their sedentary peers. However, since they can be studied more intensely and their exercise patterns are more definitively known, the strength of associations between activity and physiologic parameters is generally stronger than in observational studies of non-athletic populations. Thus, they offer a view into what is possible with good genes, good health, good nutrition, and intensive physical activity patterns. Whether "normal" aging adults are able to replicate the results achieved by these select few is a different question, which can only be answered in the context of randomized clinical trials.

With these caveats in mind, cross-sectional studies of master athletes have yielded important insights into the effect of exercise on body weight and composition in old age. For example, Pratley et al. (1995) studied master runners and non-obese (body fat <25%) sedentary controls aged 50–70 y and found no difference in mean BMI, fat free mass (FFM), or percent body fat but lower WHR in the athletes. This difference in regional fat distribution was also reflected in better metabolic parameters including lower fasting glucose, decreased area under the curve for glucose and insulin during an oral glucose tolerance test (OGTT), and increased insulin sensitivity during glucose clamp studies. Waist-to-hip ratio was the only independent predictor of glucose disposal rates in multiple regression analysis, again demonstrating the metabolic importance of the fat distribution patterns exhibited by the master athletes. It is conceivable that long-term aerobic training results in a reduced deposition of abdominal fat with aging, thereby enhancing sensitivity to insulin.

An extremely important look at the specificity of the adaptation to various exercise modalities is provided by Klitgaard's elegant investigation of elderly runners, swimmers, weight lifters and untrained young and old men (28 vs. 69 y) in Denmark (Klitgaard et al., 1990). The trained men had participated in sports in their youth and had been actively training in their current sport for 12–17 y. Muscle strength, speed of movement, muscle cross-sectional area (CT scan of the arm and leg), and mean fiber area of vastus lateralis and biceps brachii/brachialis muscles in weightlifters were the same or greater than in young controls, whereas older endurance trained athletes had declined to a similar extent as old sedentary subjects in almost all measures (Figure 6-4). For example, muscle area was 20–24% smaller with age in sedentary men, whereas the weight lifters had 18–29% larger muscle areas than their sedentary peers, making them comparable to men 40 years younger than themselves. None of the weight lifters had practiced strength training before age 50, so that this study strongly suggests that the initiation

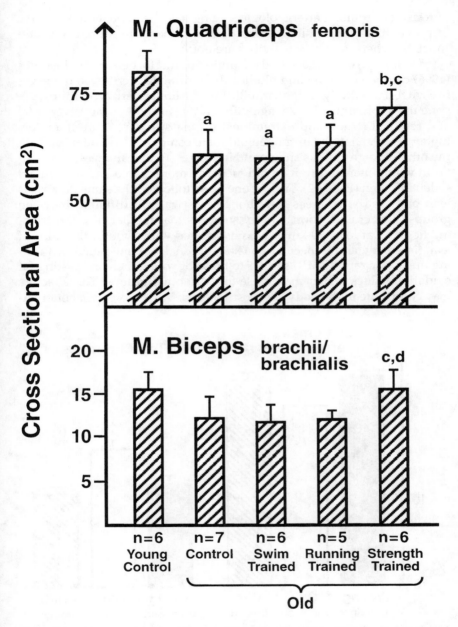

FIGURE 6-4. *Cross-sectional area of m. quadriceps femoris and the elbow flexors in young, elderly, and elderly trained subjects.* The values are means ±SEM. *n*= number of subjects. *a* = statistical difference (P < 0.05) from the young control group; *b* from the elderly control group, *c* from the swimmers, and *d* from the runners. Data from Klitgaard et al., 1990.

of resistance training after biological aging has already begun is capable of preventing or reversing age-related decrements in muscle size and function, whereas aerobic activities are not.

Using DXA to assess body composition, Horber and colleagues (1996) compared young and old healthy untrained men and old joggers in Switzerland. Body weight and BMI were similar between groups, despite the approximately 37 y age difference (31 vs. 68 y). However, total and regional (trunk and extremities) fat masses were more than 20% higher ($P < 0.02$) in the untrained old men, compared to similar levels in the other two groups, as shown in Figure 6-5. Total lean mass was similar in young men and trained old men and more than 3 kg lower in old sedentary men ($P < 0.02$). Trunk bone mass followed the same pattern as lean body mass, whereas total bone mass was not different between groups. This cross-sectional study suggests that regular physical training (jogging at least 30 km/wk) is associated with "youthful" ratios of lean tissue, fat, and trabecular bone. Additionally, trained men had resting metabolic rates (RMR) similar to those of young men and fasting fat oxidation values higher than those for both other groups. These factors may contribute to the body composition profiles observed via better en-

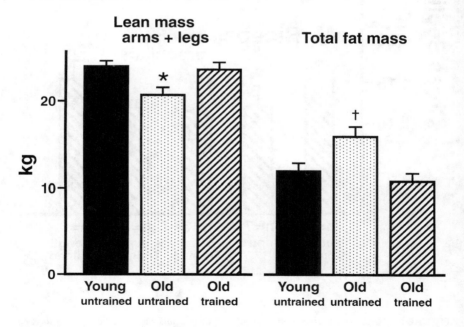

FIGURE 6-5. *Lean and fat mass in young and old untrained and old trained volunteers.* Body composition measurements obtai ned using dual energy X-ray absorptiometry (DXA). Values are given in kg. *$P < 0.01$, †$P < 0.001$. Data from Horber et al., 1996.

ergy balance and the prevention of age-related adipose tissue deposition. This study is unique in the seeming preservation of lean tissue with aerobic exercise alone, although it should be noted that details of the training history of the subjects is not provided, and they reported similar high physical activity levels 20–30 years prior to this study. It is possible that their long duration of involvement in sports or unreported muscle strengthening exercises were responsible for this difference from previous investigations. Additionally, the use of DXA for soft tissue analysis in the elderly has recently come into question, as the technique may underestimate truncal fat mass preferentially in older individuals (Snead et al., 1993), and the specificity for quantifying skeletal muscle mass inherent to CT scan imaging, urinary creatinine excretion (Wang et al., 1996) or muscle biopsy analysis, as used in Klitgaard's study (Klitgaard et al., 1990), is not possible with DXA.

Some of the limitations inherent to cross-sectional studies of master athletes can be addressed by longitudinal observations. In one such report, Pollock evaluated 24 master athletes (runners) aged 50–82 y over a 10 y period (Pollock et al., 1987). At first assessment they had body fat levels comparable to or lower than average young males (10–15%) but higher than elite young runners (5%). Despite continued training, body weight decreased (1.6 kg), body fat and relative body fat increased (1.3 kg and 2%, respectively), and fat free mass decreased (2.0 kg) by underwater weighing over the 10 y follow-up. Anthropometric measures indicated increased central adiposity and subcutaneous fat stores. Intensity of training and competition was variable among subjects but was not related to the increases in body fat. However, it is of note that three subjects who lifted weights in addition to running were the only ones to maintain their FFM over the course of observation.

It is difficult to separate the effects of aging from altered training regimens in master athletes, and it is likely that both factors explain changes in body composition over time. In a 20 y study of former Olympic oarsmen, for example, we found that body fat increased significantly from 12.3% to 15.6% between ages 24 and 44 years, but all of this change occurred during the first decade of follow-up, when training frequency was reduced from highly competitive 7 d/wk schedules to recreational rowing 3 d/wk in most subjects (Hagerman et al., 1996). Of note, the body fat of these men in middle age was far below average, and regular, non-competitive exercise was able to stabilize the changes for a decade in mid-life.

Thus, exercise training in older athletes is unable to completely offset age-related accumulation of body fat (particularly beyond 60 y of age). Overall, the cross-sectional and longitudinal observations of master athletes suggest that voluntary participation in high levels of exercise over many years attenuates the "age-related" decline in resting metabolic rate, increase in total and central fat stores, deterioration of glucose metabolism, decrease in bone mass, and perhaps loss of skeletal muscle mass and function, at least with resistive exercise. Ultimately, however, separation of the genetic factors that dictate activity levels and changes in metabolism and body composition with aging from the effects of assuming a physically active lifestyle in middle or old age can only be ascertained by randomized intervention trials such as those presented in the following sections.

Changes in Body Weight and Composition with Aerobic Exercise Interventions

Normal Older Individuals. Major reviews and meta-analyses indicate little evidence of the ability of exercise to significantly modify body weight and composition as an isolated intervention in normal elders (Ballor & Keesey, 1991; Epstein & Wing, 1980; Thompson et al., 1982). For example, King et al. (1991) reported that there were no changes in BMI or percent body fat after one year of aerobic training 3–5 d/wk at moderate-high intensity in a randomized controlled trial of 357 community-dwelling men and women aged 50–65 y. However, information on dietary intake or other components of energy expenditure is not available to further interpret these results.

In an uncontrolled trial, Schwartz and colleagues (1991) studied healthy young and old men after six months of intensive aerobic training, (5 d/wk for 45 min at 85% of heart rate reserve), during which time they were instructed not to alter their diet. Small but significant decreases in weight (2.5 kg), percent body fat (2.3%), fat mass (2.4 kg), and WHR (2%) accompanied exercise training in the old men but not in the young men, who instead had a 1.0 kg gain in FFM. However, CT scans detected greater than 20% decreases in fat deposits in subcutaneous regions of the chest and abdomen and in the internal abdominal region, along with an increase in thigh muscle area in the old men. Fat was lost preferentially from sites that were initially the largest. This study was important in revealing for the first time major changes in regional fat distribution via exercise in the absence of large losses of weight or total body fat mass. It suggests that aerobic exercise alone may improve the metabolically dangerous central deposition of fat (Bengtsson et al., 1993) even without dieting in healthy older men.

Another study using anthropometric measurements also demonstrated small losses of body weight and preferential loss of central adiposity following 9–12 mo of endurance training in healthy older men and women (Kohrt et al., 1992). It is not clear, however, that exercise of the intensity used in such studies and others with similar findings could be adhered to by individuals with chronic illness or significant obesity at baseline or that similar adaptations would take place in such individuals.

Franklin and colleagues (1978) reported that 23 men with coronary heart disease of mean age 51 y participated in an aerobic training program at low-moderate intensity (70–75% maximal heart rate for 15–30 min 3 d/wk). After 12 wk he found that body weight was unchanged, skinfold thicknesses decreased by 8%, and estimated body fat from skinfolds decreased by 1 kg (1.3%), without effect on cholesterol or glucose levels. Although the regimen did not cause musculoskeletal injuries seen in some higher intensity protocols, only 16 of the 23 subjects completed the intervention. Thus, as Pollock et al.(1971) reported regarding a vigorous walking program in middle-aged men, only small effects on body fat and no concomitant weight loss are seen with low-moderate intensity exercise regimens.

Obese Middle Aged and Older Subjects. No randomized controlled trials have used only aerobic exercise in the treatment of obesity in the elderly, and it is important to study this group specifically before making recommendations, as their ability to tolerate aerobic exercise, compliance rates, metabolic responses, and body composition changes may not be identical to younger or lean subjects. Until such data are generated, studies in young and middle-aged adults must be generalized to derive guidelines for the elderly. In one of the earliest uncontrolled series, Gwinup (1975) reported that 34 subjects started an exercise intervention of at least 30 min/d of walking and were followed for 1–2 y. Only 11 subjects (all women between ages 19–41 y) were able to comply with the study requirements, and among them, weight loss averaged 22 lb with apparently no concurrent dietary restriction. The exercise regimens actually performed by 9 of these 11 women, however, were 2–3 h of walking 7 d/wk. Thus, the practicality of this approach seems limited, particularly for older, frailer adults.

In a more recent study of middle-aged obese women, Despres et al. (1991) found that aerobic exercise resulted in reductions in abdominal adipose tissue as well as in the ratio of subcutaneous abdominal to thigh fat, indicating preferential losses of central adiposity, just as has been seen in non-obese older adults (Kohrt et al., 1992; Schwartz et al., 1991).

Overall, it appears that minimal metabolic benefit and change in body composition can be expected in weight-stable, aerobically exercising older adults. Katzel recently reported the results of a randomized trial of hypocaloric dieting vs. aerobic exercise training in obese sedentary men 46–80 y of age who were selected for being 120-160% of ideal body weight (Katzel et al., 1995). Subjects (mean age 61 y, BMI 30 kg/m^2) were randomized to 9 mo of hypcaloric dieting (300–500 kcal/d deficit) or aerobic exercise (45 min of treadmill or cycling at 70–80% of heart rate reserve for 30-45 min, 3 d/wk). Only 44 of 73 men in the diet group, 49 of 71 in the exercise group, and 18 of 26 controls completed the study. As can be seen in Figure 6-6, weight loss (average 9.5 kg), and decrease in total and abdominal obesity occurred only in the diet group. Seventy five percent of the weight lost was fat tissue and was accompanied by improvements in fasting insulin levels and glucose tolerance, cholesterol, and blood pressure. Compared to younger subjects, the older men lost significantly less weight and percent body fat. By design, the aerobic training group had no significant changes in weight, and only insulin sensitivity improved compared to controls.

Thus, the body composition, fat distribution, and metabolic changes seen in some previous exercise studies of non-obese or younger individuals were not evident (Schwartz et al., 1992). Presumably, this is because the exercisers increased their dietary intake to remain weight stable, and

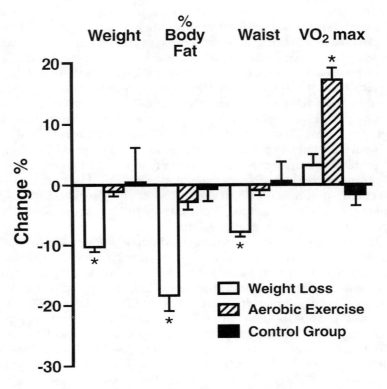

FIGURE 6-6. *Comparison of relative changes in body composition and maximal aerobic capacity after intervention in weight loss and aerobic exercise and control groups.* Values with asterisks are significantly different at P < 0.05 by ANOVA. Data are mean ±SEM. Data from Katzel et al., 1995.

lean mass was not altered by this modality of exercise. The high dropout rates in both diet and exercise groups, despite the exclusion of subjects with overt disease, medication usage, or abnormal stress tests are significant. In addition, the less robust response of the older subjects speaks to the difficulty in generalizing such findings to the larger population of obese elders.

In summary, there is no evidence to date from randomized clinical trials in obese elderly that aerobic exercise without dietary restriction can significantly lower body weight, percent body fat, central adiposity, or lipid profiles. Other reasons to advocate such exercise in this group, however, include increases in aerobic fitness (Ruoti et al., 1994) and insulin sensitivity (Hersey et al., 1994) that may occur independently of weight loss in the elderly.

Changes in Body Weight and Composition with Resistive Exercise Interventions

Normal Older Individuals. Numerous studies of normal healthy older adults indicate that high-intensity resistance training is associated with increases in FFM or muscle area and with slight decreases in percent body fat, usually with minimal alteration of total body weight(Cartee, 1994; Charette et al., 1991; Lillegard & Terrio, 1994; McCartney et al., 1995). In these studies the reported adaptive responses of skeletal muscle to hypertrophy were quite variable and were influenced by the intensity and duration of the intervention, subject characteristics, and the precision of the measurement technique. Typically, the largest changes are seen regionally in cross-sectional areas of individual muscle fibers in biopsy specimens or in CT-scan analyses of trained muscle groups, whereas whole-body measures of fat-free mass or lean mass show more modest changes (Nelson et al., 1996). In the first investigation to demonstrate significant change in muscle area with resistance training, Frontera et al. (1988) reported that 12 men in their 60's and 70's had a 28–34% increase in fiber areas in the vastus lateralis after 12 wk of knee extensor and flexor training, despite no overall changes in body weight or composition. Fiatarone et al. (1990)similarly found regional increases of 9% in muscle area by CT scan of the thigh in frail nonagenarians after 8 wk of quadriceps weight lifting training, again with no change in BMI, skinfolds, total body water by isotope dilution, or bioelectric impedance measurements. In general, studies such as those of Dupler and Cortes (1993) that used anthropometric assessment only in weight-stable populations have not been able to demonstrate changes in fat or lean compartments after strength training. Muscle cross-sectional area changes on biopsy have varied from no change to increases of 20–67% in various studies, which may be due to heterogeneous responses in individuals as well as to error in sampling techniques with this method (Cartee, 1994; Evans, 1996).

Typically, whole body changes after programs of 12–52 wk duration have been modest, with no changes in BMI, 1–2 kg gains in muscle, and 1–2% decreases in percent body fat. For example, Nelson et al. (1994) reported that one year of progressive resistance training in 40 post-menopausal women resulted in no change in body weight, BMI, sum of skinfold thicknesses, WHR, or other circumferences, compared to controls. Thigh muscle area on CT scan increased significantly by 6%, as did total body potassium (+3.3 gm), FFM by underwater weighing (1.3kg), and muscle mass estimated by 24 h creatinine excretion (+1.4kg)(Nelson et al., 1996). Thus, there was general agreement with these different estimates of muscle or fat-free body composition. Fat mass calculated by underwater weighing decreased significantly by approximately 1 kg compared to sedentary controls. By contrast, anthropometrics, DXA-estimated FFM and FM for the whole body and for appendicular regions, and bioelectric-impedance estimates of fat did not change over the year, perhaps due to insufficient sensitivity of these techniques for detecting changes specifically within the skeletal muscle compartment, where the exercise adaptation was most prominent.

This inability of anthropometric measurements to detect change in body composition after strength training is reflected in many previous studies and, therefore, should not necessarily be interpreted as lack of adaptation. Anthropometric measures are best suited for interventions that stimulate significant losses of body weight and subcutaneous fat, such as dietary intervention studies. Despite the minimal effect on total body fat in most studies of resistance training in the elderly, there is evidence of reduction in intra-abdominal fat stores in two studies. Treuth et al. (1995a) reported that 14 women (mean age = 67 y) who undertook moderate intensity progressive resistance training for 16 wk had significant reductions in CT measures of intra-abdominal fat areas (10%) as well as decreased subcutaneous fat and increased muscle (9.6%) at the midthigh area. These adaptations were seen with no overall changes in body weight, FFM or FM by underwater weighing, anthropometric indices, or dietary intake, again emphasizing the superiority of regional measurements of body composition to document adaptations to resistance training. Similar results were found after strength training in men 51–71 y old, who lost 8% of truncal fat by DXA and gained 6.6% muscle area in the thigh by MRI studies (Treuth et al., 1994). Like aerobic training (Kohrt et al., 1992; Schwartz et al., 1991), resistance training appears capable of reducing metabolically undesirable central fat deposits in the absence of weight loss or caloric restriction in the elderly.

Resistance training studies in the healthy elderly suggest favorable shifts in energy balance, even in the absence of weight loss or increases in fat-free mass. Campbell et al. (1994) have reported that total energy requirements for weight maintenance are increased approximately 15% after 12 wk of resistance training in older men and women, primarily due to increases in RMR. Treuth et al.(1995b) also described increased resting energy expenditure and fat oxidation after resistance training in postmenopausal women. Over the long term, such acute adaptations may significantly affect energy balance and contribute to the mainte-nance of a healthful body weight while minimizing fat deposition.

No studies are yet available to suggest on an epidemiological basis that resistance training will lower the prevalence of obesity or obesity-related morbidity and mortality because this type of exercise is uncom-mon in the general population, particularly among women. Thus, for now, the results of small clinical trials such as those reported above must be used to estimate benefits that may accrue with the adoption of this type of physical activity. It is clear that the age-related declines in FFM and muscle mass are not irreversible but are amenable to targeted exer-cise interventions in individuals up to 100 y of age (Fiatarone & Evans, 1993; Fiatarone et al., 1994). The benefits of using resistance training to increase muscle mass and strength in the elderly include decreased risk of injurious falls, increased bone density, better mobility, improved aer-obic capacity, increased nutritional intake, less functional dependency, better balance, improved glucose homeostasis, faster gastrointestinal transit time, less arthritic pain and immobility, relief of depressive symptoms and insomnia, and higher self-efficacy, among others (Ades et al., 1996; Fiatarone & Evans, 1990; Fluckey et al., 1994; Lohman et al., 1995; McCartney et al., 1991; Nelson et al., 1994, 1997; Singh et al., 1997a, 1997b; Stewart et al., 1988). Thus, many common geriatric syndromes beyond simple muscle atrophy may be indications for this modality of exercise.

Obese Middle Aged and Older Subjects. There are as yet no trials of resistance training as an isolated intervention to induce weight loss in obese older adults. The combination of weight lifting and hypocaloric dieting has been of increasing interest in recent years, as will be de-scribed below. However, in prior resistance training studies, which have included older individuals with a wide range of BMI values, there is no indication that obesity precludes adoption of or adaptation to training. In fact, the tolerance to resistance training is likely significantly better than to weight-bearing endurance training in obese individuals with lower extremity arthritis because of associated pain, mobility impair-ment, and exacerbation of under lying joint symptoms (Mangione et al., 1996; Oddis, 1996). The lower cardiovascular stimulation of resistance training as compared to aerobic training may also be of benefit in obese elders with many cardiovascular risk factors, overt cardiac disease, or diabetes. For example, we have safely used this form of exercise in elderly subjects with chronic congestive heart failure (Pu et al., 1997).

INTERACTION OF EXERCISE AND DIETARY MODIFICATION IN WEIGHT CONTROL FOR OLDER ADULTS

Most major reviews suggest that exercise alone exerts only modest effects on body weight and fat mass, particularly in women. In a meta-analysis of 53 such studies (up to 36 wk in duration), Ballor reported that in men aerobic exercise resulted in an average loss of 1.2 kg of body weight compared to a 1.2 kg gain in weight lifting studies (Ballor & Keesey, 1991). Body fat decreased, regardless of exercise modality, by 1.5 kg (1.7%) compared to controls. Weight training was significantly better at increasing FFM (2.2 kg), compared to 0.8 kg with cycling and no difference from controls in walking/jogging studies. In women, only walking/jogging resulted in a decrease in body weight (0.6 kg) compared to controls, as well as in significant reductions in body fat (1.3 kg, 1.7%) and no change in FFM. Losses in body weight and fat were greatest in those with high body fat initially and with the highest exercise-related energy expenditure. The gender differences seen in these studies may relate to the higher energy cost of equivalent activities in men due to their greater body mass (Gleim, 1993). Overall, substantial changes in body mass would seem to require dietary modification.

However, hypocaloric dieting alone, although effective if adhered to in creating an energy deficit and therefore loss of body weight and fat, has undesirable consequences in the elderly, including exacerbation of age-related losses of lean tissue, decreased metabolic rate, and risk for micronutrient deficiencies. Both endurance and resistance training are associated with increased energy expenditure through the cost of activity, increased basal metabolic rate, increased thermic effect of a meal, and increased lean body mass (primarily resistance), and can induce small losses of body weight and total fat as well mobilization of fat from abdominal sites in older men and women. It makes sense, therefore, that a combination of diet and exercise modalities in obese individuals may produce the largest losses of weight while attaining more desirable body composition ratios and metabolic profiles than either treatment alone. Intervention studies that have taken this approach are presented below.

Diet and Endurance Training in Obese Subjects

The combination of hypocaloric dieting and endurance training has been said to have several beneficial consequences, despite the fact that there is little evidence that combined therapy results in more short-term weight loss than dieting alone. For example, in a meta-analysis of 89 studies involving 1800 Type II diabetics conducted over the past 30 years, diet alone had a significantly greater effect on weight loss (9 kg) and glycosolated hemoglobin levels, compared to mean losses of 3.8 kg in exercise, diet and behavioral interventions (Brown et al., 1996). However, there are several reasons to consider the combination of diet and exercise for obesity in the elderly. The reduction in resting energy expenditure secondary to dieting may be prevented or attenuated by concurrent exercise (Ballor et al., 1996), although this is not uniformly seen (Ballor & Poehlman, 1993). Aerobic exercise may attenuate the losses of FFM that account for 10–50% of weight lost by hypocaloric dieting(Durrant et al., 1980). Finally, the increase in aerobic fitness itself has many physiologic and psychological consequences which cannot be achieved by dieting alone and may enhance long-term behavioral adaptations to minimize weight cycling.

There are no randomized controlled trials of weight loss comparing hypocaloric dieting to diet plus exercise in obese elders. However, two non-randomized studies have been reported in this population. Dengel and colleagues (1994a, 1994b) studied obese 60-y-old men who were non-randomly assigned by preference to one of three treatments: 1) hypocaloric dieting and behavioral modification, 2) diet plus aerobic exercise for 10 mo (3 d/wk at 50–85% of VO_2max), or 3) a control group that received brief dietary instructions only. Results were presented only for those subjects who completed the study and who lost at least 3 kg (33% of the diet group, 62% of the diet plus exercise group, and 57% of controls). Weight loss averaged 8–9 kg, body fat decreased by approximately 5%, and FFM (estimated by underwater weighing) declined by 1–2 kg, with no differences among treatment groups, as seen in Figure 6-7. Fat-free mass loss was directly related to the change in total body weight (r = 0.48) in both groups. As expected, only the exercisers exhibited an increase in aerobic capacity, but there was no difference in lipid lowering or decrease in skinfold thicknesses (preferentially truncal) between groups.

Thus, no additional benefit to weight loss, body composition, lipid profile, or fat distribution was attributable to exercise. This finding is in agreement with several other studies in younger individuals that demonstrate that loss of fat- free mass is dependent upon the total weight loss, regardless of how it is achieved. However, it should be noted from the perspective of clinical application that more than twice as many exercisers as dieters achieved the minimum study goal (loss of 3 kg), for reasons that have not been elucidated, and this may be one of the most important findings of this study. Unfortunately, the self-selec-

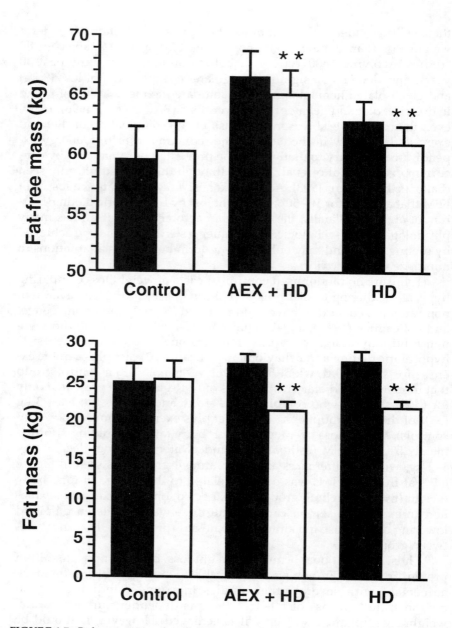

FIGURE 6-7. *Body composition changes following weight loss by hypocaloric diet vs aerobic exercise in obese older men.* Measurements made by hydrostatic weighing. Solid bars are initial values and open bars are final values after 10 months of intervention or control condition. ** indicates significant (P < 0.0001) difference from initial values within group. Values are expressed as mean ±SEM. Data from Dengel et al., 1994a.

tion of treatment assignment limits the extent to which these findings can be generalized to individuals who may be unwillingly prescribed such treatments by their physicians. Overall, the increase in aerobic fitness has independent predictive value for functional independence and mortality in the elderly (Blair et al., 1989b) and is therefore a worthy goal in obese elders who are at higher risk of death and disability than are their leaner peers.

In the only other such study of older subjects, Fox et al. (1996) reported that 41 healthy obese women of average age 66 y were non-randomly assigned to diet groups in which caloric intake was reduced by 500 or 700 kcal/d or to a diet plus exercise group with a combined deficit of 700 kcal/d. Exercise consisted of walking for 1 h 3 d/wk and resistive exercises 2 d/wk. After 24 weeks, weight loss (6.5 kg), body fat, LBM (by DXA) and fasting glucose decreased significantly over time with all treatments, whereas fat distribution (by anthropometrics), lipids, and fasting insulin levels did not change in any group. Thus exercise, even combining aerobic and resistive components, did not offer any additional benefit to these women. Interestingly, Wood et al. (1991) found that exercise increased the loss of body fat and abdominal girth and resulted in higher HDL and lower LDL/HDL ratios after one year, compared to dieting alone in overweight men, but had no additive effect in women aged 25–49. Thus, the apparent resistance of these middle-aged and older obese women to the benefits of exercise in weight control compared to trials in men and younger subjects may be due to gender-specific effects or to the less intensive nature of the energy deficit prescribed. The difficulty in making recommendations for the elderly based upon studies in individuals who do not have the disease in question (obesity) or who are much younger is evident from these studies. It is not known whether better measurements of fat distribution and muscle mass would have resulted in different conclusions from the Fox study, but at this time moderate diet and exercise interventions cannot be expected to replicate the larger shifts in body composition seen with severe caloric restriction or large expenditures of energy in physical activity.

Diet and Resistance Training in Obese Subjects

Although resistance training has been shown to reduce total and abdominal fat, dieting is a more potent way to achieve these goals. The primary purpose of combining weight lifting and diet in obese individuals is to stimulate accretion of lean mass (muscle and bone) in the face of an energy deficit. In the first report of such combined therapy, Ballor et al. (1988) reported on 41 obese young women randomly assigned to diet, exercise, diet plus exercise, or control groups for 8 wk. Dieting significantly decreased body weight, arm fat area, circumferences, skinfolds, and fat mass. Resistance training increased arm muscle area, strength, and lean body weight, and decreased percent body fat. No interaction was seen between these two treatment modalities, and the combined therapy group therefore ended up with a better body composition profile (increased lean, decreased fat) than either isolated intervention could achieve. Importantly, hypocaloric dieting (1000 kcal/d) did not appear to limit the functional adaptation or hypertrophy of muscle secondary to resistance training.

One randomized controlled trial compared resistance training to endurance training after hypocaloric dieting in obese older subjects. After 11 wk of dieting, Ballor et al. (1996) randomly allocated 18 older subjects to moderate intensity resistance or aerobic exercise training for an additional 12 wk. As can be seen in Figure 6-8, weight remained stable in the weight lifters, as the decline in fat mass was more than replaced by a gain in FFM. By contrast, the endurance-training group lost fat and FFM, which combined to produce a significant drop in total body weight. Thus, knowing that weight is being lost is insufficient to judge the metabolic benefit of an intervention when divergent adaptations in fat and lean tissue are occurring.

In terms of energy expenditure, resistance training, but not aerobic training, was associated with a tendency to increase resting energy expenditure (Ballor et al., 1996). This increase in resting energy expenditure (5%, 79 kcal/d) was not sufficient to offset the 260 kcal/d (15%) decline that had been induced by the hypocaloric diet. Finally, the thermic effect of a meal, which had also been reduced by dieting, was 8% higher after weight training and unchanged by aerobic exercise. Thus, overall more favorable body composition and energy balance changes could be attributed to resistance exercise than to aerobic exercise in this study, despite the greater increase in the energy cost of the aerobic exercise itself.

In the long term control of body weight, these body composition and resting energy expenditure adaptations seen with resistance training may be extremely important in minimizing the tendency for weight and fat to be regained after dieting (van Dale & Saris, 1989). In addition, the preservation or accretion of lean tissue and muscle strength, which is only seen with resistive exercise, assumes ever greater importance with age.

PHYSICAL ACTIVITY, DIETARY INTAKE, AND UNDERNUTRITION WITH AGING

Effect of Exercise on Energy Intake in the Older Adult

Most studies of adults of all ages indicate that energy intake is directly related to physical activity level, and inversely related to body

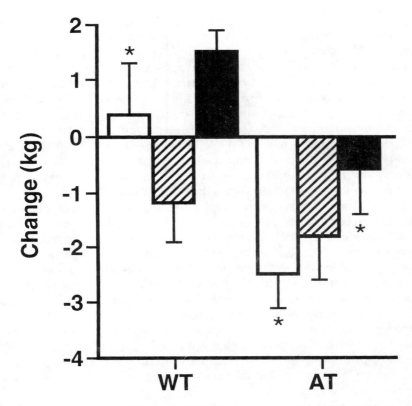

FIGURE 6-8. *Changes in body weight (open bars) fat mass (hatched bars) and fat-free mass (solid bars) following 12 weeks of exercise training.* WT = resistance training, AT = aerobic training. Measurements made by hydrostatic weighing. Values are mean ± SEM. * indicates AT group change significantly different (P < 0.05) than WT group. Data from Ballor et al., 1996.

weight or BMI. Thus, if increased energy expenditure is achieved through physical activity, it appears to be accompanied in health by increases in energy intake in order to maintain energy balance (Blair et al., 1981). Many surveys indicate that people who exercise are less likely to have nutritional deficiencies, but they are generally healthier, more likely to use multivitamin supplements, non-smokers, better educated, more financially secure, and have better social support systems than sedentary elders, so that the causal nature of these associations cannot be determined (Casper, 1995; DiPietro et al., 1993; Hanson et al., 1987). Both younger and older healthy sedentary adults as well as young or master athletes follow this pattern when *ad libitum* dietary intake is monitored. Butterworth et al. (1993) reported that highly conditioned elderly women (age 65-84 y, training aerobically on average 1.6 h/d for the past 11 y) had lower BMI and skinfold thicknesses but significantly higher intakes of energy, protein, carbohydrates, fiber, and several micronutrients by 7 d food records than did age-matched peers. Energy intake was 37.1 kcal/kg in the trained women compared to 24.1 kcal/kg in the sedentary group, and nutrient density was similar in the diets of both groups, suggesting that no changes in dietary quality accompanied the increased quantity in these trained women. However, many more of the sedentary women fell below the RDA for specific micronutrients, as compared to only one exercising woman. Thus a general increase in food quantity may be sufficient to avoid nutritional imbalances which are otherwise seen even in free-living healthy elders.

Intervention studies may not replicate the results of cross-sectional observations. For example, in an animal model using 6-, 15-, and 27-mo-old rats, Mazzeo and Horwath (1996) found that 12 wk of intensive endurance training (5 h/wk at 75% VO_2max) resulted in large fat losses and increases in lean mass (accompanied by increased food intake in the two youngest groups), but in the aged animals there was a decline in fat mass and no increase in lean mass or food intake compared to controls. Thus, this study suggests that there are differential adaptations to exercise-induced increased energy expenditure that are dependent upon age. The failure to increase food consumption appeared to limit the potential of endurance training to augment lean body mass, leaving the aged animals with lower body weight and fat mass but with similar lean mass compared to sedentary controls.

Human studies are mixed in dietary intake adaptations reported in training studies. Obese women did not increase dietary intake during endurance training in two studies (Keim et al., 1990; Nieman et al., 1990). In one of the few studies in the elderly, Butterworth and colleagues (1993) found no changes in weight or macro- or micronutrient intake by 7 d food records after a supervised 12-wk walking program (30 min/d, 5 d/wk, at 60% of maximal heart rate reserve) in women of average age 73 y, compared to a group randomized to mild flexibility classes). In contrast, several studies have shown that free-living healthy older men and women initiating aerobic or resistance training protocols maintain body weight over time periods of up to one year, despite the increased energy costs of the exercise itself, increases in resting metabolic rate that may accompany the training, and increases in spontaneous physical activity levels outside of the prescribed exercise sessions (Meredith et al., 1988; Nelson et al., 1991, 1994). Thus, whether documented or not, increases in energy intake must be occurring to prevent weight loss and allow the gains in muscle tissue seen in these studies.

The relative inaccuracy of food records compared to food weighing or metabolic studies probably accounts for some of the inconsistencies in the literature, but heterogeneous responses to exercise in the aging population cannot be ruled out. For example, (Goran & Poehlman, 1992) reported no increase in total energy expenditure by doubly-labeled water measurements after initiation of endurance training sessions in older subjects, suggesting that physical activity outside of class must have declined. Such an occurrence would minimize any tendency for exercise training to increase appetite or food intake and may also explain some of the divergent results of previous studies.

Overall, in the normal weight older adult, there is no evidence that higher physical activity levels are associated with worsening nutritional status; therefore, it would appear that normal aging does not interfere markedly with this adaptive response to exercise. In fact, because increased energy intake is associated with increased micronutrient intakes, maintenance of adequate physical activity levels may be very important for the maintenance of adequate nutrition. With aging, reduced muscle mass, metabolic rate, and energy expenditure decrease energy needs in the face of increasing requirements for certain nutrients (e.g., vitamin D, folate, B_{12}, calcium, protein), a situation which can pose serious nutritional risk (Casper, 1995; Morley, 1996).

More longitudinal studies and randomized clinical trials are clearly needed to evaluate the effect of adopting exercise on nutritional status. In the meantime, there does not appear to be risk of unintentional weight loss or malnutrition if increased energy expenditure through physical activity is promoted in normal weight healthy elders. On the other hand, if the intent is to use exercise in obese older adults to promote weight and fat loss, active instructions to change dietary patterns and caloric intake will be needed to offset the potential increase in energy intake accompanying higher levels of activity.

Exercise, Anorexia, and Weight Loss in the Frail Elderly

Obesity is rarely a concern in the frail elderly, whereas anorexia, weight loss, and diminished lean body mass (with all of its functional and metabolic consequences) assumes clinical importance. Only one study has addressed the ability of exercise to influence dietary intake in this population (Fiatarone et al., 1994). We studied 100 frail nursing home residents (average age 86 y) in a randomized controlled trial of resistance exercise and/or complete nutritional supplementation (Figure 6-9). The supplement alone had no beneficial effect on weight, body composition, or muscle function but instead was associated with a compensatory decrease in energy intake from the normal diet, so that no net increase in total energy intake occurred. Exercisers who were not supplemented had no change in total energy intake, but they had little or no access to extra food sources compared to free-living populations. In contrast, the exercisers who also had access to the supplement had a net gain in energy intake of approximately 300 kcal/d (20% above baseline), presumably as an adaptation to the increased energy needs imposed by adoption of resistive exercise training.

This finding is notable in view of the very advanced age, the heavy burden of chronic disease, medications, depression and dementia, and the functional dependency in this population, all factors associated with anorexia and weight loss in the elderly (Morley & Kraenzle, 1994). In addition to the effect of changing energy requirements on dietary intake, exercise may exert a beneficial effect on appetite via alleviation of depression. In this and other studies, we have demonstrated a significant anti-depressant effect of exercise in the elderly (Singh et al., 1997b).

The results of this study suggest that without a reversal of the con-

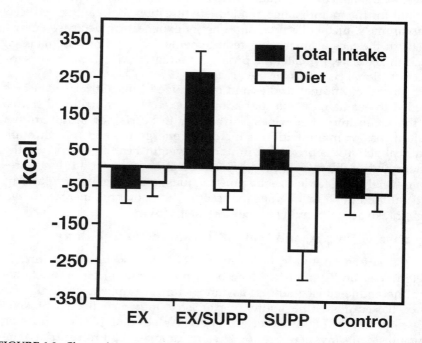

FIGURE 6-9. *Changes in energy intake after resistance training and/or nutritional supplementation in frail elderly nursing home residents.* Dietary intake calculated from 3-d food weighings, data expressed as mean ±SEM. Dietary energy intake included the energy content of meals, snacks, and supplements other than the supplement or placebo used in the study. Total energy intake included dietary energy intake plus the energy content of the study supplement. Exercise significantly blunted the decline in dietary energy intake during the trial (p=0.04). The study supplement only augmented total energy intake in subjects who also exercised. Data from Fiatarone et al., 1994.

ditions associated with extreme sedentariness (low muscle mass, resting metabolic rate, and energy expenditure in physical activity), attempts to prevent weight loss with nutritional supplementation alone may fail, which is consistent with clinical experience in this area. Resistance training, because it can modify all of these factors and also has been shown to result in higher levels of activity outside of exercise class, may offer the best chance to alter energy balance and lean tissue depletion in this vulnerable population. Further studies are needed to verify the long-term adaptations in dietary intake and energy balance in response to both aerobic and resistance training in frail elders.

PRACTICAL IMPLICATIONS

Modality of Exercise to Choose

The exercise prescription for optimum body weight and composition in the elderly should be based upon the scientific evidence of benefit of specific activities as well as on the physiologic profile, health status, and psychosocial characteristics of the older individual. Based upon the studies reviewed above, it would appear that both aerobic exercise and resistance training have benefits in this regard, but their benefits and side effect profiles are not interchangeable, and thus guidelines are needed for both safety and efficacy in the use of exercise for this purpose.

The Normal Weight Older Adult. Here the goal is to maintain body weight at a stable level with advancing years, while offsetting the typical accumulation of body fat and loss of lean tissue, including muscle and bone. General attempts to increase physical activity levels throughout the day (e.g., avoidance of mechanical aids, "labor-saving" devices, and increased walking, Table 6-1) will boost slightly total energy expenditure that otherwise may decline in old age more than energy intake, leading to slight positive energy balances which over the years result in deposition of excess energy as fat. Such general attempts to be more active will have little impact on age-related declines in resting metabolic rate, aerobic fitness, muscle strength, or lean tissue, however, so that in addition, a structured attempt to accumulate at least 3 sessions per week of aerobic activity and 2–3 sessions per week of resistive exercises is also recommended. If only one type of exercise can be committed to, it should be resistance training, since increases in resting energy expenditure, aerobic capacity, muscle strength, muscle mass, and bone density have been demonstrated with this modality of exercise, while cardiovascular exercise does not increase muscle mass or strength.

The Normal Weight Older Adult with Cardiovascular Risk Factors. The goal in these individuals is not weight loss but improved control of reversible cardiovascular risk factors including hypertension, hy-

TABLE 6-1. *Increasing energy expenditure in physical activity throughout the day.*

Walk instead of taking the car whenever possible
Park in the farthest corner of the parking lot
Always take the stairs instead of the elevator or escalator
Don't use any remote control devices
Use manual rather than power house and yard tools
Carry rather than pushing or dragging bundles
Read while riding a stationary bicycle
Use TV watching time to do calisthenics, weight lifting, or stretching

perlipidemia, glucose intolerance, diabetes, and central adiposity. Both aerobic and resistance training interventions have been shown to be of benefit in the regulation of these conditions, although there is much more extensive data on aerobic exercise; the benefits of resistive exercises are relatively recently documented (Hurley et al., 1988). Thus, personal preferences of the individual may guide the prescription.

The Obese Older Adult

Exercise alone is very unlikely to result in substantial amounts of weight loss in the obese adult, even when compliance is high. Therefore, it should always be combined with hypocaloric dietary modification for optimal results. Although the short term weight loss associated with diet plus exercise is usually not different than diet treatments alone, there are several extremely important reasons to co-administer these therapies.

First, hypocaloric dieting alone results in a decline in total energy expenditure due to decreases in resting metabolic rate, the thermic effect of feeding, and the energy cost of physical activities (as body weight is lost), as well as decreased spontaneous activity levels in animal models. This may be why weight cycling is so common and difficult to intervene upon by diet alone, since lower and lower energy intakes must be adhered to if weight loss is to be sustained over time. The simultaneous use of exercise may offset these trends by increasing resting metabolic rate and the thermic effect of meals, and by adding the energy cost of the specific activity prescribed to the total daily energy expenditure. In addition, resistance training (but not aerobic training) has been shown to result in increased spontaneous or habitual activity levels in the elderly (Fiatarone et al., 1994; Nelson et al., 1994), thus further increasing total energy expenditure. By replacing a portion of the desired energy deficit with increased energy expenditure, the allowable dietary energy intake can be liberalized slightly, which should help compliance over time.

Second, the composition of the weight loss that is incurred through hypocaloric dieting may range from 10–50% lean tissue depending upon the severity of the energy restriction. In the elderly, this is particularly worrisome because it would be occurring at a time when biological aging, chronic disease and disuse atrophy are already contributing to losses of lean tissue. Most studies of aerobic exercise in obese adults on a weight loss diet demonstrate little or no capacity to attenuate these lean tissue losses. However, resistance training has been shown in young women to change the composition of weight loss during dieting such that lean mass is gained while body weight and fat are lost (Ballor et al., 1996; Ballor et al., 1988). Therefore, assuming that these results would extend to the elderly, the preferential prescription of resistive exercise during weight loss appears prudent at this time.

Third, although hypocaloric dieting can result in substantial losses of weight and fat mass and in improvement of cardiovascular risk factor profiles in the short term, it does not result in improved aerobic capacity, muscle strength, balance, and other aspects of fitness that are seen in combined programs of diet and exercise.

Fourth, there appears to be a better adherence to other positive lifestyle modifications such as diet and smoking cessation if exercise behavior is encouraged simultaneously. This may be due to exercise-induced increases in self-efficacy which generalize to other behaviors, alleviation of coexistent depression or low self-esteem, or positive feedback from early success in reaching goals. Whatever the mechanism, the long-term efficacy of all weight loss interventions requires the adoption of lifelong behavioral changes, and exercise appears to aid in this process.

Intensity and Frequency of Exercise Required to Effect Changes in Body Composition and Weight in the Older Adult

There has been relatively little definitive information on the dose and intensity of exercise which is optimal for weight loss, but it appears that in conjunction with diet, high intensity aerobic exercise in young women is not superior to low intensity aerobic exercise if total energy expenditure is equalized by a longer duration at each session (Ballor & Poehlman, 1993). Neither regimen was able to prevent the 10% loss of fat-free mass that occurred in this study. Therefore, because most obese sedentary older adults could not sustain an aerobic training program at 80–90% of VO_2max, and given the added cardiovascular risks this would incur, lower intensity exercise is preferable for most individuals.

Metabolic parameters relevant to obesity, including glucose homeostasis, blood pressure regulation, and lipid levels have not been shown to improve significantly when training frequency is increased above three times weekly, whereas injury rates are higher with five or more training days per week (Holloszy et al., 1986; Pollock et al., 1971; Seals &

Hagberg, 1984). Therefore, a thrice weekly schedule is likely to be sustainable and effective as an adjunct to dietary restriction in obese elders.

In contrast to aerobic exercise, the benefits of resistance training (increased muscle strength, mass, and resting energy expenditure) have been observed only with high intensity progressive resistance training. If the intent of this training is to alter body composition by preserving or augmenting lean mass during diet-induced weight loss, as well as to increase resting energy expenditure, then all of the evidence suggests that a high intensity regimen (70–80% of the 1 repetition maximum as the training stimulus) 2–3 d/wk is required. Although there are as yet no studies of weight loss after combined diet and resistance training in the elderly, the results from younger populations should apply, since muscle hypertrophy and increased resting energy expenditure have been seen in a variety of elderly populations undergoing strength training.

Behavioral Issues in Control of Body Weight via Exercise in the Older Adult

The achievement and maintenance of ideal body weight and composition require lifelong patterns of healthy eating and exercise to become established. Ultimately, any therapies found successful in small efficacy studies must be shown in larger effectiveness trials to retain their potency despite the tendency for generalization to bring with it lower compliance rates and intensity of exercise than originally prescribed. Therefore, understanding adoption and adherence to exercise behavior in the elderly is as critical as the knowledge of the physiologic adaptations that exercise can induce. Unfortunately, less attention has been given to these issues of implementation, so that long-term success rates are often disappointingly low compared to the robust responses seen in short- term, high-intensity clinical trials.

Assessment of Readiness to Change

The transtheoretical model of behavior views the decisions to participate in a given behavior as stages starting with "pre-contemplation" and moving to "contemplation," "action," and "maintenance" as a new behavior is adopted. For example, presenting someone who is not even contemplating beginning an exercise regimen with a health club membership or a stationary cycle will not succeed in changing his behavior because he has not yet made the commitment to begin. However, if a crisis has moved the person to the stages of "contemplation" or "action," this might be just the motivational gift needed to allow him to achieve and maintain this new behavior. The goal of the health educator or exercise leader is to recognize the stage in which a particular individual resides and then to apply the right educational, supportive, and motivational tools at that point in time.

Exercise behavior has been shown to be very likely to be sustained long-term if one participates in it on a regular basis for at least six consecutive months (King et al., 1988, 1989). Most obese dieters never make it this far in either dietary or exercise resolutions. It makes sense, therefore, to put maximal effort behaviorally into the first 6 months of the exercise prescription if it is to be successful. Relapses are common, and relapse prevention training has been shown to decrease dropouts by anticipating common hurdles that might otherwise discourage continued participation at high levels.

Mechanisms to Enhance Adoption of and Adherence to Physical Activity in Older Adults

One of the most successful ways to initiate and sustain a new behavior is self-monitoring of progress via record keeping. These records work best initially if they are displayed publicly or monitored by leaders with feedback and rewards for progress. In older adults, particularly novices at exercise, the security of face-to-face supervision appears to be desirable initially, although this can gradually be replaced with telephone and written contact. However, many studies show that the rapid tapering of contact is associated with very low compliance rates, and therefore, during the critical 6-month initiation period, it is suggested that high levels of contact (weekly or biweekly) be maintained to ensure maximal adoption of exercise behavior. Afterwards, more internal rewards, such as success in achieving weight loss or health status goals can replace external feedback and encouragement.

Barriers to Physical Activity in Older Adults

As in younger adults, there are numerous barriers to physical activity participation in the elderly. Additionally, the elderly obese individual is one of the most difficult to enroll in sustained physical activity patterns, as they may have a lifelong pattern of sedentariness that is extremely difficult to overcome. Disinterest, perceived lack of time or access to a facility, and fear of injury or medical complication lead the list of barriers that must be overcome. Structuring pleasurable activities into the day, exercising with a partner, exercising at home, and providing medical screening and supervision provide concrete ways to overcome these barriers. It is best not to assume that all older adults are alike or that they all want to exercise in groups, for example, as King has shown that compliance is actually higher and benefits just as great in home-based exercise programs (King et al., 1991). Lack of transportation is overcome if exercise can be structured into the home environment, and this is especially important for women who are still caregivers for other family members, for those who are disabled, visually impaired, or frail and cannot safely travel from home, and for those without the financial resources to join a fitness facility.

Safety of the Exercise Prescription in the Obese or Healthy Older Adult

Evidence from numerous studies in both healthy and frail older adults suggests that exercise is safe and beneficial despite the presence of multiple chronic diseases. In general, the risk of musculoskeletal injury is greater than the risk of a cardiovascular event, but this can be minimized by using low impact activities, water exercises, or resistance training rather than weight-bearing endurance training as the mode of exercise. Adults with multiple cardiovascular risk factors should be screened by their physician prior to starting a new exercise regimen, but cardiac stress testing should be reserved for clinical indications, not merely the presence of obesity in an older adult. Low to moderate aerobic activity provides as much metabolic benefit if the duration is extended as does high intensity endurance exercise and is, therefore, preferable. In the case of resistance training, however, high intensity training is safe in the elderly and is much more effective than low intensity training at achieving skeletal muscle adaptations important for metabolism and body composition changes to occur. Osteoarthritis, diabetes, hypertension, coronary disease, and peripheral vascular disease are more common in obese elders, and attention to any changes in these conditions during exercise initiation may warrant consultation with health care providers to avoid complications.

DIRECTIONS FOR FUTURE RESEARCH

Much has been learned over the past decade about the control of body weight and composition with aging, and the "inevitable" gains in adiposity and losses of lean tissue have begun to be partitioned into biological aging, disuse, disease, nutritional imbalance, and genetic predisposition. However, there are still important gaps in our knowledge and in our ability to apply research findings in a meaningful way for the aging population. Some of the major topics that require ongoing investigation are as follows.

1) We need evidence from randomized controlled trials in obese elderly of the differential effects of aerobic and resistance exercise with and without hypoenergy diets on weight loss and body composition changes, as well as the risk/benefit ratio of each approach.

2) Research needs to determine the optimal modes and doses of exercise required at various points in the lifecycle for maintenance of a healthful body weight and composition.

3) The long-term health benefits of inducing changes in body weight and body composition in elders must be documented.

4) Better models must be developed for the maintenance of a physically active lifestyle for older adults with varying burdens of disease, levels of independence, and psychosocial characteristics.

SUMMARY

Epidemiological evidence suggests that the maintenance of a regular pattern of physical activity throughout life contributes to optimal body weight regulation, lower levels of body fat, higher levels of bone density, and perhaps attenuation of the losses of muscle mass accompanying aging. Intervention studies have shown that compliance with adequate doses of endurance or resistance training is capable of reducing body weight, body fat, and central obesity and of increasing muscle mass and bone density in older adults. However, the magnitude of such shifts is highly variable, depending upon individual characteristics and responsiveness as well as on the exact nature and duration of the exercise stimulus. The combination of a hypocaloric diet with exercise appears to be superior to either exercise or diet alone in the management of obesity, although specific randomized controlled trials in the obese elderly remain to be done. This additional benefit may be due to the ability of exercise, particularly resistive exercise, to offset the reduction in resting energy expenditure and lean body mass seen with dieting alone. Apart from its direct benefits on weight and body composition in obese elders, exercise offers a myriad of other physical, metabolic, and psychological benefits that cannot be achieved with caloric restriction. Resistance training may provide the best ratio of benefit/risk in obese older adults because it is relatively practical, safe, and specific for inducing muscle hypertrophy. Finally, exercise may enhance food intake in underweight or anorexic adults and may thus be useful in the adult "failure-to-thrive" syndrome as well.

BIBLIOGRAPHY

Ades, P. A., D. L. Ballor, T. Ashikaga, J. L. Utton, and K. S. Nair (1996). Weight training improves walking endurance in healthy elderly persons. *Ann. Intern. Med.* 124(6):568–72.

Aloia, J., S. Cohn, J. Ostuni, R. Cane, and K. Ellis (1978). Prevention of involutional bone loss by exercise. *Ann. Intern. Med.* 89:356–358.

Aloia, J., A. Vaswani, J. Yeh, and S. Cohn (1988). Premenopausal bone mass is related to physical activity. *Arch. Intern. Med.* 148:121–123.

Andres, R., D. Elahi, J.D. Tobin, and D.C. Muller (1985). Impact of age on weight goals. *Ann. Int. Med.* 103:1030–1033.

Atkinson, R., W. Dietz, and J. Foreyt (1994). *Weight Cycling*. Bethesda, MD:National Task Force for the Prevention and Treatment of Obesity.

Bailey, D. A., and R. G. McCulloch (1990). Bone tissue and physical activity. *Can. J. Sport Sci.* 15(4):229–39.

Ballor, D., and R. Keesey (1991). A meta-analysis of the factors affecting exeracise-induced changes in body mass, fat mass, and fat-free mass in males and females." *Int. J. Obes.* 15:717–726.

Ballor, D. L., and E. T. Poehlman (1993). Exercise intensity does not affect depression of resting metabolic rate during severe diet restriction in male Sprague-Dawley rats. *J. Nutr.* 123(7):1270–6.

Ballor, D. L., J. R. Harvey-Berino, P. A. Ades, J. Cryan, and J. Calles-Escandon (1996). Contrasting effects of resistance and aerobic training on body composition and metabolism after diet-induced weight loss. *Metab. Clin. Exp.* 45(2):179–83.

Ballor, D. L., V. L. Katch, M. D. Becque, and C. R. Marks (1988). Resistance weight training during caloric restriction enhances lean body weight maintenance. *Am. J. Clin. Nutr.* 47:19–25.

Barakat, H., D. Burton, and J. Carpenter (1988). Body fat distribution, plasma lipoproteins and the risk of coronary heart disease of make subjects. *Int. J. Obes.* 12:473–80.

Bengtsson, C., C. Bjorkelund, and L. Lissner (1993). Associations of serum lipid concentrations and obesity with mortality in women:20 year follow-up of participants in prospective population study in Gothenburg, Sweden. *Br. J. Med.* 307:1385–1388.

Blair, S., N. Ellsworth, W. Haskell, M. Stern, J. Farrqugar, and P. Woos (1981). Comparison of nutrient intake in middle-aged men and women runners and controls. *Med. Sci. Sports Exerc.* 13:310–315.

Blair, S., W. Kannel, and H. Kohl (1989a). Surrogate measures of physical activity and physical fitness: evidence for sedentary traits of resting tachycardia, obesity, and low vital capacity. *Am. J. Epidemiol.* 129:1145–56.

Blair, S. N., H. W. Kohl, R. S. Paffenbarger, D.G. Clark, K.H. Cooper, and L.W. Gibbons (1989b). Physical fitness and all-cause mortality: a prospective study of healthy men and women. *JAMA* 262:2395–2401.

Blair, S., J. Shaten, and K. Brownell (1993). Body weight change, all-cause mortality in the multiple risk factor intervention trial. *Ann. Intern. Med.* 119:749–757.

Block, J. E., H. Genant, K., and D. Black (1986). Greater Vertebral Bone Mineral Mass in Exercising Young Men. *West. J. Med.* 145:39–42.

Borkan, G., and A. Norris (1977). Fat redistribution and the changing body dimensions of the adult male. *Hum. Biol.* 49:494–514.

Borkan, G., D. Hults, S. Gerzof, A. Robbins, and C. Silbert (1983). Age changes in body composition revealed by computerized tomography. *J. Gerontol.* 38:673–677.

Bortz, W. M. (1982). Disuse and aging. *JAMA* 248:1203–1208.

Bortz, W. M. (1989). Redefining Human Aging. *J. Am. Geriatr. Soc.* 37(11):1092–1096.

Brown, S., S. Upchurch, R. Anding, M. Winter, and G. Ramirez (1996). Promoting weight loss in type II diabetes. *Diabetes Care* 19:613–24.

Burr, M., and K. Phillips (1984). Anthropometric norms in the elderly. *Br. J. Nutr.* 51:165–169.

Butterworth, D., D. Nieman, and B. Warren (1993). Exercise training and nutrient intake in elderly women. *J. Am. Diet Assoc.* 93:653–657.

Campbell, W. W., M. C. Crim, V. R. Young, and W. J. Evans (1994). Increased energy requirements and changes in body composition with resistance training in older adults. *Am.J. Clin. Nutr.* 60(2):167–75.

Cartee, G. D. (1994). Aging skeletal muscle: response to exercise. In: J. Holloszy (ed.) *Exercise and Sport Sciences Reviews*, Vol. 22. Philadelphia: Williams & Wilkins, pp.91–120.

Casper, R. C. (1995). Nutrition and its relationship to aging. *Exper. Gerontol.* 30(3–4):299–314.

Chapman, K. M., and R. A. Nelson (1994). Loss of appetite: managing unwanted weight loss in the older patient. *Geriatrics* 49(3):54–9.

Charette, S., L. McEvoy, G. Pyka, C. Snow-Harter, D. Guido, R. Wiswell, and R. Marcus (1991). Muscle hypertrophy response to resistance training in older women. *J. Appl. Physiol.* 70(5):, 1912–1916.

Chien, S., M. Peng, K. Chen, T. Huang, C. Chang, and H. Fang (1975). Longitudinal studies on adipose tissue and its distribution in human subjects. *J. Appl. Physiol.* 39:825–830.

Colditz, G., W. Willett, A. Rotnitzky, and J. Manson (1995). Weight gain as a risk factor for clinical diabetes mellitus in women. *Ann. Intern. Med.* 122:481–486.

Coupland, C., D. Wood, and C. Cooper (1993). Physical inactivity is an independent risk factor for hip fracture in the elderly. *J. Epidemiol. Comm. Health* 47(6):441–3.

Cummings, S.R, J.L. Kelsey, M.C. Nevitt, and K.J. O'Dowd (1985). Epidemiology of osteoporosis and osteoporotic fractures. *Epidemiol. Rev.* 7:178–208.

Dalen, N., and D. Olsson (1974). Bone mineral content and physical avtivity. *Acta Orthop. Scand.* 45:170–174.

Dalsky, G. P. (1989). The role of exercise in the prevention of osteoporosis. *Comp. Therapy* 15(9):30–7.

Dalsky, G., K. Stocke, A. Ehsani, E. Slatopolsky, W. Lee, and S. Birge (1988). Weight-bearing exercise training and lumbar bone mineral content in postmenopausal women. *Ann. Intern. Med.* 108:824–828.

Delarue, J., T. Constans, D. Malvy, A. Pradignac, C. Couet, and F. Lamisse (1994). Anthropometric values in an elderly French population. *Br. J. Nutr.* 71:295–302.

Dengel, D. R., J. M. Hagberg, P. J. Coon, D. T. Drinkwater, and A. P. Goldberg (1994a). Comparable effects of diet and exercise on body composition and lipoproteins in older men. *Med. Sci. Sports Exerc.* 26(11):1307–15.

Dengel, D. R., J. M. Hagberg, P. J. Coon, D. T. Drinkwater, and A. P. Goldberg (1994b). Effects of weight loss by diet alone or combined with aerobic exercise on body composition in older obese men. *Metab. Clin. Exp.* 43(7):867–71.

Despres, J.-P., M. Pouliot, and S. Moorjani (1991). Loss of abdominal fat and metabolic response to exercise training in obese women. *Am. J. Physiol.* 24:E159–67.

DiPietro, L. (1995). Physical activity, body weight, and adiposity: an epidemiologic perspective. In: J. Holloszy (ed.) *Exercise and Sport Sciences Reviews*. Philadelphia: Williams and Wilkins. 23:501.

DiPietro, L., D. F. Williamson, C. J. Caspersen, and E. Eaker (1993). The descriptive epidemiology of selected physical activities and body weight among adults trying to lose weight: the Behavioral Risk Factor Surveillance System survey, 1989. *Int. J. Obes. Rel. Metab. Disorders* 17(2):69–76.

Dupler, T., and C. Cortes (1993). Effects of a whole-body resistive training regimen in the elderly. *Gerontol.* 39:314–319.

Durrant, M., J. Garrow, P. Royston, S. Stalley, S. Sunkin, and P. Warwick (1980). Factors influencing the composition of the weight lost by obese patients on a reducing diet. *Br. J. Nutr.* 44:275–85.

Ellis, K. (1990). Reference man and woman more fully characterized: Variations on the basis of body size, age, sex and race. *Biol. Trace Elem. Res.* 26–27:385–400.

Enzi, G., M. Gasparo, P. Biondetti, D. Fiore, M. Semisa, and F. Zurio (1986). Subcutaneous and visceral fat distribution according to sex, age, and overweight, evaluated by cuputed tomography. *Am. J. Clin. Nutr.* 44:739–746.

Epstein, L., and R. Wing (1980). Aerobic exercise and weight. *Addict. Behav.* 5:371–388.

Evans, W. (1995). Exercise, nutrition and aging. *Clin. Geriatr. Med.* 11(4):725–734.

Evans, W. J. (1996). Reversing sarcopenia: how weight training can build strength and vitality. *Geriatr.* 51(5):46–7, 51–4.

Evans, W., and W. Campbell (1993). Sarcopenia and age-related changes in body composition and functional capacity. *J. Nutr.* 123:465–468.

Farmer, M. E., T. Harris, J. H. Madans, R. B. Wallace, J. Carnoni-Huntley, and L. H. White (1989). Anthropometric indicators and hip fracture: The NHANES I epidemiologic follow-up study. *J. Am. Geriatr. Soc.* 37:9–16.

Fiatarone, M. A., and W. J. Evans (1990). Exercise in the oldest old. *Top. Geriatr. Rehab.* 5:63–77.

Fiatarone, M., and W. Evans (1993). The etiology and reversibility of muscle dysfunction in the elderly. *J. Gerontol.*

Fiatarone, M. A., E. C. Marks, N. D. Ryan, C. N. Meredith, L. A. Lipsitz, and W. J. Evans (1990). High-intensity strength training in nonagenarians. Effects on skeletal muscle. *JAMA* 263:3029–3034.

Fiatarone, M. A., E. F. O'Neill, N. D. Ryan, K. M. Clements, G. R. Solares, M. E. Nelson, S. R. Roberts, J. K. Kehayias, L. A. Lipsitz, and W. J. Evans (1994). Exercise training and nutritional supplementation for physical frailty in very elderly people. *N. Engl. J. Med.* 330:1769–1775.

Fischer, J., and M. A. Johnson (1990). Low body weight and weight loss in the aged. *J. Am. Diet. Assoc.* 90(12):1697–706.

Fleg, J., and E. Lakatta (1988). Role of muscle loss in age-associated reduction in VO₂max. *J. Appl. Physiol.* 65:1147–1151.

Fluckey, J. D., M. S. Hickey, J. K. Brambrink, K. K. Hart, K. Alexander, and B. W. Craig (1994). Effects of resistance exercise on glucose tolerance in normal and glucose-intolerant subjects. *J. Appl. Physiol.* 77(3):1087–92.

Flynn, M., G. Nolph, A. Baker, W. Martin, and G. Krause (1989). Total body potassium in aging humans: a longitudinal study. *Am. J. Clin. Nutr.* 50:713–717.

Folsom, A., S. Kay, and T. Sellers (1993). Body fat distribution and 5–year risk of death in older women. *JAMA* 269:483–487.

Forbes, G. (1992). Exercise and lean weight: the influence of body weight. *Nutr. Rev.* 50:157–61.

Fox, A. A., J. L. Thompson, G. E. Butterfield, U. Gylfadottir, S. Moynihan, and G. Spiller (1996). Effects of diet and exercise on common cardiovascular disease risk factors in moderately obese older women. *Am. J. Clin. Nutr.* 63(2):225–33.

Franklin, B. A., I. Besseghini, and L. H. Golden (1978). Low intensity physical conditioning: effects on patients with coronary heart disease. *Arch. Phys. Med. Rehab.* 59(6):276–80.

Frontera, W., V. Hughes, K. Lutz, and W. Evans (1991). A cross-sectional study of muscle strength and mass in 45– to 78–yr-old men and women. *J. Appl. Physiol.* 71:644–650.

Frontera, W. R., C. N. Meredith, K. P. O'Reilly, H. G. Knuttgen, and W. J. Evans (1988). Strength conditioning in older men: skeletal muscle hypertrophy and improved function. *J. Appl. Physiol.* 64:1038–1044.

Gleim, G. (1993). Exercise is not an effective weight loss modality in women. *J. Am. Coll. Nutr.* 12(4):363–367.

Going, S., D. Williams, and T. Lohman (1994). Aging and body composition: Biological changes and methodological issues. *Exerc. Sports Sci. Rev.* 22:411–458.

Goran, M., and E. Poehlman (1992). Endurance training does not enhance total energy expenditure in healthy elderly persons. *Am. J. Physiol.* 263:E950–E957.

Grisso, J. A., J. L. Kelsey, B. L. Strom, G.Y. Chiu, G. Maislin, L.A. O'Brien, S. Hoffman, and F. Kaplan (1991). Risk factors for falls as a cause of hip fracture in women. *N. Engl. J. Med.* 324:1326–31.

Gwinup, G. (1975). Effects of exercise alone on the weight of obese women. *Arch. Intern. Med.* 135:676–680.

Hagerman, F., R. Fielding, M. Fiatarone, J. Gault, D. Kirkendall, K. Ragg, and W. Evans (1996). A 20–year longitudinal study of Olympic oarsmen. *Med. Sci. Sports Exerc.* 28:1150–1156.

Hamdy, R., J. Anderson, K. Whalen, and L. Harvill (1994). Regional differences in bone density of young men involved in different exercises. *Med. Sci. Sports Exerc.* 26(7):884–888.

Hanson, B. S., I. Mattisson, and B. Steen (1987). Dietary intake and psychosocial factors in 68–year-old men. A population study. *Comprehensive Gerontology. Section B, Behavioural, Social & Applied Sciences* 1(2):62–7.

Harris, M. I., W. C. Hadden, W. C. Knowler, and P. H. Bennett (1987). Prevalence of diabetes and impaired glucose tolerance and plasma glucose levels in U.S. Population Aged 20–74 yr. *Diabetes* 36:523–34.

Harris, T., G. M. Kovar, R. Suzman, J. C. Kleinman, and J. J. Feldman (1989). Longitudinal study of physical ability in the oldest-old. *Am. J. Public Health* 79:698–702.

Heikkinen, J., Kurttula-Matero, E. Kyllonen, J. Vuori, T. Takala, and H. K. Vaananen (1991). Moderate Exercise Does Not Enhance the Positive Effect of Estrogen on Bone Mineral Density in Postmenopausal Women. *Calcif. Tissue Int.* [Suppl] 49:S83–S84.

Hersey, W. C., J. E. Graves, M. L. Pollock, R. Gingerich, R. B. Shireman, G. W. Heath, F. Spierto, S. D. McCole, and J. M. Hagberg (1994). Endurance exercise training improves body composition and plasma insulin responses in 70– to 79–year-old men and women. *Metab. Clin. Exp.* 43(7):847–54.

Higgins, M., R. D'Agostino, W. Kannel, J. Cobb, and J. Pinsky (1993). Benefits and adverse effects of weight loss. Observations from the Framingham Study [published erratum appears in *Ann. Intern. Med.* 119(10):1055, 1993]. *Ann. Intern. Med.* 119(7):758–63.

Holloszy, J. O., J. Schultz, J. Kusnierkiewicz, J. M. Hagberg, and A. A. Ehsani (1986). Effects of exercise on glucose tolerance and insulin resistance. *Acta Med. Scand. (Suppl.)* 711:55–65.

Horber, F. F., S. A. Kohler, K. Lippuner, and P. Jaeger (1996). Effect of regular physical training on age-associated alteration of body composition in men. *Eur. J. Clin. Invest.* 26(4):279–85.

Hubert, H., D. Block, and J. Fries (1993). Risk factors for physical disability in an aging cohort: The NHANES I Epidemiologic Followup Study. *J. Rheumatol.* 20(3):480–488.

Huddleston, A. L., D. Rockwell, and D. N. Kulund (1980). Bone Mass in Lifetime Tennis Players. *JAMA* 244:1107–1109.

Hurley, B., J. Hagberg, A. Goldberg, D. Seals, A. Ehsani, R. Brennan, and J. Holloszy (1988). Resistive training can reduce coronary risk factors without altering VO$_2$max or percent body fat. *Med. Sci. Sports Exerc.* 20:150–154.

Imamura, K., H. Ashida, T. Ishikawa, and M. Fujii (1983). Human major psoas muscle and scrospinalis muscle in relation to age: A study by computed tomography. *J. Gerontol.* 38:678–681.

Katzel, L. I., E. R. Bleecker, E. G. Colman, E. M. Rogus, J. D. Sorkin, and A. P. Goldberg (1995). Effects of weight loss vs aerobic exercise training on risk factors for coronary heart disease in healthy, obese, middle-aged and older men. A randomized controlled trial [see comments]. *JAMA* 274:, 1915–21.

Keim, N., T. Barbieri, and A. Belko (1990). The effects of exercise on energy intake and body composition in overweight women. *Int. J. Obes.* 14:335–346.

King, A., B. Frey-Hewitt, D. Dreon, and P. Wood (1989). Diet vs. exercise in weight maintenance: the effects of minimal intervention strategies on long-term outcomes in men. *Arch. Intern. Med.* 149:2741–2746.

King, A., W. Haskell, C. Taylor, H. Kraemer, and R. DeBusk (1991). Group- vs home-based exercise training in healthy older men and women: A community-based clinical trial. *JAMA* 266:1535–1542.

King, A., C. Taylor, W. Haskell, and R. Debusk (1988). Strategies for increasing early adherence to and long-term maintenance of home-based exercise training in healthy middle-aged men and women. *Am. J. Cardiol.* 61:628–632.

Kissebah, A., and G. Krakower (1994). Regional adiposity and morbidity. *Physiol. Rev.* 74(4):761–811.

Klitgaard, H., M. Mantoni, S. Schiaffino, S. Ausoni, L. Gorza, C. Laurent-Winter, P. Schnohr, and B. Saltin (1990). Function, morphology and protein expression of ageing skeletal muscle: a cross-sectional study of elderly men with different training backgrounds. *Acta Physiol. Scand.* 140:41–54.

Kohrt, W. M., K. A. Obert, and J. O. Holloszy (1992). Exercise training improves fat distribution patterns in 60– to 70–year-old men and women. *J. Gerontol.* 47(4):M99–105.

Kohrt, W. M., D. B. Snead, E. Slatopolsky, and S. J. Birge, Jr. (1995). Additive effects of weight-bearing exercise and estrogen on bone mineral density in older women. *J. Bone Min. Res.* 10(9):1303–11.

Krolner, B., B. Toft, S. P. Nielsen, and E. Tondevold (1983). Physical Exercise as Prophylaxix Against Involutional Vertebral Bone Loss: a Controlled Trial. *Clin. Sci.* 64:541–546.

Krotkiewski, M. and e. al. (1983). Impact of obesity on metabolism in men and women: importance of regional adipose tissue distribution. *J. Clin. Invest.* 72:1150–1162.

Larsson, L. (1983). Histochemical characteristics of human skeletal muscle during aging. *Acat Physiol. Scand.* 117:469–471.

Larsson, L., B. Sjodin, and J. Karlsson (1978). Histochemical and biochemical changes in human skeletal muscle with age in sedentary males, age 22–65 years. *Acta Physiol. Scand.* 103:31–39.

Lauritzen, J. B., P. A. McNair, and B. Lund (1993). Risk factors for hip fractures. A review. *Danish Med. Bull.* 40(4):479–85.

Lexell, J., K. Henriksson-Larsen, B. Wimblod, and M. Sjostrom (1983). Distribution of different fiber types in human skeletal muscles: Effects of aging studied in whole muscle cross sections. *Muscle Nerve* 6:588–595.

Ley, C., B. Lees. and J. Stevenson (1992). Sex- and menopause-associated changes in body-fat distribution. *Am. J. Clin. Nutr.* 55:950–954.

Lillegard, W. A., and J. D. Terrio (1994). Appropriate Strength Training. *Med. Clin. N. Am.* 78(2):457–77.

Lohman, T., S. Going, and R. Pamenter (1995). Effects of resistance training on regional and total bone mineral density in premenopausal women:a randomized prospective study. *J. Bone Min. Res.* 10(7):1015–1024.

Losonczy, K., T. Harris, J. Huntley, E. Simonsick, R. Wallace, N. Cook, A. Ostfeld, and D. Blazer (1995). Does weight loss from middle age to old explain the inverse weight mortality relation in old age? *JAMA* 141:312–321.

Mangione, K. K., K. Axen, and F. Haas (1996). Mechanical unweighting effects on treadmill exercise and pain in elderly people with osteoarthritis of the knee. *Phys. Therapy* 76(4):387–94.

Manson, J., G. Colditz, M. Stampfer, W. Willett, B. Rosner, R. Monson, F. Speizer, and C. Hennekens (1990). A prospective study of obesity and risk of coronary heart disease in women. *N. Engl. J. Med.* 322:882–889.

Manson, J., D. Nathan, A. Krolewski, M. Stampfer, W. Willett, and C. Hennekens (1992). A prospective study of exercise and incidence of diabetes among U.S. male physicians. *JAMA* 268(1):63–67.

Manson, J., E. Rimm, M. Stampfer, G. Colditz, W. Willett, A. Krolewski, B. Rosner, C. Hennekens, and F. Speizer (1991). Physical activity and incidence of non-insulin-dependent diabetes mellitus in women. *Lancet* 338:774–778.

Mazess, R. (1982). On aging bone loss. *Clin. Orthop.* 165:239–252.

Mazzeo, R. S., and S. M. Horvath (1986). Effects of training on weight, food intake, and body composition in aging rats. *Am. J. Clin. Nutr.* 44(6):732–8.

McCartney, N., A. Hicks, J. Martin, and C. Webber (1995). Long-term resistance training in the elderly: effects on dynamic strength, exercise capacity, muscle, and bone. *J. Gerontol.* 50A(2):B97–B104.

McCartney, N., R. McKelvie, D. Haslam, and N. Jones (1991). Usefulness of weightlifting training in improving strength and maximal power output in coronary artery disease. *Am. J. Cardiol.* 67:939–945.

Meredith, C. N., W. R. Frontera, and W. J. Evans (1988). Effect of diet on body composition changes during strength training in elderly men. *Am. J. Clin. Nutr.* 47:767.

Meredith, C. N., M. J. Zackin, W. R. Frontera, and W. J. Evans (1987). Body composition and aerobic capacity in young and middle-aged endurance-trained men. *Med. Sci. Sports Exerc.* 19:557–563.

Montgomery, I., J. Trinder, S. Paxton , D. Harris, G. Fraser, and I. Colrain (1988). Physical exercise and sleep: the effect of the age and sex of the subjects and type of exercise. *Acta Physiol. Scand.* 133(Supplement 574):36–40.

Morley, J. (1996). Anorexia in older persons: Epidemiolgy and optimal treatment. *Drugs & Aging* 8:134–155.

Morley, J. E. (1986). Nutritional Status of the Elderly. *Amer. J. Med.* 81:679–695.

Morley, J. E., and D. Kraenzle (1994). Causes of weight loss in a community nursing home. *J. Am. Geriatr. Soc.* 46:583–585.

Morley, J.E., Z. Glick, and L.Z. Rubenstein (1995). *Geriatric Nutrition: A Comprehensive Review (2nd ed.).* New York, NY: Lippincott-Raven.

Nelson, M., M. Fiatarone, J. Layne, I. Trice, C. Economos, R. Fielding, R. Ma, R. Pierson, and W. Evans (1996). Analysis of body-composition techniques and models for detecting change in soft tissue with strength training. *Am. J. Clin. Nutr.* 63:678–86.

Nelson, M., M. Fiatarone, C. Morganti, I. Trice, R. Greenberg, and W. Evans (1994). Effects of high-intensity strength training on multiple risk factors for osteoporotic fractures. *JAMA* 272:1909–1914.

Nelson, M., E. Fisher, F. Dilmanian, G. Dallal, and W. Evans (1991). A 1–y walking program and increased dietary calcium in postmenopausal women: effects on bone. *Am. J. Clin. Nutr.* 53:1394–11.

Nelson, M., J. Layne, A. Nuernberger, M. Allen, J. Judge, D. Kaliton, and M. Fiatarone (1997). Home-based exercise training in the frail elderly: Effects on physical performance. *Med. Sci. Sports Exerc.* (abstract) 29:S110.

Nevitt, M. C., S. R. Cummings, S. Kidd, and D. Black (1989). Risk factors for recurrent nonsyncopal falls: A prospective study. *JAMA* 261:2663–2668.

Nichols, J., K. Nelson, K. Peterson, and D. Sartoris (1995). Bone mineral density responses to high-intensity strength training in active older women. *J. Aging Phys. Act.* 3:26–38.

Nieman, D., L. Onasch, and J. Lee (1990). The effects of moderate exercise training on nutrient intake in mildly obese women. *J. Am. Diet Assoc.* 90:1557–1562.

Notelovitz, M., D. Martin, R. Tesar, F. Y. Khan, C. Probart, C. Fields, and L. McKenzie (1991). Estrogen and Variable-Resistance Weight Training Increase Bone Mineral in Surgically Menopausal Women. *J. Bone Min. Res.* 6(6):583–590.

Oddis, C. V. (1996). New perspectives on osteoarthritis. *Am. J. Med.* 100(2A):10S-15S.

Ohlson, L., B. Larsson, K. Svardsudd, L. Welin, H. Eriksson, L. Wilhelmsen, P. Bjorntorp, and G. Tibblin (1984). The influence of body fat distribution on the incidence of diabetes mellitus: 13.5 years of follow-up of the participants in the study of men born in, 1913. *Diabetes* 34:1055–1058.

Orlander, J., K. Kiessling, L. Larsson, J. Karlsson, and A. Aniansson (1978). Skeletal muscle metabolism and ultrastructure in relation to age in sedentary men. *Acta Physiol. Scand.* 104:249–261.

Orwoll, E. S., D. C. Bauer, T. M. Vogt, and K. M. Fox (1996). Axial bone mass in older women. Study of Osteoporotic Fractures Research Group. *Ann. Intern. Med.* 124(2):187–96.

Owens, J. F., K. A. Matthews, R. R. Wing, and L. H. Kuller (1992). Can physical activity mitigate the effects of aging in middle-aged women? *Circulation* 85(4):1265–70.

Pamuk, E., D. Williamson, M. Serdula, J. Madans, and T.E. Byers (1993). Weight loss and subsequent death in a cohort of US adults. *Ann. Intern. Med.* 119:744–748.

Pate, R. R., M. Pratt, S. N. Blair, W. L. Haskell, et.al. (1995). Physical Activity and Public Health: A Recommendation From the Centers for Disease Control and PRevention and the American College of Sports Medicine. *JAMA* 273(5):402–407.

Pocock, N., J. Eisman, T. Gwinn, P. Sambrook, P. Kelly, J. Freund, and M. Yeates (1989). Muscle Strength, Physical fitness and Weight but not Age Predict Femoral Neck Bone Mass. *J. Bone Min. Res.* 4:441–448.

Pollock, M. L., C. Foster, D. Knapp, J. L. Rod, and D. H. Schmidt (1987). Effect of age and training on aerobic capacity and body composition of master athletes. *J. Appl.Physiol.* 62(2):725–31.

Pollock, M., H. Miller, R. Janeway, A. Linnerud, B. Robertson, and R. Valentino (1971). Effects of walking on body composition and cardiovascular function of middle-aged men. *J. Appl. Physiol.* 30:126–30.

Pratley, R., J. Hagberg, E. Rogus, and A. Goldberg (1995). Enhanced insulin sensitivity and lower waist-to-hip ratio in master athletes. *Am. J. Physiol.* 268:E484–E490.

Prentice, A. M., K. Leavesley, P. R. Murgatroyd, W. A. Coward, C. J. Schorah, P. T. Bladon, and R. P. Hullin (1989). Is severe wasting in elderly mental patients caused by an excessive energy requirement? *Age Ageing* 18(3):158–67.

Prior, J. C., Y. M. Vigna, S. I. Barr, S. Kennedy, M. Schulzer, and D. K. Li (1996). Ovulatory premenopausal women lose cancellous spinal bone: a five year prospective study. *Bone* 18(3):261–7.

Pruitt, L. A., R. D. Jackson, R. L. Bartels, and H. J. Lehnhard (1992). Weight-Training Effects on bone Mineral Density in Early Postmenopausal Women. *J. Bone Min. Res.* 7(2):179–185.

Pu, C., M. Johnson, D. Forman, L. Piazza, and M. Fiatarone (1997). High-intensity progressive resistance training in older women with chronic heart failure. *Med. Sci. Sports Exerc.* (abstract) 29:S148.

Puig, T., B. Marti, M. Rickenbach, S. F. Dai, C. Casacuberta, V. Wietlisbach, and F. Gutzwiller (1990). Some determinants of body weight, subcutaneous fat, and fat distribution in 25–64 year old Swiss urban men and woman. *Sozial- und Praventivmedizin* 35(6):, 193–200.]

Ray, W. A., M. R. Griffen, W. Schaffner, N. K. Baugh, and L. J. Melton (1987). Psychotropic drug use and the risk of hip fracture. *N. Engl. J. Med.* 316(7):313–19.

Richelson, L., H.W. Wahner, L.I. Melton, III, and B.L. Riggs (1984). Relative contributions of aging and estrogen deficiency to postmenopausal bone loss. *N. Engl. J. Med.* 311:1273–1275.

Rico, H., M. Revilla, R. Hernandez, J. Gonzales-Riola, and L. Villa (1993). Four-compartment model of body composition of normal elderly women. *Age Ageing* 22:265–268.

Riggs, B., H. Wahner, W. Dunn, R. Mazess, K. Offord, and L. Melton (1981). Differential changes in bone mineral density of the appendicular and axial skeleton with aging: relationship to spinal osteoporosis. *J. Clin. Invest.* 67:328–335.

Riggs, B., H. Wahner, L. Melton, L. Richelson, H. Judd, and K. Offord (1986). Rates of bone loss in appendicular and axial skeletons of women: evidence of substantial vertebral bone loss before menopause. *J. Clin. Invest.* 77:1487–1491.

Roberts, S. B., P. Fuss, W. J. Evans, M. B. Heyman, and V. R. Young (1993). Energy expenditure, aging and body composition. *J. Nutr.* 123(2 Suppl):474–80.

Roberts, S. B., P. Fuss, M. B. Heyman, W. J. Evans, R. Tsay, H. Rasmussen, M. A. Fiatarone, J. Cortiella, G. E. Dallal, and V. R. Young (1994). Control of Food Intake in Older Men. *JAMA* 272(20):1601–1606.

Roberts, S., V. Young, P. Fuss, M. Heyman, M. Fiatarone, G. Dallal, J. Cortiella, and W. Evans (1992). What are the dietary energy needs of elderly adults? *Int. J. Obes.* 16:969–976.

Romieu, I., W. C. Willett, M. J. Stampfer, G. A. Colditz, L. Sampson, B. Rosner, C. H. Hennekens, and F. E. Speizer (1988). Energy intake and other determinants of relative weight. *Am. J. Clin. Nutr.* 47(3):406–12.

Rumpel, C., T. Harris, and J. Madans (1993). Modifications of the relationship between the quetelet index and mortality by weight-loss history among older women. *Ann. Epidemiol.* 3:343–350.

Ruoti, R. G., J. T. Troup, and R. A. Berger (1994). The effects of nonswimming water exercises on older adults. *J.Orthopaedic & Sports Physical Therapy* 19(3):140–5.

Santora, A. C.(1987). Role of nutrition and exercise in osteoporosis. *Am. J. Med.* 82(1B):73–9.

Schwartz, R. S., K. C. Cain, W. P. Shuman, V. Larson, J. R. Stratton, J. C. Beard, S. E. Kahn, M. D. Cerqueira, and I. B. Abrass (1992). Effect of intensive endurance training on lipoprotein profiles in young and older men. *Metab. Clin. Exp.* 41(6):649–54.

Schwartz, R. S., W. P. Shuman, V. Larson, K. C. Cain, G. W. Fellingham, J. C. Beard, S. E. Kahn, J. R. Stratton, M. D. Cerqueira, and I. B. Abrass (1991). The effect of intensive endurance exercise training on body fat distribution in young and older men. *Metab. Clin. Exp.* 40(5):545–51.

Seals, D., and J. Hagberg (1984). The effects of exercise training on human hypertension: A review. *Med. Sci. Sports Exerc.* 16:207–215.

Seidell, J. C., M. Cigolini, J. P. Deslypere, J. Charzewska, B. M. Ellsinger, and A. Cruz (1991). Body fat distribution in relation to physical activity and smoking habits in 38–year-old European men. The European Fat Distribution Study. *Am. J. Epidemiol.* 133(3):257–65.

Shephard, R. J. (1994). Physical activity and reduction of health risks: how far are the benefits independent of fat loss? *J. Sports Med. Phys. Fitness* 34(1):91–8.

Shimokata, H., R. Andres, P. Coon, D. Elahi, D. Muller, and J. Tobin (1988). Studie in the distribution of body fat. II. Longitudinal effects of changes in weight. *Int. J. Obes.* 13:455–464.

Singh, N. A., K. M. Clements, and M. A. Fiatarone (1997a). A Randomised controlled trial of the effect of exercise on sleep. *Sleep* 20(2):95–101.

Singh, N. A., K. M. Clements, and M. A. Fiatarone (1997b). A randomized controlled trial of progressive resistance training in depressed elders. *J. Gerentol.* 52A(1):M27–35.

Smidt, G., S. Lin, K. O'Dwyer, and P. Blanpied (1992). The effect of high-intensity trunk exercise on bone mineral density of postmenopausal women. *Spine* 17(3):280–285.

Snead, D., S. Birge, and W. Kohrt (1993). Age-related differences in body composition by hydrodensitometry and duel-energy X-ray absorptiometry. *J. Appl. Physiol.* 74:770–775.

Steen, B. (1988). Body composition and aging. *Nutr. Rev.* 46:45–51.

Stevens, J., R. Knapp, J. Keil, and R. Verdugo (1991). Changes in body weight and girths in black and white adults studied over a 25 yr interval. *Int. J. Obes.* 15:803–808.

Stewart, K., M. Manson, and M. Kelemen (1988). Three-year participation in circuit weight training improves muscular strength and self efficacy in cardiac patients. *J. Cardiopulmonary Rehabil.* 8:292–296.

Thompson, J., G. Jarvic, and R. Lahey (1982). Exercise and obesity: etiology, physiology and intervention. *Psych. Bull.* 91:55–79.

Thune, I., T. Brenn, E. Lund, and M. Gaard (1997). Physical activity and the risk of breast cancer. *N. Engl. J. Med.* 336:1296–75.

Treuth, M., G. Hunter, T. Szabo, R. Weinsier, M. Goran, and L. Berland (1995a). Reduction in intra-abdominal adipose tissue after strength training in older women. *J. Appl. Physiol.* 78(4):1425–1431.

Treuth, M., G. Hunter, R. Weinsier, and S. Kell (1995b). Energy expenditure and substrate utilization in older women after strength training: 24–h calorimeter results. *J. Appl. Physiol.* 78(6):2140–2146.

Treuth, M., A. Ryan, R. Pratley, M. Rubin, J. Miller, B. Nicklas, J. Sorkin, S. Harman, A. Goldberg, and B. Hurley (1994). Effects of strength training on total and regional body composition in older men. *J. Appl. Physiol.* 77:614–20.

Tuomilehto, J., L. Jalkanen, J. T. Salonen, and A. Nissinen (1985). Factors associated with changes in body weight during a five-year follow-up of a population with high blood pressure. *Scandinavian Journal of Social Medicine* 13(4):173–80.

Tzankoff, S. P., and A. H. Norris (1978). Longitudinal changes in basal metabolic rate in man. *J. Appl. Physiol.* 33:536–539.

van Dale, D., and W. Saris (1989). Repetitive weight loss and weight regain: effects on weight reduction, resting metabolic rate, and lipolytic activity before and after exercise and/or diet treatment. *Am. J. Clin. Nutr.* 49(3):409–416.

Wagnar, E. H., A. Z. Lacroix, D. M. Buchner, and E. B. Larson (1992). Effects of physical activity on health status in older adults. *Annual Review of Public Health* 13:451–468.

Wang, Z., D. Gallagher, M. Nelson, D. Matthews, and S. Heymsfield (1996). Total-body skeletal muscle mass: evaluation of 24–h urinary creatinine excretion by computerized axial tomography. *Am. J. Clin. Nutr.* 63:863–869.

Willett, W., J. Manson, M. Stampfer, G. Colditz, B. Rosner, F. Speizer, and C. Hennekens (1995). Weight, weight change, and coronary heart disease in women. *JAMA* 273(6):461–465.

Wood, P. D., M. L. Stefanick, P. T. Williams, and W. L. Haskell (1991). The effects on plamsa lipoproteins of a prudent weight-reducing diet, with or without exercise, in overweight men and women. *N. Engl. J. Med.* 325:461–466.

DISCUSSION

NADEL: You stated that aerobic training in older people did not result in a body-weight change, but you referred to one study in which improvements in the plasma lipid profile occurred, which would appear to be important for people in their 70s. Is there a benefit to aerobic training as opposed to resistive training as the training mode of choice for people in their 60s or 70s?

FIATARONE: Resistance training has similar effects on plasma lipids, but there are far fewer studies of resistance training than there are of aerobic training. For a young to young-old person who has many atherogenic risk factors and is somewhat overweight, then you certainly want to emphasize weight loss, and the best way to do that is probably a combination of diet and either resistance or aerobic training. Resistance training is important in people who cannot do aerobic training, and that includes many older obese patients, whether they are 60 or 90. So you don't have to give up. If a patient says, " I can't walk 45 min/d," a physician can say, "Go to the gym, sit down, do 45 min of weight lifting, and you will get the same benefit in terms of metabolic profile and weight loss." In fact, it appears that the increases in resting metabolic rate and in the thermic effect of feeding are greater for resistance training than for aerobic training. So the long-term adaptations enabling a person to maintain a reasonable body weight seem to be favored by resistance training. There is no evidence in the literature that aerobic training works better for weight control than does resistance training as an augmentation to diet.

NADEL: The loss of motor units with age affects not only muscle mass but also the precision of movement. Does a lifetime of resistance training affect the rate of motor unit decline?

FIATARONE: Muscle biopsies from older resistance-trained men show that their muscle fibers are indistinguishable from those of 20–y-olds. So at least from the peripheral endpoint, it appears that resistance training does minimize aging-associated deficits in muscle fibers. However, training effects on the neural aspects of strength are unclear. A loss of alpha motor neurons probably causes atrophy of skeletal muscle fibers. The theory is that alpha motor neuron dropout is diminished with physical training, but there is no evidence to support this hypothesis.

NADEL: The interventions that I would like you to comment on are growth hormone, protein supplementation, and estrogen replacement therapy.

FIATARONE: So far, there is no evidence that growth hormone can specifically increase muscle mass, and there is no evidence that it can improve muscle function. There is a trial in AIDS patients showing that treadmill time is improved with a particular growth-hormone secreta-gogue, but it is not clear what is driving that change in treadmill time. You can certainly decrease body fat mass with growth hormone. The tolerance to these agents is quite low, although the newer ones are better than growth hormone in terms of dropout.

As for protein supplementation, we have been interested in whether augmented protein intake improves performance or muscle function after exercise, and the data are disappointing. There is one study by Frontera et al. (1988) in which the investigators supplemented half the men who were weight lifting with a high-energy protein supplement. The men who got the supplement had a much greater energy intake—and extra 500–700 kcal/d, and they gained more muscle fat than did the people who were not supplemented. However, their improvement in muscle strength was similar to that for the controls. Because it was not clear if the improvement in muscle and fat was due to the extra energy or to the protein, in a second study, two groups consumed either 0.8 or 1.6 g of protein/kg/d. The high protein intake had no benefit on muscle mass accretion or any other variable that was measured. There is no other study showing, as far as I know, that excessive protein intake augments performance or muscle function. There is obviously a big industry that promotes protein supplements, but there is no evidence to prove that they are useful. Furthermore, the typical American diet certainly contains ample protein to supply the protein needs, whether you believe those needs to be 1 or 1.4 g of protein/kg/d.

Your third question was about resistance training or exercise and estrogen replacement. I have not been involved in such studies, but I believe one experiment on bone combined the two and found a positive and additive effect of the two treatments. There are a couple of studies of hormone replacement therapy as a way to decrease visceral adiposity or the loss of lean tissue around the perimenopausal years, and estrogen appears promising in these areas as well.

GUTIN: How about testosterone therapy for older men?

FIATARONE: Of all the hormones, testosterone is probably the best bet for improving muscle mass and muscle function compared to resistance training alone. A good study in the *NEJM* in 1996 looked at men who were given weight lifting alone, testosterone alone, the combination of the two, or nothing, and the people who got the combined intervention improved more than did the weight lifters alone both in terms of muscle mass accretion and function. Even the testosterone-alone group had gained muscle mass without any resistance training, which is certainly not what happens with growth hormone. You do not see functional gains with growth hormone unless you are actually training the muscle. Is the risk worth that benefit? Certainly for men who are hypogonadal, we would treat them because there is a very clear syndrome of osteopenia and muscle atrophy and dysfunction in men with secondary gonadal failure. Should we treat normal men who have fairly normal levels of testosterone in order to prevent sarcopenia? I don't have the answer to that.

SATTERWHITE: In regard to testosterone's positive effects on muscle mass and strength, what are your thoughts on the theory that in addition to an increase in protein accretion in muscle, testosterone enhances motor unit recruitment? In other words, does testosterone treatment lead to an increase in the number of motor units recruited in a maximal effort or to an increase in the firing pattern of these units which may increase power output? Also, women do not improve muscle performance quite as much as when they use testosterone. Is this perhaps due to fewer testosterone receptors on muscle cells in women?

FIATARONE: I don't know anything about testosterone's effect on neural mechanisms.

KENNEY: One of the factors that determines cold tolerance, regardless of age, is the combination of body geometry (including the ratio of surface area to mass) and relative composition—especially of the limbs. In the limbs, adipose tissue and muscle act in series to provide insulation to cold. With respect to your own or others' resistance-training studies, are there really changes in geometry of the limbs, e.g., cross-sectional limb area, in people over the age of 70 that accompany the changes in tissue composition of the limbs?

FIATARONE: We have found increases of 5–10% in cross-sectional area of muscle, usually with no change in the fat area. We haven't looked at geometry as a separate index, but there is certainly an expansion of the muscle compartment; whether that changes the overall geometry, I am not sure. We are doing a study now where we are examining the arm for the first time with CT scans, as we normally have done just the leg. We have a study now of 100 women who have been resistance training for a year; they have incredibly small muscle areas with lots of surrounding fat.

LAMB: What is the evidence that older people will adhere to a resistance-training program any better than they do to an aerobic-training program?

FIATARONE: It is very hard to get people to engage in an intensive or even moderately intensive aerobic exercise program if they are experiencing knee pain, we have found that individuals with very severe disabilities can complete high-intensity weight-lifting programs. In home-based studies on-going for as long as 2 y, even in the frail elderly we have found adherence rates for participating in home weight-lifting programs to be on the order of 85%. On the other hand, in our 12-wk trials with aerobic training, particularly when people are asked to perform stationary cycling, which is so boring, they all drop out as soon as the 12 wk are over; nobody ever goes back to that stationary cycle. But the weight lifters almost all want to continue. In fact, in most of our programs we have had to expand from 6 mo to a year to two because nobody will drop out. We study a lot of older women who obviously are all novices at weight lifting, and their acceptance of it is very high.

M. WILLIAMS: Short bursts of aerobic exercise, e.g., 3–4 min each, combined with resistance training may give older people the benefits of both aerobic and resistance exercise. Have you done any studies looking at circuit training involving both aerobics and resistance-type training?

FIATARONE: There are no such studies in the literature. We are currently doing a study combining traditional high-resistance weight training with power training and aerobic training on a seated stepper machine in hopes of inducing all of the benefits of each type of training. I think the intolerance to aerobic activity is primarily a function of intolerable weight-bearing activity that mostly can be attributed to pain in the knees. That is where we find most of our problems, even when using seated steppers. Knee arthritis is very prevalent in older people, and it creates a major limitation to walking or cycling or stepping. We found that after some weeks of weight lifting, knee pain from osteoarthritis is often reduced, presumably by improving knee stability with enhanced quadriceps strength; after knee pain subsides, you can probably add aerobic training. This is what we do in the nursing home, where we have people who can barely walk; we do weight lifting first, and once they are able to actually stand up and bear their body weights, we think about aerobic training. That is also probably a good approach to training obese elders, who are often intolerant to weight-bearing exercise.

HOUTKOOPER: What can you tell us about ethnic or racial differences in adaptations of older people to different types of exercise programs?

FIATARONE: Very little, because almost everyone has studied white people. Unfortunately, there is epidemiologic evidence that nonwhites are typically more sedentary than whites. I can recall only one study of black diabetics participating in aerobic exercise; there was a fairly good adherence rate, but it required a very intensive behavioral intervention.

DESPRES: You referred to Leslie Katzel's paper published in *JAMA* in 1995. I don't know about the reaction of the media in the United States, but in Canada, it was tremendous. The media representatives asked us about our current position because we had been saying for years that exercise is good. Now, despite the high prevalence of abdominal-obese individuals with risk factors, this paper said that exercise is not good for them, and that to reduce cardiovascular disease risk and reduce weight, they should be encouraged to diet rather than to exercise. It should, however, be emphasized that, in this study, the investigators did not want the exercise-trained group to lose weight, so they increased their energy intake. What is your own experience when you exercise elderly subjects, i.e., do you see a compensatory adaptation in their food intake?

FIATARONE: When we put people on an aerobic-training program for a year, they remain weight stable, which means they must be increasing their energy intake to compensate for their greater energy expenditure. We don't see such compensation in the nursing home, where the patients have no access to extra food; we have to give it to them. But our free-living subjects are able to maintain weight. If they are in a metabolic unit, we must feed them 15% more energy to keep them from losing weight. So, in real life, what would probably happen is that people would not consume sufficient extra energy, there would be a slight energy deficit, and there would probably be a mobilization of visceral fat. That is what the literature suggests, i.e., you don't get a huge fat loss, but more of it is visceral than anywhere else, and that's what's important. So exercise is not useless, but if you want a more potent fat-loss effect, you clearly have to add hypoenergy dieting.

MELBY: How would aerobic versus resistive exercise act to improve insulin resistance in the elderly population?

FIATARONE: With aerobic training, there is an improvement in glycogen storage and in insulin sensitivity, especially in glucose-intolerant subjects. We've measured a 10% improvement in glucose disposal rate using a euglycemic clamp and a 40% increase in glut-4 receptors after a 12-wk program of traditional aerobic training. With resistance training that increases the size of the muscle compartment, which is the major storage area for glucose, glucose tolerance would improve. There are a couple of studies now suggesting that the benefits of resistance training are probably of the same magnitude as seen with aerobic training. The improvements with weight loss are more dramatic in obese people, but if somebody is a lean, insulin-resistant person or doesn't have a great need for weight loss, exercise of either type will probably be efficacious. There has been more work done with aerobic training, but because the specificity of resistance training is toward muscle enlargement, my feeling is that maybe that's a more potent approach to training.

MELBY: I wonder if it might be just as important to maintain the skeletal muscle mass for the disposal of circulating free fatty acids, which may be elevated with the excess intra-abdominal body fat that accompanies aging.

FIATARONE: Resistance training may be a more potent form of training than just doing aerobic exercise.

EICHNER: You emphasized that the relationship between mortality rate and body weight was U-shaped, and you seemed to suggest that there were no data supporting a linear relationship. But did not the Harvard Alumni study suggest a linear relationship, i.e., that the thinner men lived longer.

FIATARONE: There are data showing that lean people who have always been lean will live longer than obese people who lose weight. The largest database is the Build study, the Metropolitan Life Insurance database. Ideal body mass index certainly seems to be different, depending on what age group you look at. In the nurses' health study that includes about 25,000 women, the ideal body mass index for the prevention of cardiovascular events is about 19–20 kg/m^2. However, physical activity was not estimated in that study; that is unfortunate because activity is a big confounder and may explain some of the "protective" effects of these very low BMIs. It is likely that these leaner women were more physically active, which may have contributed to their very low mortality rates. The evidence clearly is that the ideal body mass index shifts to the right as one ages.

7

Exercise, Body Composition, and Health in Children

BERNARD GUTIN, PH.D.
MATTHEW HUMPHRIES, M.S.

INTRODUCTION

We will begin by summarizing what is known from non-experimental studies about the relations of exercise and body composition to health of children, with a focus on preclinical markers for future coronary artery disease (CAD) and non-insulin dependent diabetes mellitus (NIDDM), because they are the health problems most closely associated with obesity. We will then clarify what is known about the determinants of physical activity and the role of exercise in the etiology of childhood obesity. Next, we will review experimental studies of exercise and physical training, including some field studies in school environments. After suggesting some practical implications for physicians, teachers, dietitians, parents, and those who influence public policy, we will end with some suggestions for future research.

Wherever possible, we will focus on research that used children as subjects. However, with respect to many of the specific topics involved, little or nothing is known from studies of youths; indeed, many important questions have not yet been fully answered in adults. Where data on children are limited, we will review what is known from research on adults. Because the growth and maturation of youths may interact with other factors, extrapolations of findings from adults to children need to be treated as hypotheses to be tested directly in subsequent studies with children.

We will give special emphasis to recent studies, especially those that have used new techniques of body composition and energy expenditure assessment. For example, dual x-ray absorptiometry is easily administered to children and provides reliable measurement of total body fat (Gutin et al., 1996b), and it provides information on three compartments of total body mass, i.e., bone mineral content, fat-free soft tissue, and fat mass. With respect to regional deposition of fat, important new information has been provided by studies that have used computed tomography scanning or magnetic resonance imaging to distinguish visceral adipose tissue from subcutaneous abdominal adipose tissue (Brambilla et al., 1994; Caprio et al., 1996a,b; Owens et al., 1997; Yanovski et al., 1996). Magnetic resonance imaging is especially appropriate for repeated measures on children because it does not involve any radiation exposure.

With respect to measurement of energy expenditure, our understanding of some components of 24 h energy expenditure has improved in recent years due to increased use of metabolic chambers. However, the restriction of subjects to the chamber precludes investigation of energy expenditure during free-living physical activity. The development of the doubly labeled water procedure has improved assessment of free-living energy expenditure and physical activity (Goran, 1997). In this procedure, the youth drinks an initial dose of water in which the hydrogen and oxygen are labeled and gives urine samples before and after a 10–14 d period. The isotopes are stable and involve no radiation, so the procedure is quite safe (Jones & Leatherdale, 1991). The labeled oxygen is eliminated from the body as both carbon dioxide and water, while the labeled hydrogen is eliminated only as water. Thus, the elimination rate of the labeled hydrogen is a measure of water flux, the elimination rate of the labeled oxygen is a measure of both water and carbon dioxide flux, and the difference between the two is a measure of carbon dioxide flux, which is converted to energy expenditure by standard indirect calorimetric calculations (Montoye et al., 1996). Then resting energy expenditure, as measured in the laboratory with indirect calorimetry, is subtracted from 24 h energy expenditure to derive the energy used in physical activity.

Definitions of some key terms to be used in this chapter may be useful. Although a distinction can be drawn between the terms *physical activity* and *exercise*, for purposes of this chapter they will be used interchangeably. However, our definitions of *cardiovascular fitness* and *cardiovascular health* do need explication.

By *cardiovascular fitness* we refer to the ability of the body to take in oxygen, transport it around the body, utilize it at the tissue level, and remove various waste products. In field studies, performance in endurance events is frequently used to measure cardiovascular fitness. In the laboratory, the peak oxygen consumption attained during tasks such as treadmill running is ordinarily considered the best measurement of this parameter. However, there are several reasons to recognize the value of submaximal indices of fitness as well. First, children, especially those who are obese and unfit, may not put forth the effort needed to achieve a "true" maximal oxygen consumption or maximal score on an endurance event. Since the peak oxygen consumption value is ordinarily found at the maximal work rate achieved, maximal oxygen consumption can be considered a maximal performance test as well as a physiologic index of oxygen transport capacity. Second, performance of such an all-out task may be debilitating and unpleasant for the unfit and obese child, thereby endangering the retention of the child in a study that requires repeated measurements of fitness. Third, endurance run time may be predicted equally well by a submaximal, truly physiologic index, such as ventilatory breakpoint, as by maximal oxygen consumption (Palgi et al., 1984). Fourth, submaximal indices such as ventilatory breakpoint and submaximal heart rate are sensitive to the influence of physical training (Mahon & Vaccaro, 1989), even when maximal oxygen consumption is not changed (Gutin et al., 1995; Stewart & Gutin, 1976).

We consider *cardiovascular health* to be made up of a number of factors, as illustrated in Figure 7-1. Many of these are in the nature of preclinical markers of adult disease, but there is reason to believe that the processes leading to the "adult" diseases actually begin in childhood. Although there is some reason to hypothesize that exercise may influence all the factors in the Figure 7-1, by no means is there definitive evidence of such causal links. Indeed, it is likely that exercise will eventually be shown to have little direct effect on some of these factors. The key point is that a favorable change in one of the factors (i.e., body composition), which is not accompanied by an adverse impact on any others, represents a net improvement in cardiovascular health. Moreover, we consider health to be a continuum, with the obese-unfit youth who has elevated CAD/NIDDM risk factors at one end and the fit-lean youth with low risk levels at the other end. Thus, a youth might have normal levels of CAD/NIDDM risk factors but only be in the middle of the continuum. If he/she undertakes an exercise program that improves cardiovascular fitness, that would be construed as promoting health.

In considering the relation of exercise to health in youths, it is necessary to note that exercise poses some risks in the form of sports injuries. In fact, Aaron and LaPorte (1997) suggest that many of the pur-

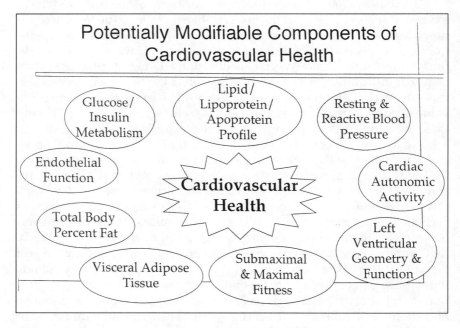

FIGURE 7-1. *Potentially Modifiable Components of Cardiovascular Health. Modified from Gutin and Owens, 1996.*

ported benefits of regular exercise are myths and that on balance exercise is harmful rather than beneficial to the health of youngsters. This notion must be kept in mind as we consider the relations among exercise, body composition, and health in this chapter.

EXERCISE, BODY COMPOSITION, AND HEALTH: NON-EXPERIMENTAL DESIGNS

The CAD/NIDDM Metabolic Syndrome

Many of the health problems associated with obesity, such as CAD and NIDDM, manifest themselves in the form of morbidity and mortality during the adult years. However, the origins of these problems can be traced to childhood. For example, CAD risk factors measured in childhood predict development of coronary lesions in young adults (Tracy et al., 1995), suggesting that some of the damage produced by these risk factors begins in youths and that lifestyle interventions to reduce risk factors early in life may be warranted. Such interventions are more likely to be effective if they are built upon a clear understanding of the etiological processes they are designed to influence.

Because lifestyle habits are to some degree formed early in life and track into adulthood (Kemper & van Mechelen, 1995), effective early intervention may have life-long impact. In the United Kingdom, it was shown that active adults tended to have been active as children, and sedentary adults who had been active as children were more likely to be persuaded to become active (James, 1996). In addition, body weight lost in weight control intervention programs is more likely to be sustained in children than in adults (Epstein et al., 1995a).

The links among various risk factors for CAD and NIDDM (i.e., hypertension, dyslipidemia, and hyperinsulinemia) indicate the presence of an underlying metabolic syndrome sometimes named syndrome X or the insulin resistance syndrome (Després et al., 1997; Reaven, 1988). Because the components of the syndrome are risk factors for CAD and NIDDM, we will refer to it as the CAD/NIDDM risk syndrome. In adults, it is clear that obesity, particularly central abdominal obesity, and physical inactivity are associated with this syndrome (Després et al., 1997; Williams, 1994). Moreover, recent studies in children have shown that poor cardiovascular fitness, excess body fatness, and elevated CAD/NIDDM risk factors are all interrelated, even in children as young as 5–6 y of age (Boreham et al., 1997; Gutin et al., 1990; Gutin et al., 1994; Kwiterovich, 1993; Webber et al., 1995).

Moreover, it is not clear to what degree the hyperinsulinemia found in this syndrome serves as a stimulus to growth (Horswill et al., 1997) and to what extent it is caused by the obesity. Since weight loss can lead to reduced insulin levels (e.g., Knip & Nuutinen, 1993), at least to some degree the excess fat seems to be a cause of the hyperinsulinemia.

Because child obesity and poorer fitness have increased in prevalence over the last 10–15 y (Kuntzleman, 1993; Troiano et al., 1995), the implications for the future public health are worrisome. Black females are at especially high risk for obesity and associated health problems (Pi-Sunyer, 1991); even in childhood, black girls are fatter than white girls (Obarzanek et al., 1994). One illustration of the seriousness of the secular trend to increased obesity is the 10-fold increase in the incidence of NIDDM (i.e., what used to be called "adult-onset diabetes") among youngsters in Cincinnati over the same period of time during which obesity was increasing (Pinhas-Hamiel et al., 1996). Support for the positive influence of exercise is provided by the results of prospective studies that found favorable changes in CAD risk in those children who improved the most in physical fitness (Hofman & Walter, 1989; Shea et al., 1994).

It is unclear to what degree physical activity and fitness exert their favorable influence on CAD/NIDDM risk factors by helping the child avoid excess fatness and to what degree fitness and fatness exert independent effects. There is some evidence that activity and fatness can exert independent influences on risk factors. For example, Suter & Hawes (1993) found activity (measured by questionnaire) to be associated with a favorable blood lipid profile, independent of fatness (measured with skinfolds) in 10–15 y olds, and Shea et al. (1994) found that systolic blood pressure increased less over a 2-y period in children who increased the most in cardiovascular fitness, independent of changes in body fatness. The possible importance of exercise intensity was highlighted in a study that found that non-resting energy expenditure (measured with doubly labeled water), adjusted for weight to provide an index of overall physical activity, was unrelated to CAD risk factors. However, the time spent in moderately intense activity (measured with self-report) was related to favorable LDL cholesterol levels even after controlling for percent body fat (Craig et al., 1996). This suggests that intensity of activity may be a more important determinant of risk than the energy spent in activity. Indirect support for the importance of high intensity training is provided by an adult study (Hurley et al., 1988) that showed strength training to improve CAD/NIDDM risk status, despite no change in maximal oxygen consumption and percent body fat. The mechanism for the favorable effect of high intensity exercise may involve the improved insulin action elicited by any form of muscle contraction.

Some evidence also suggests that activity and fitness in children do tend to exert much of their favorable effect on CAD/NIDDM risk factors through their influence on fatness. For example, in a sample of 1092 third grade children, obesity was associated with higher systolic blood pressure and total cholesterol, whereas self-reported physical activity levels were not related to the risk factors (McMurray et al., 1995). We found that both low maximal oxygen consumption (expressed in mL/kg of body weight) and high percent body fat (measured with dual x-ray absorptiometry) were correlated with unfavorable CAD/NIDDM risk factor levels in 7–10 y olds (Gutin et al., 1994); these results are shown in Table 7-1. Especially noteworthy were the magnitudes of the rank correlations between fasting insulin and percent fat and maximal oxygen consumption. However, when multiple regression was applied, only percent fat explained a significant independent proportion of the variance in the risk factors. After controlling for body fatness and aerobic fitness, the black 7–11 y olds had higher insulin levels than the whites, which is consistent with the higher incidence of NIDDM in blacks (Cowie et al., 1993).

We followed up this study with one in which weight was controlled experimentally rather than statistically; that is, cardiovascular fitness was expressed as submaximal heart rate during the weight-supported task of supine cycling (Gutin et al., 1997c), thus dissociating fitness from weight (and fatness). Table 7-2 shows that, after controlling for age and gender, percent fat was significantly related to unfavorable levels of systolic blood pressure, triglycerides, HDL cholesterol, the ratio of total to HDL cholesterol, and insulin; however, cardiovascular fitness was not significantly correlated with any of the risk factors.

TABLE 7-1. *Spearman rank correlations between fatness, fitness, and risk factors. The atherogenic index was an integrated value derived from total cholesterol, HDL cholesterol, apoprotein A-I, and apoprotein B; a higher value indicates poorer risk status. Modified from Gutin et al., 1994.*

	Percent Fat	Peak Oxygen Consumption	Waist/Hip Ratio
Peak Oxygen Consumption	$-0.76^{\#}$		
Waist/Hip Ratio	-0.01	-0.11	
Atherogenic Index	0.38^{**}	-0.27^{*}	0.20
Triglycerides	$0.48^{\#}$	-0.41^{**}	-0.03
Insulin	$0.78^{\#}$	$-0.72^{\#}$	0.04
Glucose	-0.32^{**}	$0.49^{\#}$	0.08
Systolic Blood Pressure	0.25	-0.18	0.02
Diastolic Blood Pressure	-0.08	0.03	-0.13

* $p < 0.05$
** $p < 0.01$
\# $p < 0.001$

TABLE 7-2. *Partial correlations (controlling for age and gender) between fatness, weight-independent fitness, and risk factors in 7-13 y old children. Modified from Gutin et al. (1997c).*

	Percent Fat	Submaximal HR
Percent Fat		0.15
Systolic Blood Pressure	0.32**	0.01
Diastolic Blood Pressure	−0.01	0.05
Triglycerides	0.42**	0.04
Total Cholesterol	0.16	0.17
HDL-Cholesterol	−0.31**	−0.04
LDL-Cholesterol	0.18	0.19
Total Cholesterol/HDL-Cholesterol	0.37**	0.05
(Log) Insulin	0.50**	0.22
Glucose	0.23	0.09
Glycohemoglobin	−0.01	0.06

** $p < 0.01$

Left Ventricular Geometry and Function

In adults, higher left ventricular mass is predictive of future cardiovascular morbidity (Devereux et al., 1994). However, there is some evidence that elevated left ventricular mass is also associated with higher levels of physical activity in youths (Treiber et al., 1993). Because physical activity is associated with lower levels of cardiovascular disease (US-DHHS, 1996), there is an apparent paradox involved. This may be resolved by hypothesizing that different components of left ventricular mass are influenced differently by different stimuli (Messerli & Ketelhut, 1993). That is, hypertension imposes an afterload on the heart, which results in greater wall thickness, whereas aerobic exercise produces a greater venous return (preload), thereby increasing cavity size. When we compared left ventricular dimensions in 8–12 y old distance runners and non-runners, the data were consistent with this hypothesis; i.e. the runners had significantly larger internal dimensions but somewhat (not significantly) thinner walls (Gutin et al., 1988). However, Rowland et al. (1994) failed to find differences in cardiac dimensions in prepubertal runners and non-runners. Thus, more work is needed with larger numbers of subjects to clarify this matter.

In adults and children, obesity is related to elevated left ventricular mass and relative wall thickness, i.e., the ratio of wall thickness to cavity size (Devereux et al., 1994; Treiber et al., 1993). We recently investigated the extent to which body composition explained variation in left ventricular geometry in 62 children, 7–13 y of age (Gutin et al., 1998). In addition to left ventricular mass and relative wall thickness, we investigated mid-wall fractional shortening, an index of left ventricular systolic function that identifies individuals at elevated risk for future cardiovascular mortality who are otherwise undetected by conventional endocardial shortening indices (deSimone et al., 1996). As shown in Table 7-3, we found that greater percent fat was associated with unfavorable levels of left ventricular mass (normalized to height$^{2.7}$), relative wall thickness, and mid-wall fractional shortening. One mechanism through which body composition may influence left ventricular variables is via the hyperinsulinemia that is associated with obesity (Sasson et al., 1993), so we explored the role of plasma concentrations of insulin in the fasted children. Although (Ln)insulin was significantly correlated with left ventricular mass in a bivariate analysis, in the multiple regression analysis that included fat mass it did not retain independent explanatory power. These results suggest that unfavorable left ventricular geometry and function may be associated with the CAD/NIDDM metabolic syndrome, including body fatness.

Endothelial Dysfunction

Endothelial dysfunction is a relatively early event in atherogenesis (Meredith et al., 1993). More specifically, low levels of endothelium-dependent arterial dilation are associated with various manifestations of cardiovascular disease in adults and children (Celermajer, 1997), leading us to investigate this matter further in 7–13 y old children (Treiber et al., 1997). Endothelium-dependent arterial dilation was determined by measuring with an echocardiograph the difference in diameter of the superficial femoral artery at baseline and after release of a tourniquet applied to the leg for 5 min. Better endothelial function, as represented by a greater amount of dilation in response to the increased blood flow that occurs when the tourniquet is released, was associated with lower percent fat and better cardiovascular fitness, as measured via heart rate response to supine cycling. These results support the idea that fitness and fatness play a role in the early stages of the atherogenic process.

TABLE 7-3. *Partial correlation (age controlled) coefficients (and probability values) for body composition and insulin versus left ventricular (LV) variables in 7-13 y old children. Modified from Gutin et al. (1998).*

	Percent Fat	Fat Free Mass	Fat Mass	Insulin
LV Mass	0.36**	0.76**	0.58**	0.27*
LV Mass/Height$^{2.7}$	0.34**	0.38**	0.42**	0.25
Relative Wall Thickness	0.34**	−0.41**	0.42**	0.20
Midwall Fractional Shortening	−0.37**	−0.40**	−0.40**	−0.18

* $p < 0.05$
** $p < 0.01$

Fat Patterning

In adults, fat stored in the abdominal region, especially in the visceral compartment, is more clearly associated with CAD/NIDDM risk factors and the development of NIDDM than is fat stored in other parts of the body (Wei et al., 1997; Williams, 1994), although noncentral obesity is by no means metabolically benign (Young & Gelskey, 1995). Moreover, Hunter et al. (1997) reported that in adult men free-living physical activity was inversely correlated with visceral adipose tissue, even after controlling for subcutaneous abdominal adipose tissue.

Our early studies of 5–11 y olds (Gutin et al., 1990; 1994) detected no association between fat patterning and risk factors. Asayama et al. (1995) studied 6–12 y old Japanese children and found that indices of general adiposity and fat patterning (i.e., waist/hip and waist/thigh circumferences) were correlated with CAD risk factors in boys; however, in girls only the indices of fat patterning were correlated with the risk factors. The Bogalusa Study, which can detect weak relationships as statistically significant because large numbers of children are studied, found a tendency for central, but not peripheral, skinfold thickness to be related to CAD/NIDDM risk factors (Freedman, 1995).

An important limitation of child studies that used anthropometry or dual x-ray absorptiometry is that they could not distinguish subcutaneous abdominal adipose tissue from the more deleterious visceral adipose tissue (Després et al., 1997). In adults, various measures of central fat deposition, including the waist/hip ratio or waist circumference alone, may be related to risk factors. However, in children, very little of the abdominal fat is in the visceral adipose tissue compartment relative to the amount in subcutaneous abdominal adipose tissue (Brambilla et al., 1994; Fox et al., 1993; Goran et al., 1995b; Owens et al., 1997). Therefore, at an early stage in the development of the CAD/NIDDM syndrome (i.e., in childhood), it may be necessary to measure visceral adipose tissue directly in order to uncover its relation to other risk factors.

A study that used magnetic resonance imaging in obese children (Brambilla et al., 1994) found that visceral adipose tissue, but not subcutaneous abdominal adipose tissue, was significantly related to LDL cholesterol and triglycerides. Furthermore, a study involving obese and non-obese adolescent girls found that visceral adipose tissue was significantly correlated with triglycerides, HDL cholesterol, and insulin in the obese girls only (Caprio et al., 1996a). On the other hand, a study of non-obese 7–10 y old girls found no significant relationship between visceral adipose tissue and triglycerides, HDL cholesterol, or insulin (Yanovski et al., 1996). Therefore, the visceral adipose tissue-risk factor relationship appears to be more pronounced in obese than in lean children.

We recently examined the relationships among these factors in 7–11 y old children (Owens et al., 1997). Although all the children were obese, thereby limiting generalizations to this population, the range of fatness was quite broad (27–61% fat). Total body percent fat and fat mass were determined using dual x-ray absorptiometry, whereas visceral adipose tissue and subcutaneous abdominal adipose tissue were measured using magnetic resonance imaging. Table 7-4 shows the bivariate correlations between the body composition variables and the risk factors. Multiple regressions revealed that for most of the lipid and lipoprotein parameters (triglycerides, HDL cholesterol, the ratio of total to HDL cholesterol, LDL particle size, and apolipoprotein B), visceral adipose tissue was the only predictor variable retained in the final models. The negative relationship between LDL particle size and visceral adipose tissue is noteworthy because of the evidence that small, dense LDL particles are relatively more atherogenic than larger, more buoyant particles (Stampfer et al., 1996). For non-lipid risk factors (such as insulin and systolic blood pressure), total fat mass rather than visceral adipose tissue was retained as a significant predictor in the regression models.

The role of ethnicity in fat patterning of prepubertal children was investigated by Goran et al. (1997). They found that, after controlling for subcutaneous abdominal adipose tissue, white children, especially the girls, had significantly higher levels of visceral adipose tissue. This is consistent with findings in white and black women (Conway et al.,

TABLE 7-4. *Correlations between adiposity measures and cardiovascular risk factors in obese 7-11 y old children. Modified from Owens et al. (1997).*

Variable	n	VAT	SAAT	% Body Fat	Total Fat Mass
Triglycerides	60	0.46[**]	0.22	0.06	0.18
Total Cholesterol	62	0.08	−0.03	0.01	−0.06
HDL Cholesterol	62	−0.40[**]	−0.32[*]	−0.08	−0.28[*]
TC/HDLC	62	0.45[**]	0.35[**]	0.12	0.29[*]
LDL Cholesterol	60	0.02	−0.01	0.04	−0.03
LDL Particle Size	41	−0.32[*]	−0.21	−0.01	−0.13
Apoprotein A-I	62	−0.05	−0.09	−0.09	−0.09
Apoprotein B	62	0.32[*]	0.32[*]	0.15	0.29[*]
Insulin	56	0.34[*]	0.40[**]	0.35[**]	0.49[*]
Systolic Blood Pressure	64	0.21	0.28[*]	0.15	0.33[**]
Diastolic Blood Pressure	64	−0.19	−0.11	−0.04	−0.07
LV mass/height$^{2.7}$	53	0.26	0.36[**]	0.25	0.37[**]

* $p < 0.05$
** $p < 0.01$
VAT = visceral adipose tissue
SAAT = subcutaneous abdominal adipose tissue
TC/HDLC = ratio of total cholesterol to HDL cholesterol
LV = left ventricular

1995). Thus, to some degree the greater prevalence of obesity in black females might be mitigated by there having lower levels of fatness in the most atherogenic region.

Indices of Clotting and Fibrinolysis

Some hemostatic indices have emerged as risk factors for cardiovascular disease and stroke (Kannel et al., 1987; Panchenko et al., 1995; Shimomura et al., 1996). Fibrinogen, synthesized in the liver, helps control blood viscosity through red cell aggregation, and in adult studies has been found to be positively related to visceral fat and body mass index (Cigolini et al., 1996; Meilahn et al., 1996). Plasminogen activator inhibitor-1 (PAI-1), also produced in the liver, inhibits the action of tissue-type plasminogen activator and contributes to thrombus formation (Shimomura et al., 1996). Positive relations between PAI-1 concentrations and upper body fat distribution have been observed in women (Meilahn et al., 1996; Vague et al., 1989). Cigolini et al. (1996) observed positive associations between PAI-1 concentrations and visceral fat. Less information is available about the relationship of adiposity to D-Dimer, an end product of fibrin breakdown (Panchenko et al., 1995).

With respect to what is known about these relations in children, there is some evidence that general fatness is positively associated with fibrinogen and PAI-1 concentrations (Bao et al., 1993; Legnani et al., 1988), but no studies have reported D-Dimer concentrations, and no information is available concerning the relationship between hemostatic variables and visceral adipose tissue. Therefore, we examined these relationships in a group of 7–11 y old obese children who varied from 27–61% fat (Ferguson et al., 1998). Insulin was included in the analysis because it is one possible mechanism through which fatness may influence hemostatic activity (Schneider & Sobel, 1991).

As shown in Table 7-5, all three hemostatic indices were associated with various adiposity measurements, suggesting that clotting/fibrinolysis is another pathway through which body composition influences the early etiology of cardiovascular disease.

Bone Density

Bone density is an aspect of body composition that plays a major role in the ability of bone to resist fracture when placed under strain (Cummings et al., 1990). Since accretion of bone mass is especially great during the early years of life, it is important to understand the factors that influence its development during childhood. It is likely that the peak levels of bone mass achieved early in life reduce the chances that the older person will eventually decline to a point where osteoporotic

TABLE 7-5. *Correlations between plasma hemostatic factors, adiposity measures, and insulin. Modified from Ferguson et al. (1998)*

Variable	Fibrinogen	PAI-1	D-Dimer	% Fat	VAT	SAAT	Fat Mass	Fat Free Mass
% Fat	0.42**	0.08	0.40*	—	0.40**	0.78#**	0.85#**	0.25
VAT	0.21	0.49**	0.16	0.40**	—	0.55**	0.51**	0.47**
SAAT	0.40**	0.32*	0.37*	0.78#**	0.55**	—	0.94**	0.65**
Fat Mass	0.42**	0.28	0.40**	0.85#**	0.51**	0.94**	—	0.71**
Fat Free Mass	0.23	0.50**	0.27	0.25	0.47**	0.65**	0.71**	—
BMI	0.41**	0.24	0.43**	0.78#**	0.48**	0.93**	0.93**	0.62**
Insulin	0.11	0.61#**	0.13	0.42#**	0.58#**	0.59#**	0.63#**	0.68#**

* $p < 0.05$
** $p < 0.01$
\#   Spearman Correlation Coefficient

fractures result; that is, like CAD and NIDDM, osteoporosis might be termed a pediatric disease (Chesnut, 1989).

Exercise and cardiovascular fitness are lifestyle factors that have been shown to influence bone density in adults (Gutin & Kasper, 1992). However, the influence of these factors on bone density in children is less clear, perhaps because of the way that cardiovascular fitness is measured and expressed. Since fitness is customarily measured in tasks that involve moving the body weight (e.g., treadmill walking/running) and/or is expressed in relation to body weight (e.g., maximal oxygen consumption per unit of body weight), fitness and weight (or fatness) are closely and inversely correlated (Gutin et al., 1994), making it difficult to determine their independent effect on factors such as bone density. For example, Rice et al. (1993) found that peak oxygen consumption per unit of body weight did not explain variance in bone density in adolescent girls. Since body weight was the single factor that explained the most variance in bone density, its presence in the denominator of the fitness variable may have obscured the potential positive relationship of fitness to bone density. We conducted a study (Gutin et al., submitted) in which we experimentally disentangled fitness from weight by measuring fitness in a weight-supported task (supine cycling); the results of the final regression models are shown in Table 7-6. Cardiovascular fitness explained a significant proportion of the variance in total body bone density and bone mineral content, after controlling for age, gender, ethnicity, fat-free soft tissue, and fat mass. Thus, there is reason to believe that activity and fitness may play a role in the prevention of fractures throughout life.

Summary of Non-Experimental Studies

The evidence reviewed is consistent with the notions that several major "adult" health problems actually have their origins in childhood

TABLE 7-6. *t-ratios of final multiple regression models for bone density and bone mineral content). The proportions of the variance explained by the models (R-square) are also given. Modified from Gutin et al. (submitted).*

	Bone Density	Bone Mineral Content
Age	2.67**	3.76**
Fat Free Soft Tissue	3.06**	4.78**
Fat Mass	0.10	2.85**
Gender	−0.72	0.93
Ethnicity	3.13**	2.59**
Exercise Heart Rate	−2.08*	−2.04*
Total R-square	0.688	0.812

* $p < 0.05$
** $p < 0.01$

and that excess body fat, especially visceral fat, is associated with pre-clinical markers for some of these diseases. However, causal inferences drawn from the results of non-experimental designs must be considered very tentative until supported by experimental studies that determine the extent to which changes in fatness are followed by changes in the fatness-related preclinical markers. These studies will be reviewed later in this chapter.

DETERMINANTS OF PHYSICAL ACTIVITY

Research dealing with free-living activity as a behavioral outcome is limited by lack of satisfactory measurement instruments (Sallis et al., 1996). As more objective methods of activity assessment are developed, such as doubly labeled water, our understanding of this topic may expand. Because cardiovascular fitness is related to habitual physical activity (Pate et al., 1990), and because systematic increases in activity (i.e. physical training) lead to increases in cardiovascular fitness (e.g., Savage et al., 1986; Yoshizawa et al., 1997), fitness information provides an indirect index of physical activity.

A complete review of this topic may be found in an excellent paper by Sallis et al. (1996); only a brief summary of the literature is possible in this chapter. Based on their review and other recent papers, the following conclusions may be drawn. (1) Boys are more active than girls (Trost et al., 1996). This is supported by data showing that even as young as 5–6 y of age boys are more fit than girls (Gutin, 1990). (2) Whites seem to be more active in aerobic activities than blacks or Mexican-Americans, which is consistent with recent data (Pivarnik et al., 1995; Trowbridge et al., 1997) showing that even after controlling for body fatness, black youths were lower in cardiovascular fitness than were whites. (3) Physical activity tends to decline during the teen years, especially in girls (Pate et al., 1994), contributing to the greater increase in body fatness that occurs in girls (Bar-Or & Baranowski, 1994). (4) Confidence in one's abilities to perform exercise (i.e. physical self-efficacy) is a strong predictor of future physical activity in adolescents (Reynolds et al., 1990). (5) Peers, siblings, and parents are influences on physical activity, probably through some combination of modeling, prompting, and reinforcement. (6) Youths are more active in the winter than in other seasons, on weekends compared to weekdays, and outdoors compared to indoors. Although television viewing is associated with obesity (Gortmaker et al., 1996), it has not been clearly shown to be associated with decreased physical activity. (7) Children are more likely to engage in intermittent, rather than sustained, bouts of high-intensity exercise (Sallo & Silla, 1997).

THE ETIOLOGY OF CHILDHOOD OBESITY

Overview

Although there is clear evidence that genetic factors play a role in obesity, it is also apparent that non-genetic factors are important, especially in technologically advanced societies (Bouchard, 1994). Regardless of whether the underlying impetus is genetic or environmental, variations in body energy stores are necessarily due to variations in one or more components of energy expenditure or intake.

Because of the complexity of these processes and the difficulty of measuring many of the involved variables precisely, little definitive information is available from prospective studies of the role of energy expenditure and diet in the natural history of obesity. Although improved techniques for measurement of total body and regional fatness and energy expenditure have begun to provide some valuable data, shortcomings inherent in diet assessment still limit our ability to determine the role of diet in weight control and health.

In light of the important role of visceral adipose tissue in the CAD/NIDDM risk syndrome starting in childhood, it is important to clarify how free-living physical activity influences its development. Unfortunately, no information is yet available about this matter in people of any age.

Resting Energy Expenditure

Total energy expenditure is comprised of resting metabolic rate, the thermic effect of food, and physical activity; resting metabolic rate constitutes 60–70% of the total, the thermic effect of food approximately 10% and physical activity the remainder (Ravussin & Swinburn, 1992).

In order to capture most of the thermic effect of food it is necessary to measure postprandial metabolism while the child remains relatively motionless for several hours, a daunting task for both the subjects and investigators. Moreover, the thermic effect of food is the component of energy expenditure that is least reproducible (Ravussin & Swinburn, 1992). Therefore, it has not been extensively studied, and its role in the etiology of childhood obesity is unclear. Although some adult studies suggest that the thermic effect of food may be blunted in obese people (Segal et al., 1987), cross-sectional studies of children do not provide a consistent picture concerning differences between lean and obese populations (e.g., Bandini et al., 1990; Maffeis et al., 1993), and no prospective studies in children have been reported.

Resting metabolic rate has been more extensively studied. Some cross-ethnic comparisons support the idea that resting metabolic rate can account for obesity in some populations. For example, one possible reason for the greater prevalence of obesity among blacks and their greater difficulty in losing weight (Kumanyika, 1993) is an inherent tendency to have a lower resting metabolic rate, as has been shown in some studies of adults and children (Foster et al., 1997; Kaplan et al., 1996; Morrison et al., 1996). However, the cross-sectional nature of these investigations precludes firm conclusions of causality; prospective studies in children of different ages are needed to elucidate the nature of these relationships.

A prospective study in adult Pima Indians showed that relatively low resting metabolic rates measured in a chamber, adjusted for fat mass and fat-free mass, led to accumulation of excess weight (Ravussin et al., 1988). However, child studies have not provided clear evidence that low levels of energy expenditure account for accretion of excess weight.

A cross-sectional study found that children of obese parents had relatively low resting metabolic rate (Griffiths & Payne, 1976), suggesting that they were at increased risk for development of obesity. However, when these children were followed-up 12 y later (Griffiths et al., 1990), the children of the obese parents were not found to be more obese than the children of nonobese parents. Moreover, two larger-scale doubly labeled water studies (Goran et al., 1995a; Davies et al., 1995b) failed to find any evidence that children of obese parents had defects in any aspect of energy expenditure.

Cross-sectional studies comparing obese and nonobese children, in which the influence of body composition was taken into account statistically, have found the groups to have similar resting and 24-h metabolic rates (Bandini et al., 1990; DeLany et al., 1996; Fontvieille et al., 1992; Maffeis et al., 1993). Two recent doubly labeled water studies of children (Goran et al., 1998; Wells et al., 1996) failed to show that resting energy expenditure predicted body fatness 2–4 y later.

Physical Activity

We will divide the treatment of this topic into two sections. In this section, we review cross-sectional and prospective cohort studies dealing with the role of exercise in the natural history of fatness. We will see that difficulties in how physical activity is expressed make it impossible to draw definitive conclusions. In the next section, we will review experimental studies in which youngsters have begun exercise programs; such research designs permit clearer causal connections to be discerned.

Although physical activity constitutes a relatively small portion of total energy expenditure on average, it has potential importance in explaining obesity development for several reasons. First, it is largely volitional. Second, its great individual variability provides an opportunity for it to explain a large portion of the variance in total energy expenditure. Third, activity can increase fat-free mass, the main determinant of resting metabolic rate (Ravussin & Swinburn, 1992), with long- term consequences of energy balance. Fourth, people spend most of the day in a postprandial state, during which the thermic effect of food may be potentiated by exercise (Segal & Gutin, 1983). Fifth, exercise training can influence substrate utilization, thereby playing a role in how ingested nutrients are partitioned into fat and fat-free mass.

It is problematic to determine from non-experimental studies whether or not exercise and body fatness are related because of the difficulty of knowing how to express physical activity. If it is expressed as energy expenditure, then it might be concluded that obese youths are *more* active than nonobese youths, as was found in a doubly labeled water study by Bandini et al. (1990). However, differences in mechanical work done must be considered when interpreting data on energy expenditure during activity; that is, a heavier child uses more energy to move the body a given distance. Thus, if a lean and an obese child display the same free-living activity energy expenditure, it represents less movement in the obese child. Consequently, it is necessary to adjust activity energy expenditure for body weight to determine if variations in movement are associated with fatness. The problem concerns the exponent to use in making this adjustment. If an exponent of one is used (i.e., energy expenditure is simply divided by weight), then an overcorrection may result, automatically creating a negative correlation with fatness (Prentice et al., 1996). Unfortunately, the correction factor varies for different children, depending on how much of their activity involves carrying the body weight (e.g. walking/running) and how much involves activities in which the body weight is supported and most of the work is external (e.g. cycling). The variety of procedures used to try to correct for body weight may account for the discrepant findings of cross-sectional doubly labeled water studies (e.g. Davies et al., 1995a, 1995b; Goran et al., 1996).

Unfortunately, perhaps for some of these same reasons, prospective studies that have used doubly labeled water methodology have not provided a clear picture either. One study (Roberts et al., 1988) suggested that greater activity energy expenditure led to less weight gain during the first year of life in a small group of infants, but two larger-scale studies (Goran et al., 1998; Wells et al., 1996) failed to show that activity energy expenditure predicted body fatness 2–4 y later.

The statistically sophisticated study by Goran et al. (1998) illustrates the complexity of the matter. They estimated activity to be the difference between total 24 h energy expenditure and resting energy expenditure, expressed either in absolute terms or adjusted (by regression) for fat-free mass. Therefore, the energy cost of transporting the fat mass was included in the activity energy expenditure, but fat mass was not included in the adjustment. This presumably led to an inflated baseline activity energy expenditure in the fatter children. The children who were fattest at baseline were the ones whose rate of increase in fatness was the greatest over time. Thus, an inflated baseline activity level for them may have obscured the potential contribution of low levels of actual movement to gain in fatness.

Time-motion studies, even those that depend on self or parental report (which is less objective than energy expenditure measurements), may provide a more direct index of how much exercise the child does. Cross-sectional studies of this nature show that active children are less fat (e.g. Goran et al., 1996) even while ingesting more energy (Deheeger et al., 1997); however, it is impossible to tell whether the activity caused less fatness or whether lower fatness caused the greater activity. A clearer picture emerges from recent epidemiological studies in which the exercise levels of children were estimated by the parents in relation to other children of the same age. It was found that exercise and family history of obesity were principal risk factors for later development of childhood obesity (Mo-suwan & Geater, 1996) or higher levels of body mass index (Klesges et al., 1995). Another recent study, which used the Caltrac movement sensor to measure activity, found that preschoolers who were classified as inactive were 3.8 times as likely as active children to have an increasing triceps skinfold slope during the average of 2.5 y of follow-up (Moore et al., 1995).

To the degree that aerobic fitness can be accepted as a proxy for physical activity, recent results of a 3-y longitudinal study of 7–12 y olds (Janz & Mahoney, 1997) are pertinent. It was found that those children who increased the most in maximal oxygen consumption were those who increased the most in fat-free mass and left ventricular mass but who increased the least in skinfold fatness.

Another factor to consider is the intensity of the exercise. In adults, Tremblay et al. (1990) found that when total energy expenditure during physical activity was held constant statistically, people who engaged in high intensity exercise were leaner and had less central fat deposition. However, little is known about the role of different exercise intensities in the etiology of childhood fatness.

Exercise may also influence accumulation of fat by improving the use of lipids as a substrate for energy (Mayers & Gutin, 1979; Saris, 1995) because fat oxidation has been identified as a risk factor for weight gain in adult Pima Indians (Zurlo et al., 1992). People who oxidized less fat than carbohydrate over the course of the day, as indicated by lower respiratory exchange ratios, were more likely to gain weight and fat mass;

i.e., the unoxidized fat was more likely to go into storage. This effect was independent of 24 h energy expenditure measured in the metabolic chamber. Non-obese black females with a family history of obesity also have lower levels of lipid oxidation at rest and during exercise than do white females, as well as lower resting energy expenditure and higher insulin levels, all of which may predispose them to the eventual onset of obesity (Chitwood et al., 1996). Consistent with this hypothesis are recently reported data showing that obese children, during the dynamic phase of fat deposition, had a decreased degree of lipolysis in response to epinephrine infusion (Bougnères et al., 1997). However, Le Stunff and Bougnères (1993) found *increased* lipid oxidation in obese children, even in the early stages of obesity. Maffeis et al. (1996) also observed greater lipid oxidation in obese children, perhaps as a compensatory mechanism for their higher levels of fat intake. The ability of lipid oxidation to predict future changes in fatness of children has not yet been elucidated in prospective studies. Perhaps reduced lipid oxidation plays a role only prior to the onset of obesity, especially in those whose fat intake is not especially high, after which lipid oxidation increases as part of a feedback loop to prevent further accretion of fat.

In light of the recent discovery in mice that the hormone leptin decreases energy intake and increases energy expenditure, some investigations of these relations have been undertaken in children. Caprio et al. (1996b) found in children and young adults that leptin was closely correlated with subcutaneous abdominal adipose tissue ($r = .84$, $p < .001$) and somewhat less closely correlated with visceral adipose tissue ($r = .59$, $p < .001$); in addition, acute increases in insulin concentrations did not affect circulating insulin levels. Lahlou et al.(1997) found that serum leptin levels were positively correlated with fasting insulin levels, adiposity, and weight gain the previous year, but were not associated with resting energy expenditure. Moreover, leptin was not related to lower energy intake; indeed the obese children ingested 2–3 times more energy (measured with self-reports) than did the lean children. Salbe et al.(1997) examined cross-sectional relations among these factors in 5-y-old Pima Indian children. They found that leptin concentrations, which were closely correlated to percent body fat ($r = .84$), were also correlated with physical activity level (the ratio of total to resting energy expenditure, measured with doubly labeled water), after adjustment for body fat ($r = .26$, $p < .01$). Nagy et al., (1997) found black and white girls to have higher leptin levels than did black and white boys; however, these differences were no longer significant after controlling for total body composition, visceral adipose tissue, and subcutaneous abdominal adipose tissue. These results indicate that in children leptin is a marker of adiposity but does not suppress energy intake or halt fat deposition, suggesting some type of leptin resistance. Perhaps the most important lesson to derive is that predictions from mouse studies concerning relations that may exist in humans must be made with great caution.

Diet

Accurate and reliable quantitative information about energy and macronutrient intake would be valuable, but such data are difficult to obtain, especially in children. Cross-sectional studies using diet recall methods have generally not found a relationship between body fatness and energy intake (Miller et al., 1990). This is counter-intuitive, in light of the fact that obese adults and children have relatively high fat-free mass along with their elevated fat mass, and consequently have elevated resting energy expenditure (Segal & Gutin, 1983), the largest component of 24 h energy expenditure. Assuming that the energy costs of thermoregulation and growth are small (Davies et al., 1995b), 24 h energy expenditure must equal energy intake. Using the doubly labeled water procedure to validate self- reported measures of energy intake, researchers have found that obese adults (Schoeller et al., 1990) and adolescents (Bandini et al., 1990) tend to underreport energy intake to a greater degree than lean people do. More objective and expensive means of collecting diet data, such as direct observation, might influence the youth's diet behavior and are very intrusive; thus this methodology is not feasible for most studies. Consequently, methodological considerations make it difficult to draw any clear conclusions about the role of total free-living energy intake in the etiology of obesity.

With respect to fat intake, most (Eck et al., 1992; Gazzaniga & Burns, 1993; Maffeis et al., 1996; Nguyen et al., 1996; Stubbs et al., 1995), but not all (Muecke et al., 1992), studies support the idea that diets high in fat are associated with body fatness or gain in weight. Lissner et al. (1997) found that a high-fat diet led to greater 6 y weight gain in women who were sedentary but not in those who were physically active. Thus, it may be the synergistic effect of a high-fat diet and sedentary behavior that is a key determinant of obesity. Prospective studies testing this hypothesis have not yet been reported in children.

Summary

Because of the difficulty of measuring activity and diet, compounded by the uncertainty of what is meant by "physical activity", few definitive conclusions are warranted. Perhaps the most reasonable conclusion is similar to one reached in a study of 10 y weight changes in a national cohort of adults (Williamson et al., 1993); i.e., that low physical activity leads to weight gain, while weight gain leads to further diminution of activity. This would imply that interventions that either decrease fatness or increase activity would turn the cycle in the other, more favorable, direction.

EXPERIMENTAL STUDIES OF EXERCISE AND PHYSICAL TRAINING

Overview

Although cross-sectional and longitudinal cohort studies can provide a foundation for hypotheses concerning the relations among exercise, body composition, and health, only controlled experiments can apply rigorous tests of the hypotheses. For example, knowing that there is a cyclic relationship between inactivity, weight gain, more inactivity, etc., in free-living children may be less important than knowing what happens when a child purposefully increases his/her activity level. This section will first review the literature on the influence of physical training on energy expenditure, diet, body composition, and CAD/NIDDM risk factors. Then we will describe the methodology and results of a recently completed study in our laboratory that provides new information concerning these factors.

Indirect support for the value of exercise early in life comes from experimental studies on animals that have shown physical training to prevent obesity (Oscai, 1989) and to greatly attenuate development of the CAD/NIDDM risk syndrome (Reaven et al., 1988). Although it is reasonable to formulate hypotheses from animal studies, the complexity of the growing human requires that the hypotheses be tested directly in children at different stages of maturity.

A simple model of what might occur when a youth begins an exercise program is that the energy expenditure of the exercise is added to the youth's customary daily energy expenditure, leading to an increase in 24 h energy expenditure. If energy intake is also uninfluenced by the physical training, the physical training will produce an energy deficit, reduction in body energy stores, and favorable changes in all the CAD/NIDDM risk factors related to obesity.

But what if children who participate in a vigorous physical training program decrease their normal daily physical activities (e.g., walking or cycling to school) or increase time spent in sedentary activity (e.g., watching television), with the result that their 24 h energy expenditure is similar to that of children who do not participate in the physical training? Furthermore, what if the interaction of physical training with different types of diets sometimes causes energy intake to increase more than energy expenditure, thereby leading to a positive rather than a negative energy balance? What if the links between fatness and risk factors in children noted in cross-sectional research are partly or largely coincidental rather than causal, such that improvements in the former do not necessarily lead to improvements in the latter? Finally, what if different types or intensities of physical training influence these factors in different ways in youths of various types (e.g., those with positive or negative family histories of obesity or those with varying levels of maturity, gender, or ethnicity)?

It is clear that this matter is far from simple. As a result, definitive answers to these questions are not available regarding people of any age, especially children. We will attempt to piece together what is known in order to arrive at some hypotheses (and perhaps some conclusions) concerning the effects of exercise.

Energy Expenditure and Diet

Restriction of energy intake (i.e., dieting) allows a person immediately to produce a relatively large daily energy deficit compared to what would be appropriate for exercise alone. For example, many obese youths can reduce energy intake by 1000 kcal/d, while it would be difficult and perhaps dangerous for an unfit youth to try to increase physical activity by that amount. Thus, dieting is more effective for short-term weight loss.

However, dieting leads to a reduction of resting metabolism in proportion to decreases in fat-free mass (Maffeis et al., 1992), thus setting the stage for the dieter to regain the lost weight when the diet stops (Schwingshandl & Borkenstein, 1995). In contrast, when exercise is used for weight loss, reductions in fat-free mass are minimized (Ballor & Poehlman, 1994), supporting the logic of incorporating exercise into programs designed for long-term weight control. While adult studies suggest that aerobic training by itself does not ordinarily alter fat-free mass or resting energy expenditure (Poehlman et al., 1991), little is known about the effect of physical training in growing children.

To our knowledge, no direct experimental information is available concerning the effect of physical training on the thermic effect of food in children, largely because of the laborious nature and questionable value of its measurement. There is evidence that mild exercise may potentiate the thermic effect of food in some populations (Segal & Gutin, 1983). If this were true in children, engaging in regular physical training in a postprandial state (i.e. most waking hours) would provide an additional boost to metabolism.

Another aspect of resting metabolism is the elevated resting energy expenditure following each exercise session. Although this factor tends to be relatively modest following exercise at intensities that are typically prescribed (e.g., 50–70% of peak oxygen consumption), there seems to be an exponential relationship between exercise intensity and post-exercise energy expenditure (Brehm & Gutin, 1986; Broeder et al., 1991). Thus, this factor might make a greater contribution to 24 h energy expenditure for youths who train at a relatively high intensity (Treuth et al., 1996). The higher resting metabolism found in some aerobically trained people (Poehlman et al., 1991) may be partially due to the interaction of the effects of the last exercise session with subsequent eating and may be lost after a few days of training cessation (Herring et al., 1992). However, if the person exercises at a high intensity every day or two, then resting metabolism may be continuously elevated.

The third component of 24 h energy expenditure that may be influenced by physical training is energy expenditure during the hours when the person is not engaged in the training itself. Using the doubly labeled water procedure for objective measurement of 24 h energy expenditure, combined with laboratory measurement of post-prandial metabolic rate in the laboratory, Goran and Poehlman (1992) found in elderly people that physical training did not result in increased 24 h energy expenditure, despite increases in resting energy expenditure; this suggests that the subjects compensated for energy used in the physical training by reducing their free-living activity. Conversely, when exercise was added to dieting in 21–50 y old obese women, either no change (Kempen et al., 1995) or an increase (Racette et al. 1995b) in energy expenditure during physical activity occurred.

In another study that used doubly labeled water to measure 24 h energy expenditure, adolescents who began a training program exhibited a 12% increase in daily energy expenditure, only half of which could be explained by the energy cost of the training itself (Blaak et al., 1992). Because heart rate monitoring and activity diaries suggested that no change had occurred in spontaneous activity, the authors speculated that the training may have increased resting metabolism by increasing post-exercise energy expenditure and the increase in fat-free mass elicited by the training. The thermic effect of food may have also been increased, partially because the children may have increased their energy intake in response to the training. An increase in energy intake does seem to have occurred because the trained group did not decline significantly in percent fat during the short training period of 4 wk.

Thus, elderly people may find strenuous physical training taxing, such that they reduce free-living activity, while younger people find it stimulating and maintain or even increase free-living activity.

Some recent experimental studies of short-term exercise-diet interactions have provided interesting (and surprising) findings. Although this area of investigation has mainly used adult subjects, important implications for youths may be drawn.

When different types of foods have been offered in controlled laboratory studies, the combination of exercise and low-fat (high carbohydrate) meals resulted in a negative energy balance for 24–48 h periods, as would be expected. However, offering high-fat foods after a bout of exercise eliminated or completely reversed the energy deficit expected from the exercise (King & Blundell, 1995; Tremblay et al., 1994a). Thus, if youths who begin a physical training program are offered high-fat foods by parents, school personnel, and peers, then perhaps the daily bouts of exercise will be followed by excess energy intake, with the paradoxical result that body energy stores are not reduced, and may even be increased.

Another factor is exercise intensity. In a laboratory study of lean young men, a bout of high-intensity (but not low-intensity) exercise led to a short-term negative energy balance for the day (King et al., 1994). This may be one mechanism through which high-intensity physical training would be more effective than low-intensity training. It is important to note that these studies were carried out in lean men. Some adult studies showed that lean subjects increased energy intake to compensate for several weeks of increased activity (Woo & Pi-Sunyer, 1985), whereas obese subjects did not, with the result that steady fat loss resulted in the obese subjects (Woo et al., 1982). In a less controlled setting, Racette et al. (1995a) found that adding exercise to a dieting regimen seemed to enhance the compliance of the women to the prescribed diet.

There is a paucity of information concerning the effect of physical training on diet in youths. Based on the adult data, we might expect that lean, but not obese, youths will increase their energy intake in response to training, but this may be influenced by the fat intake of their diets; the greater the proportion of fat in the diet, the more likely they are to increase energy intake.

Effects on Cardiovascular Fitness

The extent to which cardiovascular fitness can be enhanced by physical training in normal children seems limited, especially if cardiovascular fitness is expressed as maximal oxygen consumption (Payne & Morrow, 1993). However, when other indices of cardiovascular fitness were used, such as heart rate during submaximal exercise (Gutin et al., 1995; Stewart & Gutin, 1976) or ventilatory breakpoint (Mahon & Vaccaro, 1989), clear improvements were seen, suggesting that indices of fitness measured during submaximal exercise may be more sensitive to the effects of physical training than is maximal oxygen consumption. The importance of carrying out the training over a long enough period to see its true impact is illustrated by a study of 4–6 y old Japanese girls (Yoshizawa et al., 1997). It was found that performing a 915 m endurance run 6 d/wk produced significant improvement in maximal oxygen consumption after 12 and 18 mo of training; however, the differences after only 6 mo of training did not yet achieve statistical significance.

Relatively little is known about the role of exercise intensity in children for improving cardiovascular fitness. Massicotte and Macnab (1974) found somewhat better improvements in cardiovascular fitness when the training intensity was relatively high. However, all groups trained for 12 min/session, so that total work accomplished was confounded with training intensity. The short duration of the exercise sessions and of the entire physical training program (6 wk) also limits the conclusiveness of the results. Savage et al. (1986), who took the approach of holding total work constant while varying intensity, found that the high-intensity training increased cardiovascular fitness more effectively than low-intensity training.

Effects on Body Composition

Epstein et al. (1996) presented a careful analysis of studies of exercise in the treatment of child and adolescent obesity, concluding that: (1) exercise alone was ineffective; (2) exercise plus diet was more effective for weight and fitness than diet alone; and (3) programs emphasizing lifestyle change rather than formal physical training sometimes produced better long-term effects on weight. In a clever use of alternative reinforcement approaches, Epstein et al. (1995b) showed that reinforcing children for reducing sedentary behaviors was more effective for reduction of percent fat than reinforcing them for increased physical activity or a combination of the two.

The two exercise-alone studies reviewed by Epstein et al. (1996) were conducted in schools, making it difficult to control and document the physical training stimulus. We have recently shown in a more controlled environment that training, without dietary intervention, did reduce body fatness in obese children (Gutin et al., 1995; Gutin et al., 1997a; described below), suggesting that on average the children did not decrease free-living activity or increase energy intake to compensate for the energy used in the physical training.

The influence of different types, amounts, and intensities of exercise has not been studied extensively in youths. With respect to body fatness, Bar-Or & Baranowski (1994) concluded that there are too few data available to even make a recommendation concerning intensity. In adults, Tremblay et al. (1994b) found that high intensity training was more effective in reducing body fatness than was somewhat lower intensity training. If total energy used during the exercise sessions is the critical parameter, then simply lengthening the low-intensity sessions can allow the youth to use the same amount of energy as would be used in a high-intensity session. Savage et al. (1986) used this approach with prepubertal boys and found skinfold fat to decline similarly in the low- and high-intensity groups, even though the high-intensity training resulted in a clearer improvement in cardiovascular fitness.

Even when the energy expenditure during the training itself is controlled, there are reasons to suspect that higher intensities may be more efficacious in reducing fatness if the intervention continues for a longer period than the typical 2–4 mo. First, the exponential relationship between exercise intensity and post-exercise metabolism may gradually lead to greater loss of fat as a result of high intensity training. Second, if high intensity training increases cardiovascular fitness more effectively, as shown by Savage et al. (1986), then the youth would be able progressively to use up more energy in a given amount of training time, eventually leading to greater fat loss.

In light of the role of visceral adipose tissue in the CAD/NIDDM risk syndrome, it is important to clarify how training influences this fat depot. Adult studies that used computed tomography or magnetic resonance imaging to measure visceral adipose tissue found that training reduced visceral adipose tissue more than it reduced fat deposits in other areas of the body (Ross & Rissanen, 1994; Schwartz et al., 1991). Using dual x-ray absorptiometry and anthropometry (which cannot distinguish visceral from subcutaneous adipose tissue), we found no tendency for physical training to reduce central fatness more than peripheral fatness in 7–11 y old obese girls (Gutin et al., 1995). To our knowledge, no studies of the effects of training on visceral adipose tissue in children or adolescents have been reported (other than the one from our laboratory described below).

Effects On Obesity-Related CAD/NIDDM Risk Factors

Studies of physical training and CAD/NIDDM risk factors in youths have generally failed to provide clear evidence that the training was effective (Armstrong & Simons-Morton, 1994), leading some to conclude that regular exercise does not improve these aspects of cardiovascular health of children (Rowland, 1996). However, a conclusive judgement on this matter may not yet be warranted (Gutin & Owens, 1996) because of limitations of these studies, including: (1) the training dose may have been insufficient in magnitude or inadequately controlled; (2) the number of subjects may have been too small, and (3) the subjects may have been so healthy that no improvement in risk factors would be expected. For example, Alpert and Wilmore (1994) concluded that training studies that used hypertensive youths were more likely to show reduced blood pressure than were studies using normotensive youths.

In adults who have been sedentary and/or obese for many years, the CAD/NIDDM syndrome has had time to develop to dangerous levels; thus, interventions such as physical training may have a greater potential to reduce risk factors than would be true in youths.

Hansen et al. (1991) reported the effect on blood pressure of adding 3 d/wk of physical education to a normal 2 d/wk program, in a project that had relatively few limitations; it included randomized control groups for children who were normotensive or hypertensive at baseline, had sample sizes that were relatively large (64–69 youths/group), was conducted for a relatively long period of 8 mo, and included all subjects in the statistical analyses regardless of their degree of compliance with the treatment regimens. It was found that after 3 mo of the intervention the groups did not differ significantly in fitness or blood pressure. However, after 8 mo the exercise groups had increased significantly in fitness and declined significantly in systolic and diastolic blood pressure. This study provides solid support for the hypothesis that extra physical education can reduce blood pressure in both hypertensive and normotensive youths 9-11 y of age.

A 2 y study of obese Japanese children, which involved 7 d of aerobic exercise per week, found substantial decreases in skinfold fatness and increased HDL cholesterol after 1 and 2 y (Sasaki et al., 1987). Such a long duration for a training study helps to clarify the actual long-term effect of regular exercise. Others have showed that weight loss led to reduced insulin (Knip & Nuutinen, 1993) and that obese adolescents who engaged in a diet plus exercise treatment reduced their fatness and other CAD/NIDDM risk factor levels more than the group that used diet alone (Becque et al., 1988; Rocchini et al., 1987).

We conducted a small study of the effects of a 10-wk intervention period of supervised physical training or lifestyle education in obese 7–11 y old black girls (Gutin et al., 1996a). The lifestyle education group engaged in weekly behavior modification sessions dealing with healthy eating and exercise habits. The physical training group showed a significant increase in cardiovascular fitness and a significant decrease in percent body fat, while the lifestyle education group declined significantly more in dietary energy and percent of energy intake from fat. Fasting insulin did not change significantly in either group. Blood glucose was reduced more in the lifestyle education group than in the exercise group, and glycohemoglobin declined from baseline in both groups. The lipid/lipoprotein changes were similar in the two groups, showing declines in the ratio of total to HDL cholesterol and in plasma triglyceride concentrations and increases in the ratio of LDL cholesterol to apoprotein B, which indicates a favorable decrease in small, dense LDL (Sniderman et al., 1980). Thus, the interventions were similarly effective in improving some CAD/NIDDM risk factors, perhaps through different pathways; i.e., the physical training improved fitness and fatness, while the lifestyle education improved diet.

Another aspect of cardiovascular health that may be influenced by exercise and body composition is cardiac autonomic traffic; a high ratio of sympathetic to parasympathetic activity is an index of poorer cardiovascular and metabolic health in adults and children (Akinci et al., 1993; Algra et al., 1993; Javorka et al., 1988; Rollins et al., 1992) . Early research in this area involved blocking the action of sympathetic and/or parasympathetic receptors with drugs, an invasive procedure. Techniques for measuring the beat-to-beat variability in electrocardiogram intervals—i.e., heart period variability (also called heart rate variability) —allows information concerning autonomic traffic to be derived via non-pharmacologic methods. The potential clinical importance of exercise training is illustrated by a study in which dogs who trained for 6 wk increased their parasympathetic activity substantially and were afforded protection against the ventricular fibrillation associated with acute myocardial ischemia (Hull et al., 1994). Some, but not all, adult studies showed physical training to improve the balance of sympathetic to parasympathetic activity. Since obesity and low levels of cardiovascular fitness are associated with lower levels of parasympathetic activity, we reasoned that the effect of physical training might be seen most clearly in youths who were both unfit and obese at baseline. Thus, we randomized 35 obese children to a control group or a group that engaged in 4 mo of physical training, for 5 d/wk, 40 min/d. Table 7-7

TABLE 7-7. *Means (SE) of change scores after 4 mo of physical training or control treatment and p-values for comparisons of groups in 7–11 y old children. Modified from Gutin et al. (1997b).*

	Physical Training Group n=17	Control Group n=18	p-value
Submaximal Heart Rate	−3.3 (2.0)	+5.3 (2.7)	<0.01
Percent fat	−4.1 (1.0)	−0.6 (0.7)	<0.01
Resting Heart Rate	−3.5 (2.2)	+1.8 (3.1)	ns (<0.09)
RMSSD	+9.8 (6.8)	−6.4 (5.6)	<0.05
LFP	−21.2 (48.2)	−10.2 (36.3)	ns
LFP, percent of total power	−7.6 (3.6)	+2.4 (3.3)	<0.03
HFP	−29.1 (65.2)	−71.7 (58.2)	ns
HFP, percent of total power	+0.5 (4.5)	−4.0 (3.7)	ns
LFP/HFP	−0.7 (1.3)	+0.4 (1.1)	<0.01

RMSSD = Root Mean Square of Successive Differences—This is a time domain index of parasympathetic activity
LFP = Low frequency Power—This is a frequency domain index of combined sympathetic and parasympathetic activity
HFP = High Frequency Power—This is a frequency domain index of parasympathetic activity
LFP/HFP = The ratio of LFP/HFP is an index of sympathetic-parasympathetic balance

shows that, compared to the control group, the training group reduced submaximal heart rate, percent body fat and the ratio of sympathetic to parasympathetic activity (Gutin et al., 1997b), indicating an improved cardiac autonomic balance.

Efficacy of Controlled Physical Training for Obese Children: Study from The Georgia Prevention Institute

We conducted a study that determined the effect of physical training, without dietary intervention, on various aspects of cardiovascular health in 74 obese 7–11 y olds (mean of 44% fat). Cardiovascular fitness was measured via heart rate response to supine cycling, a task that rendered fitness independent of body weight and fatness. Vigorous physical activity was measured with a 7 d recall, diet with 4 d of recalls, total body composition with dual x-ray absorptiometry, visceral and subcutaneous abdominal adipose tissue with magnetic resonance imaging, resting and exercise blood pressures with an automated monitor, and left ventricular parameters with echocardiography. A variety of variables were derived from a fasting blood sample (e.g., lipids, lipoproteins, LDL particle size, insulin, glucose, glycohemoglobin, and fibrinogen). Classes were offered 5 d/wk, and the attendance was 80%. The mean heart rate was 157 bpm for the 40-min sessions, and the children expended 226 kcal/session; thus a substantial training dose was imparted to the children. After 4 mo the measurements made at baseline were repeated, the two groups switched assignments (i.e., group 1 engaged in training for the first 4 mo and did not train for the next 4 mo, while group 2 did the opposite), and the measurements were made again at the 8 mo time point. Time-by-group analyses of variance were applied to determine the effects of the training and detraining.

Figure 7-2 shows the results over 8 mo for percent fat, the primary outcome variable. The time x group interaction was significant, and the pattern was as predicted; i.e., group 1 declined in percent fat during the period of training and increased somewhat during the next 4 mo, while group 2 remained stable during the first 4 mo and declined during the 4 mo when they engaged in the training. The time by group interaction was also significant for bone mineral density, with greater increases during the 4 mo periods of training than during the periods of no training.

We collected magnetic resonance imaging data only at baseline and the 4 mo time points; the body composition results are shown in Table 7-8. Both groups increased in visceral adipose tissue, but the increase of the control group was significantly greater than that of the physical training group. The difference between groups in subcutaneous abdominal adipose tissue was also significant (Owens et al., 1998).

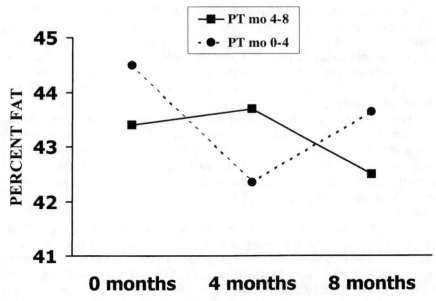

FIGURE 7-2. *Training, detraining, & percent fat in obese children.*

TABLE 7-8. *Mean change scores for the PT and control groups after 4 mo of intervention, and p-values for comparison of changes. Modified from Owens et al. (1998).*

| Variable | PT Group (n = 35) | | Control Group (n = 39) | | |
	Mean	SE	Mean	SE	p
Total body mass, kg	+1.1	0.4	+2.0	0.2	0.1
Fat Mass, kg	−0.8	0.5	+0.9	0.3	<0.01
Fat-Free Mass, kg	+1.9	0.3	+1.1	0.2	0.03
Percent Fat	−2.2	0.6	0	0.4	<0.01
VAT, cm^3	+1.3	8.3	+20.9	4.3	0.02
SAAT, cm^3	−16.2	27.1	+48.9	19.9	0.03
Submax HR, bpm	−3.8	1.8	+0.2	1.4	0.04
Total Energy Expenditure, kcal	+102	32	+13	39	0.09
MVPA, kcal	+81	53	−96	48	0.02

Abbreviations:
MVPA = moderate to vigorous physical activity
VAT = visceral adipose tissue
SAAT = subcutaneous abdominal adipose tissue
HR = heart rate

As predicted, vigorous activity increased and submaximal heart rate decreased during periods of training, and changed in the opposite directions during periods of no training. Since there were no significant differences in moderate physical activity or in energy or macronutrient intake between periods of training and no training, the body composition changes must be attributed to the vigorous activity represented by the physical training.

With respect to other risk factors, no significant time-by-group interactions were found for: most hemodynamic variables, left ventricular geometry and function, and some lipid parameters. The exceptions were insulin, triglycerides, and the ratio of total cholesterol to high density lipoprotein cholesterol, for which the pattern was as predicted, i.e., reductions during training but not during the 4 mo periods of no training.

Thus, the physical training, without any dietary intervention, had the favorable effect of improving total body composition while preventing the natural increase in visceral adipose tissue that occurs as children mature. In addition, some aspects of the CAD/NIDDM metabolic syndrome were favorably influenced. However, many of the other obesity-associated risk factors were not significantly influenced by the training, perhaps because the changes in fitness and body composition produced in 4 mo were relatively modest in magnitude.

Summary of Experimental Studies of Exercise and Physical Training

Several conclusions may be drawn concerning the experimental studies of exercise reviewed. When obese youths begin a physical training program that does not include any dietary intervention, they do not completely compensate for the energy expenditure involved in the training by reducing their free-living energy expenditure at other times of day or by increasing their energy intake. Consequently, they tend to reduce fat mass, and because the training also enhances fat-free mass (including bone density), their overall body composition is favorably influenced. With respect to fat patterning, our study shows that even in children, who have relatively small amounts of visceral adipose tissue compared to adults, physical training can attenuate the maturity-associated increases in this especially atherogenic fat depot.

One way of interpreting these results is that exercise can enhance body composition, but does not alter many other risk factors during the early stages of CAD and NIDDM. However, the cross-sectional and longitudinal cohort studies described earlier in this chapter suggest that youths who are more fit and less fat over long periods of time exhibit more favorable CAD/NIDDM risk profiles. Therefore, it is possible that more profound changes in body composition that might be produced by longer periods of training, or combinations of training with low-fat diets, can have a significant impact on obesity-related risk factors.

SCHOOL-BASED INTERVENTION STUDIES

In the studies reviewed above, physical training was generally imposed on the subjects to see what effect was produced. Moreover, the data were often analyzed only for those subjects who met a pre-established criterion for exposure to the training (e.g., 3 d/wk). Such studies are necessary to determine the efficacy of physical training, just as a study of the pharmacologic action of a drug analyzes only data for people who actually take the drug. However, when a program is offered to children in field settings, the degree to which the youths actually perform the exercise varies. Moreover, the net effectiveness of the intervention is dependent on both the efficacy of the exercise and the adherence to the exercise prescription, just as the effectiveness of a prescribed medication depends both on its efficacy for those who take it and the degree of patient adherence to the prescribed regimen. In practical terms, the effectiveness of the strategies used to promote adherence to the prescribed exercise is as important as the efficacy of the exercise itself (Epstein et al., 1996).

Several studies have been implemented in school settings to study the influence of various interventions on exercise, fitness, body composition, and other CAD/NIDDM risk factors; these studies have generally sought to influence both physical activity and diet, so it is difficult to tease out the unique effects of the exercise. Some have also addressed smoking prevention or cessation, but we will not comment on this aspect of the studies. Because of the large number and complexity of such studies, we will describe only a few that illustrate the current state of the art.

School-based programs that intend to use exercise to influence cardiovascular health must involve several steps, beginning with changing the activity habits and fitness of the youths. If the activity habits are changed, the issue still remains as to whether the changes actually improve body composition and obesity-related risk factors.

One study that showed favorable results for some aspects of cardiovascular health (Arbeit et al., 1992) involved all the children in the fourth and fifth grades of two control and two intervention schools. The intervention schools utilized a reduced-fat school lunch program, physical education classes that concentrated on personal and aerobic fitness, and cardiovascular risk factor screening techniques. The exercise program included 12 didactic lessons designed to improve the knowledge and attitudes of the children concerning the role of exercise in cardio-vascular health, as well as a year-long fitness program incorporated into the physical education curriculum. The program was successful in decreasing the 1 mi run/walk times of fifth grade boys, but the favorable trend for the girls did not achieve significance. The subjects who improved their run/walk times also showed significant decreases in triceps and subscapular skinfolds and in systolic blood pressure. At the end of the program, significant cross-sectional correlations were found between run/walk times and favorable levels of skinfolds (in the boys), resting heart rate (in the girls), and HDL cholesterol (both genders).

Donnelly et al. (1996) reported a study that used relatively sophisticated measurement methods, such as hydrodensitometry for body composition and a treadmill test for maximal oxygen consumption. In the 2 y study, the intervention was designed to enhance physical activity within the physical education program. Students were trained 3 d/wk for 30–40 min in activities that utilized the larger muscle groups. The intervention schools also adopted a modified school lunch program and special classes for educating students about healthy nutrition. In year two of the program, classroom physical activity (as measured with a direct observation system) was 6% greater in the intervention school, but out-of-school physical activity (as measured with a 1 d recall) was 20% lower in the intervention school. Consistent with the absence of significant differences between the schools in total energy expenditure or intake, no significant differences were seen for maximal oxygen consumption or percent fat; the absence of treatment effects on body composition was also true when a subset of relatively fat youths was analyzed. There were also no significant differences between control and intervention groups for blood parameters such as cholesterol, triglycerides, insulin, or glucose. However, significant differences were seen between groups for HDL cholesterol and the total to HDL cholesterol ratio, with the intervention group exhibiting more favorable changes.

The CATCH study (Luepker et al., 1996) was the largest and most rigorous school-based field trial reported to date. It was a multi-site effort that at baseline involved 5106 third-graders from ethnically diverse groups in four states. This study set out to modify the school lunch programs, to increase the amount of moderate to vigorous physical activity in physical education classes, and to improve knowledge about healthy eating and exercise. One particular strength was that it lasted for a 3 y period. The intervention schools were able to reduce the percentage of fat in the school lunches, and the intervention subjects reported a significantly lower intake of energy and fat. The time spent in moderate to vigorous physical activity during classes (by direct observation) and the daily vigorous physical activity (by self-report) were significantly greater in the intervention schools; however, the total daily physical activity reported by the youths and the 9 min run time did not differ significantly for the intervention and control groups. At the end of the 3 y period, no significant differences between groups were found for height, weight, body mass index, percent fat, blood pressure, total cholesterol, HDL cholesterol, or apolipoprotein B. Thus, the study was successful in modifying diet and moderate to vigorous physical activity but failed to show individual benefits for the reduction of fatness or CAD risk.

These studies suggest that it is feasible to make favorable changes in school physical education and nutrition programs, which sometimes lead to improved fitness and CAD risk status. However, the results have not been at all conclusive, showing how difficult it is to improve cardiovascular health of children through school-based health promotion interventions.

PRACTICAL IMPLICATIONS

To what degree does scientific evidence support the concept that parents, health professionals, and formulators of public policy can play important roles in prevention and treatment of childhood obesity and associated health problems? First, it appears that already in childhood, body composition is associated with unfavorable levels of a number of preclinical markers for "adult" diseases such as CAD and NIDDM, providing support for the idea that these diseases have their origins in childhood. The marked increase in childhood obesity and NIDDM over the last 10–15 y suggests that the stage is being set for a great deal of excess morbidity and mortality in the future. Moreover, it appears that inadequate physical activity is at least part of the explanation for the development of obesity. Secondly, there is evidence that children, especially obese children, who do engage in vigorous physical activity, even without dietary intervention, can improve their body composition. Thirdly, it appears that adding exercise to a low-fat and/or low-energy diet for obese youths adds to the effectiveness of the regimen. Fourthly, it appears that family members and school environments can play a role in enhancing moderate and vigorous physical activity.

A recent large-scale study in Thailand (Mo-suwan & Geater, 1996) casts an interesting light on the roles of activity and diet in preventing childhood obesity. They found that for young children a family history of obesity and a low exercise level (as estimated by the parents in relation to other children of the same age) were the main risk factors for later development of childhood obesity. The authors concluded that increasing exercise was clearly the most appropriate intervention to prevent obesity in Thailand because the risk of nutritional deficiency is still high, and a mass intervention program focusing on reduction of energy intake might make the situation worse. In light of the fact that obesity and perhaps poor nutrition are more prevalent in lower social classes in the United States, a similar situation might exist here.

Although cross-sectional and longitudinal cohort studies support the hypothetical chain that goes from greater physical activity to better body composition to enhanced CAD/NIDDM risk status, controlled and randomized interventions have only partly supported this line of reasoning. This may be because at this early stage in the development of the CAD/NIDDM risk syndrome the relationships shown in the non-experimental studies are not causal in the directions hypothesized or because the exercise dose imparted to the youths was insufficient in intensity, volume, or duration. In the next section we suggest some research strategies that might help resolve this issue. Until the matter is definitely resolved, the causal hypothesis is biologically plausible. Even if childhood and adolescence turn out to be stages of life wherein exercise is incapable of improving many of the CAD/NIDDM risk factors, it has been shown to improve body composition and fitness, factors that influence how active and fat the youths will be in the future (i.e., as adults). Because adult activity and body composition have been shown to improve CAD/NIDDM risk status, as described in the recent Surgeon-General's report on physical activity and health (USDHHS, 1996), a prudent course of action is to encourage exercise for the present, as well as the future, cardiovascular health of children.

Families can play a role by modeling regular exercise behavior, providing incentives, and providing transportation to active environments (e.g., dance classes, gyms). Schools can play a role by altering their curriculums to insure that physical education classes include vigorous activity and concept development concerning active lifestyles. Communities can provide more supervised play areas and programs, especially in low socioeconomic neighborhoods where physical activity tends to be low because the danger of violence keeps children indoors. The hours of 3 to 6 p.m. on weekdays seem like an especially valuable target for such health promotion programs to be offered in schools. In recent decades, cities have been planned around the needs of automobiles rather than public health, thereby limiting physical activity. In the United Kingdom it was found that rearranging auto traffic patterns to limit traffic in the vicinity of their homes was effective in encouraging children to play outside (James, 1996).

Notwithstanding all these potential benefits of exercise to cardiovascular health, the admonitions of Aaron and LaPorte (1997) must be kept in mind. That is, we must minimize the adverse impact of exercise on health, mainly in the form of sports injuries, in order to assure that its net effect is positive.

DIRECTIONS FOR FUTURE RESEARCH

First, we need more information concerning the optimal exercise dose for body composition and other aspects of health. Relatively little is known about how much or what intensity of exercise is most efficacious in altering cardiovascular health in people of any age, and especially little is known about this matter in children. In fact, with respect to lipids, Armstrong and Simons-Morton (1994) could find no empirical dose-response data on adolescents at all. The same can be said about visceral adipose tissue. We might hypothesize that if higher intensity physical training results in greater improvements in cardiovascular fitness (Savage et al., 1986) or greater losses of fat for the reasons suggested above, then it may eventually result in greater changes in associated CAD/NIDDM risk factors. In terms of volume of exercise needed, it is logical, but not yet definitely demonstrated, that greater amounts of activity and associated energy expenditure (e.g., 2 h/d vs. 1 h/d in an after-school program, or 12 mo vs 2 mo of physical training) are more likely to reduce body fatness than are lesser amounts of activity. It is conceivable that adult guidelines for exercise prescription are inadequate for children. For example, 30 min/d of controlled exercise may not be enough to compensate for the large reductions in activity and fitness brought about by factors such as the reduction of school physical education, the danger of spending time outdoors during non-school hours, and the evolving dominance of sedentary activities such as television, video games, and computers.

In deciding how to alter lifestyle to improve body composition, it is necessary to consider both exercise and diet together. Therefore, efficacy studies of interactions between different training doses and different types of diets are needed to provide a stronger scientific foundation for community interventions. Several lines of evidence support the hypothesis that a combination of exercise and a low-fat (high-carbohydrate) diet may be optimal for reduction of fatness. First, non-experimental studies suggest that high-fat diets and low physical activity are synergistic for the development of obesity. Second, the controlled laboratory studies suggest that exercise plus a high-fat diet do not lead to the expected energy deficit over a 1–2 d period. Also, studies show that higher carbohydrate diets stimulate the thermic effect of food to a greater degree, which is perhaps synergistic with physical activity.

An issue related to the concept of exercise intensity, about which very little is known, is the role of strength training in weight control programs. It does seem clear that resistance training can help youths to improve their muscular strength and endurance (Payne et al., 1997), helping their performance and future participation in sports and dance activities. Since strength training usually involves taking the muscle group close to, or all the way to, momentary failure, it is high in intensity, even though the overall energy expended may not be as high as in aerobic training sessions. The high intensity of the exercise, and the resulting increases in muscle (i.e., lean) tissue, lead to favorable changes in body composition. Moreover, the intense muscular activity may enhance insulin action and improve CAD/NIDDM risk status, independent of body fatness or cardiovascular fitness (Hurley et al., 1988).

Relatively little is known about how gender, ethnicity, and pubertal status interact with exercise and diet to influence body composition and associated CAD/NIDDM risk factors. Such information would help in the design of interventions targeted to the appropriate groups and outcome variables.

SUMMARY

It is clear that already in young children, excess body fatness, especially visceral adipose tissue, is linked to unfavorable levels of preclinical markers for "adult" diseases such as CAD and NIDDM. Data from cross-sectional and non-experimental longitudinal studies suggest that exercise and fitness during childhood have favorable effects on these preclinical markers, with much of the effect mediated by the influence of exercise on body composition. However, randomized trials of controlled physical training over periods up to 4 mo have produced mixed results, with many failing to provide evidence of favorable changes in these preclinical markers.

One way to reconcile these somewhat discrepant results is to postulate that the non-experimental studies allow the uncovering of cause-effect relations that emerge after several years of exposure to the detrimental effects of inactivity or excess fatness, while short-term experimental studies do not produce an increase in activity over a long enough period for favorable changes in the preclinical markers to take place. This concept is supported by the few controlled intervention studies that were carried out over relatively long periods of 8 mo to 2 y (Hansen et al., 1991; Sasaki et al., 1987). The other possibility is that exercise has a limited or negligible causal effect on preclinical markers during childhood (Rowland, 1996) and the relations found in the non-experimental studies are due to the common influence of some other factor, such as a genetic predisposition to be both active/fit and to have favorable levels of the markers. Longer-term experimental studies are needed to clarify the true impact of exercise.

With respect to the etiology and treatment of obesity, it is likely that exercise acts synergistically with low-fat diets to prevent obesity and to treat it effectively. Controlled interventions that have included both of these factors have generally been more successful than either alone. This may be because the low-fat and low-energy diets immediately lead to a substantial energy deficit, while the exercise adds somewhat to the energy deficit, preserves fat-free mass, and facilitates long-term retention of the weight loss. Although it is clear that visceral adipose tissue is associated with the CAD/NIDDM risk syndrome starting in childhood, almost nothing is known about its etiology or the degree to which exercise or diet can influence it during childhood.

The secular trend toward greater obesity over the last two decades (Troiano et al., 1995) suggests that past public health efforts to improve activity and diet behaviors have been overcome by societal trends toward less activity and/or greater intake of high-fat foods. To date, programs that have taken a public health approach in school and community settings have had only modest success in altering diet, exercise, and preclinical markers of adult diseases. However, the recent report of the Surgeon General (USDHHS, 1996) shows that the scientific evidence linking physical activity to health is convincing. Perhaps this increasing recognition of the importance of physical activity will energize funding agencies to sponsor more research on these topics, providing an improved foundation for the development of more effective interventions. In the meanwhile, there is enough known to encourage parents, health professionals, teachers, and legislatures to implement measures that may increase physical activity of our children, thereby contributing to their present and future health.

BIBLIOGRAPHY

Aaron, D.J., and R.E. Laporte (1997). Physical activity, adolescence, and health: an epidemiological perspective. In J. Holloszy (ed.) *Exercise and Sport Sciences Reviews Vol. 25.* Baltimore: Williams & Wilkins, pp. 391–405.

Akinci, A., A. Celiker, E. Baykal, and T. Tezuc (1993). Heart rate variability in diabetic children: Sensitivity of the time- and frequency-domain methods. *Pediatr. Cardiol.* 14:140–146.

Algra, A., J. Tijssen, J. Roelandt, and J. Pool (1993). Heart rate variability from 24-hour electrocardiography and the 2-year risk for sudden death. *Circulation* 88:180–185.

Alpert, B.S., and J.H. Wilmore (1994). Physical activity and blood pressure in adolescents. *Ped. Exerc. Sci.* 6:361–380.

Arbeit M.L., C.C. Johnson, D.S. Mott, D.W. Harsha, T.A. Nicklas, L.S. Webber and G.S. Berenson (1992). The Heart Smart Cardiovascular School Health Promotion: behavior correlates of risk factor change. *Prev. Med.* 21:18–32.

Armstrong, N., and B. Simons-Morton (1994). Physical activity and blood lipids in adolescents. *Ped. Exerc. Sci.* 6:381–405.

Asayama K., H. Hayashibe, K. Dobashi, Y. Kawada, and S. Nakazawa (1995). Relationships between biochemical abnormalities and anthropometric indices of overweight, adiposity and body fat distribution in Japanese elementary school children. *Int. J. Obes.* 19:253–259.

Ballor, D.L., and E.T. Poehlman (1994). Exercise-training enhances fat-free mass preservation during diet-induced weight loss: a meta-analytical finding. *Int. J. Obes.* 18:35–40.

Bandini, L., D. Schoeller, H. Cyr, and W. Dietz (1990). Validity of reported energy intake in obese and nonobese adolescents. *Am. J. Clin. Nutr.* 52:421–425.

Bao, W., S.R. Srinivasan, and G.S. Berenson (1993). Plasma fibrinogen and its correlates in children from a biracial community: The Bogalusa Heart Study. *Fibrinolysis* 2:211–214.

Bar-Or, O., and T. Baranowski (1994). Physical activity, adiposity, and obesity among adolescents. *Pediatr. Exerc. Sci.* 6:348–360.

Becque, M., V. Katch, A. Rocchini, C. Marks, and C. Moorehead (1988). Coronary risk incidence of obese adolescents: reduction by exercise plus diet interventions. *Pediatrics* 81:605–612.

Blaak, E.E., K.R. Westerterp, O. Bar-Or, L.J.M. Wouters, and W.H.M. Saris (1992). Total energy expenditure and spontaneous activity in relation to training in obese boys. *Am. J. Clin. Nutr.* 55:777–782.

Bouchard, C. (1994). Genetics of obesity: overview and research directions. In: C. Bouchard (ed.) *The Genetics of Obesity*. Boca Raton:CRC Press, pp. 223–233.

Bougnères, P., C. Le Stunff, C. Pecqueur, E. Pinglier, P. Adnot, and D. Ricquier (1997). In vivo resistance to lipolysis to epinephrine. *J. Clin. Invest.* 99:2568–2573.

Boreham, C.A., J. Twisk, M.J. Savage, G.W. Cran, and J.J. Strain (1997). Physical activity, sports participation, and risk factors in adolescents. *Med. Sci. Sports Exerc.* 29:788–793.

Brambilla, P., P. Manzoni, S. Sironi, P. Simone, A. Del Maschio, B. di Natale, and G. Chiumello (1994). Peripheral and abdominal adiposity in childhood obesity. *Int. J. Obes.* 18:795–800.

Brehm, B.A., and B. Gutin (1986). Recovery energy expenditure for steady state exercise in runners and nonexercisers. *Med. Sci. Sports Exerc.* 18:205–210.

Broeder, C.E., M. Brenner, Z. Hofman, J.M. Paijmans, E.L. Thomas, and J.H. Wilmore (1991). The metabolic consequences of low and moderate intensity exercise with or without feeding in lean and borderline obese males. *Int. J. Obes.* 15:95–104.

Caprio, S., L.D. Hyman, S. McCarthy, R. Lange, M. Bronson, and W.V. Tamborlane (1996a). Fat distribution and cardiovascular risk factors in obese adolescent girls: importance of the intraabdominal fat depot. *Am J. Clin. Nutr.* 64:12–17.

Caprio, S., W.V. Tamborlane, D. Silver, C. Robinson, R. Leibel, S. McCarthy, A. Grozman, A. Belous, D. Maggs, and R.S. Sherwin (1996b). Hyperleptinemia: an early sign of juvenile obesity. Relations to body fat depots and insulin concentrations. *Am. J. Physiol.* 271:E626–E630.

Celermajer, D.S. (1997). Endothelial dysfunction: Does it matter? Is it reversible? *J. Am. Coll. Cardiol.* 30:325–333.

Chesnut, C.H. (1989). Is osteoporosis a pediatric disease? Peak bone mass attainment in the adolescent female. *Pub. Health Rep.* Sept-Oct:50–54.

Chitwood, L.F, S.P. Brown, M.J. Lundy, and M.A. Dupper (1996). Metabolic propensity toward obesity in black vs white females: responses during rest, exercise and recovery. *Int. J. Obes.* 20:455–462.

Cigolini M., G. Targher, I.A. Bergamo Andreis , M. Tonoli , G. Agostino, and G. De Sandre (1996). Visceral fat accumulation and its relation to plasma hemostatic factors in healthy men. *Arterioscler. Thromb. Vasc. Biol.* 16:368–374.

Conway, J.M., S.Z. Yanovski, N.A. Avila, and V.S. Hubbard (1995). Visceral adipose tissue differences in black and white women. *Am. J. Clin. Nutr.* 61:765–771.

Cowie, C., M. Harris, R. Silverman, E. Johnson, and K. Rust (1993). Effect of multiple risk factors on differences between blacks and whites in the prevalence of non-insulin-dependent diabetes mellitus in the United States. *Am. J. Epidemiol.* 137:719–732.

Craig, S.B., L.G. Bandini, A.H. Lichtenstein, E.J. Schaefer, and W.H. Dietz (1996). The impact of physical activity on lipids, lipoproteins, and blood pressure in preadolescent girls. *Pediatrics* 98:389–395.

Cummings, S.R., D.M. Black, M.C. Nevitt, W.S. Browner, J.A. Cauley, H.K. Genant, S.R. Mascioli, J.C. Scott, D.G. Seeley, P. Steiger and T.M. Vogt (1990). Appendicular bone density and age predict hip fracture in women. *JAMA* 263:665–668.

Davies, P., J. Gregory, and A. White (1995a). Physical activity and body fatness in pre-school children. *Int. J. Obes.* 19:6–11.

Davies, P.S., J.C. Wells, C.A. Fieldhouse, J.M. Day, and A. Lucas (1995b). Parental body composition and infant energy expenditure. *Am. J. Clin. Nutr.* 61:1026–1029.

Deheeger, M., M.F. Rolland-Cachera, and A.M. Fontvieille (1997). Physical activity and body composition in 10 year old French children: linkages with nutritional intake. *Int. J. Obes.* 21:372–379.

DeLany, J.P., D.W. Harsha, J. Kime, J. Kumler, L. Melancon, and G.A. Bray (1996). Energy expenditure in lean and obese pre-pubertal children. *Obes. Res.* 3:S67–S72.

Després, J-P. (1997). Visceral obesity, insulin resistance, and dyslipidemia: contribution of endurance exercise training to the treatment of the plurimetabolic syndrome. In J. Holloszy (ed.) *Exercise and Sports Sciences Reviews, Vol 25*. Baltimore: Williams & Wilkins, pp. 271–300.

Devereux, R., F. de Simone, A. Ganau, M. Roman (1994). Left ventricular hypertrophy and geometric remodeling in hypertension: stimuli, functional consequences and prognostic implications. *J. Hypertens.* 12:S117–S127.

Donnelly, J.E., D.J. Jacobsen, J.E. Whatley, J.O. Hill, L.L. Swift, A. Cherrington, B. Polk, Z. Tran, and G. Reed (1996). Nutrition and physical activity program to attenuate obesity and promote physical and metabolic fitness in elementary school children. *Obes. Res.* 4:229–243.

Eck, L.H., R.C. Klesges, C.L. Hanson, and D. Slawson (1992). Children at familial risk for obesity: an examination of dietary intake, physical activity and weight status. *Int. J. Obes.* 16:71–78.

Epstein, L.H., K.J. Coleman, M.D. Myers (1996). Exercise in treating obesity in children and adolescents. *Med. Sci. Sports Exerc.* 28:428–435.

Epstein, L.H., A.M. Valoski, M.A. Kalarchian, and J. McCurley (1995a). Do children lose and maintain weight easier than adults: A comparison of child and parent weight changes from six months to ten years. *Obes. Res.* 3:411–417.

Epstein, L.H., A.M. Valoski, L.S. Vara, J. McCurley, L. Wisniewski, M.A. Kalarchian, K.R. Klein, and L.R. Shrager (1995b). Effects of decreasing sedentary behavior and increasing activity on weight change in obese children. *Health Psych.* 2:109–115.

Ferguson, M.A., B. Gutin, S. Owens, M. Litaker, R. Tracy, and J. Allison (1998). Fat distribution and hemostatic measures in obese children. *Am. J. Clin. Nutr.* (in press).

Fontvieille, A.M., J. Dwyer, and E. Ravussin (1992). Resting metabolic rate and body composition of Pima Indian and Caucasian children. *Int. J. Obes.* 16:535–542.

Foster, G.D., T.A. Wadden, and R.A. Vogt (1997). Resting energy expenditure in obese African American and Caucasian women. *Obes. Res.* 5:1–8.

Fox, K., D. Peters, N. Armstrong, P. Sharpe, and M. Bell (1993). Abdominal fat deposition in 11–year-old children. *Int. J. Obes.* 17:11–16.

Freedman, D.S. (1995). The importance of body fat distribution in early life. *Am. J. Med. Sci.* 310:S72–S76.

Gazzaniga, J.M., and T.L. Burns (1993). Relationship between diet composition and body fatness, with adjustment for resting energy expenditure and physical activity, in prepubescent children. *Am. J. Clin. Nutr.* 58:21–28.

Goran, M.I. (1997). Nutrition Society Medal Lecture: Energy expenditure, body composition, and disease risk in children and adolescents. *Proceedings of the Nutrition Society* 56:1–16.

Goran, M.I., and E.T. Poehlman (1992). Endurance training does not enhance total energy expenditure in healthy elderly persons. *Am. J. Physiol.* 263:E950–E957.

Goran, M.I., M.H. Carpenter, A. McGloin, R. Johnson, J.M. Hardin, R.L. Weinsier (1995a). Energy expenditure in children of lean and obese parents. *Am. J. Physiol.* 268:E917–E924.

Goran, M.I., G. Hunter, and R. Johnson (1996). Physical activity related energy expenditure and fat mass in young children. *Int. J. Obes.* 20:1–8.

Goran, M.I., M. Kaskoun, and W.P. Shuman (1995b). Intra-abdominal adipose tissue in young children. *Int. J. Obes.* 19:279–283.

Goran, M.I., T.R. Nagy, M.S. Treuth, C. Trowbridge, C. Dezenberg, A. McGloin, and B.A. Gower (1997). Visceral fat in white and African American prepubertal children. *Am. J. Clin. Nutr.* 65:1703–1708.

Goran, M.I., R. Shewchuk, B.A. Gower, T.R. Nagy, W.H. Carpenter, and R. Johnson (1998). Longitudinal changes in fatness in Caucasian children: no effect of childhood energy expenditure. *Am. J. Clin. Nutr.* 67:309–16.

Gortmaker, S.L., A. Must, A.M. Sobol, K. Peterson, G.A. Colditz, and W.H. Dietz (1996). Television viewing as a cause of increasing obesity among children in the United States, 1986–1990. *Arch. Pediatr. Adolesc. Med.* 150:356–362.

Griffiths, M., and P.R. Payne (1976). Energy expenditure in small children of obese and non-obese parents. *Nature* 260:698–700.

Griffiths, M., P.R. Payne, A.J. Stunkard, J.P.W. Rivers, and M. Cox (1990). Metabolic rate and physical development in children at risk of obesity. *Lancet* 336:76–78.

Gutin, B., and M.J. Kasper (1992). Can vigorous exercise play a role in osteoporosis prevention? a review. *Osteoporosis Int.* 2:55–69.

Gutin, B., and S. Owens (1996). Is there a scientific rationale supporting the value of exercise for the present and future cardiovascular health of children? *Ped. Exerc. Sci.* 8:294–302.

Gutin, B., C. Basch, S. Shea, I. Contento, M. DeLozier, J. Rips, M. Irgoyen, and P. Zybert (1990). Blood pressure, fitness, and fatness in 5– and 6–year-old children. *JAMA* 264:1123–1127.

Gutin, B., N. Cucuzzo, S. Islam, C. Smith, R. Moffatt, and D. Pargman (1995). Physical training improves body composition of black obese 7– to 11–year-old girls. *Obes. Res.* 3:305–312.

Gutin, B., N. Cucuzzo, S. Islam, C. Smith, and M.E. Stachura (1996a). Physical training, lifestyle education, and coronary risk factors in obese girls. *Med. Sci. Sports Exerc.* 28:19–23.

Gutin, B., S. Islam, T. Manos, N. Cucuzzo, C. Smith, and M. Stachura (1994). Relation of percentage of body fat and maximal aerobic capacity to risk factors for atherosclerosis and diabetes in black and white seven-to eleven-year-old children. *J. Pediatr.* 125:847–852.

Gutin, B., M. Litaker, S. Islam, T. Manos, C. Smith, and F. Treiber (1996b). Body composition measurement in 9–11-y-old children by dual-energy X-ray absorptiometry, skinfold-thickness measurements, and bioimpedance analysis. *Am. J. Clin. Nutr.* 63:287–292.

Gutin, B., N. Mayers, J. Levy, and M. Herman (1988). Physiologic and echocardiographic studies of age-group runners. In: E. Brown and C. Branta (eds.) *Competitive Sports for Children and Youths*. Champaign: Human Kinetics, pp. 117–128.
Gutin, B., S. Owens, S. Riggs, M. Ferguson, S. Moorehead, F. Treiber, W. Karp, W. Thompson, J. Allison, M. Litaker, K. Murdison, and N-A. Lee (1997a). Effect of physical training on cardiovascular health in obese children. In N. Armstrong, B. Kirby, and J. Wellsman (eds.) *Children and Exercise XIX*. London: E & FN Spon, pp. 382–389.
Gutin, B., S. Owens, G. Slavens, S. Riggs, and F. Treiber (1997b). Effect of physical training on heart period variability in obese children. *J. Pediatr.* 130:938–943.
Gutin, B., S. Owens, F. Treiber, S. Islam, W. Karp, and G. Slavens (1997c). Weight-independent cardiovascular fitness and coronary risk factors. *Arch. Pediatr. Adol. Med.* 151:462–465.
Gutin, B., S. Owens, F. Treiber, S. Riggs, and S. Islam (submitted). Cardiovascular fitness is associated with higher levels of total bone density in children.
Gutin, B., F. Treiber, S. Owens, G. Mensah (1998). Relations of body composition to left ventricular geometry and function in children. *J. Pediatr.* (in press).
Hansen, H., K. Froberg, N. Hyldebrandt, and J. Nielson (1991). A controlled study of eight months of physical training and reduction of blood pressure in children: the Odense schoolchild study. *Int. J. Obes.* 18:795–800.
Herring, J.L., P.A. Mole, C.N. Meredith, and J.S. Stern (1992). Effect of suspending exercise training on resting metabolic rate in women. *Med. Sci. Sports Exerc.* 24:59–65.
Hofman, A., and H.J. Walter (1989). The association between physical fitness and cardiovascular risk factors in children in a five-year follow-up study. *Int. J. Epidemiol.* 18:830–835.
Horswill, C.A., W.B. Zipf, C.L. Kien, and E.B. Kahle (1997). Insulin's contribution to growth in children and the potential for exercise to mediate insulin's action. *Ped. Exerc. Sci.* 9:18–32.
Hunter, G.R., T. Kekes-Szabo, S.W. Snyder, C. Nicholson, I. Nyikos, and L. Berland (1997). Fat distribution, physical activity, and cardiovascular risk factors. *Med. Sci. Sports Exerc.* 29:362–369.
Hull, S.S., E. Vanoli, P.B. Adamson, R.L. Verrier, R.D. Foreman, and P.J. Schwartz (1994). Exercise training confers anticipatory protection from sudden death during acute myocardial ischemia. *Circulation* 89:548–552.
Hurley, B.F., J.M. Hagberg, A.P. Goldberg, D.R. Seals, A.A. Ehsani, R.E. Brennan, and J.O. Holloszy (1988). Resistive training can reduce coronary risk factors without altering VO2max or percent body fat. *Med. Sci. Sports Exerc.* 20:150–154.
James, W.P.T. (1996). Chapter discussion. In: D.J. Chadwick and G. Cardew (eds.) *The Origins and Consequences of Obesity*. Chichester: Wiley, pp. 252–253.
Janz, K.F., and L.T. Mahoney (1997). Three-year follow-up of changes in aerobic fitness during puberty: the Muscatine study. *Res. Quart. Exerc. Sport* 68:1–9.
Javorka, K., J. Buchaned, J. Javorkova, M. Zibolen, and M. Minarik (1988). Heart rate and its variability in juvenile hypertronics during respiratory maneuvers. *Clin. Exp. Hyper.-Theory & Practice* 10:391–409.
Jones, P., and S. Leatherdale (1991). Stable isotopes in clinical research: safety reaffirmed. *Clin. Sci.* 80:277–280.
Kannel W.B., P.A. Wolf, W.P. Castelli, and R.B. D'Agostino (1987). Fibrinogen and risk of cardiovascular disease: the Framingham Study. *JAMA* 258:1183–1186.
Kaplan, A.S., B.S. Zemel, and V.A. Stallings (1996). Differences in resting energy expenditure in prepubertal black children and white children. *J. Pediatr.* 129:643–647.
Kempen, K.P.G., W.H.M. Saris, and K.R. Westerterp (1995). Energy balance during an 8–wk energy-restricted diet with and without exercise in obese women. *Am. J. Clin. Nutr.* 62:722–729.
Kemper, H., and W. van Mechelen (1995). Physical fitness and the relationship to physical activity. In: H Kemper (ed.) *The Amsterdam Growth Study*. Champaign: Human Kinetics, pp. 174–188.
King, N.A., and J.E. Blundell (1995). High-fat foods overcome the energy expenditure induced by high-intensity cycling or running. *Europ. J. Clin. Nutr.* 49:114–123.
King, N.A., V.J. Burley, and J.E. Blundell (1994). Exercise-induced suppression of appetite: effects on food intake and implications for energy balance. *Europ. J. Clin. Nutr.* 48:715–724.
Klesges, R.C., L.M. Klesges, L.H. Eck, and M.L. Shelton (1995). A longitudinal analysis of accelerated weight gain in preschool children. *Pediatrics* 95:126–130.
Knip, M., and O. Nuutinen (1993). Long-term effects of weight reduction on serum lipids and plasma insulin in obese children. *Am. J. Clin. Nutr.* 57:490–493.
Kumanyika, S. (1993). Ethnicity and obesity development in children. *Ann. NY Acad. Sci.* 699:81–92.
Kuntzleman, C.T. (1993). Childhood fitness: what is happening? What needs to be done? *Prev. Med.* 22:520–532.
Kwiterovich, P.O. (1993). Prevention of coronary disease starting in childhood: what risk factors should be identified and treated? *Coronary Artery Dis.* 4:611–630.
Lahlou, N., P. Landais, D. De Boissieu, and P-E. Bougnères (1997). Circulating leptin in normal children and during the dynamic phase of juvenile obesity: relation to body fatness, energy metabolism, caloric intake, and sexual dimorphism. *Diabetes* 46:989–993.

Legnani C., M. Maccaferri, P. Tonini, A. Cassio, E. Cacciari, and S. Coccheri (1988). Reduced fibrinolytic response in obese children: association with high baseline activity of the fast acting plasminogen activator inhibitor (PAI-1). *Fibrinolysis* 2:211–214.

Le Stunff, C. and P.F. Bougnères (1993). Time course of increased lipid and decreased glucose oxidation during early phase of childhood obesity. *Diabetes* 42:1010–1016.

Lissner, L., B.L. Heitman, and C. Bengtsson (1997). Low-fat diets may prevent weight gain in sedentary women: prospective observations from the population study of women in Gothenburg, Sweden. *Obes. Res.* 5:43–48.

Luepker, R.V., C.L. Perry, S.M. McKinlay, P.R. Nader, G.S. Parcel, E.J. Stone, L.S. Webber, J.P. Elder, H.A. Feldman, C.C. Johnson, S.H. Kelder, and M.W. Wu (1996). Outcomes of a field trial to improve children's dietary patterns and physical activity. *JAMA* 275:768–776.

Maffeis, C., L. Pinelli, and Y. Schutz (1996). Fat intake and adiposity in 8 to 11–year-old children. *Int. J. Obes.* 20:170–174.

Maffeis, C., Y. Schutz, R. Micciolo, L. Zoccante, and L. Pinelli (1993). Resting metabolic rate in six- to ten-year-old obese and nonobese children. *J. Pediatr.* 122:556–562.

Maffeis, C., Y. Schutz, and L. Pinelli (1992). Effect of weight loss on resting energy expenditure in obese prepubertal children. *Int. J. Obes.* 16:41–47.

Mahon, A.D., and P. Vaccaro (1989). Ventilatory threshold and VO$_2$max changes in children following endurance training. *Med. Sci. Sports Exerc.* 21:425–431.

Massicotte, D.R., and R.B.J. Macnab (1974). Cardiorespiratory adaptations to training at specified intensities in children. *Med. Sci. Sports* 6:242–246.

Mayers, N., and B. Gutin (1979). Physiological characteristics of elite pre-pubertal cross country runners. *Med. Sci. Sports* 11:172–176.

McMurray, R.G., J.S. Harrell, A.A. Levine, and S.A. Gansky (1995). Childhood obesity elevates blood pressure and total cholesterol independent of physical activity. *Int. J. Obes.* 19:881–886.

Meilahn E.N., J.A. Cauley, R.P. Tracy, E.O. Macy, J.P. Gutai, and L.H. Kuller (1996). Association of sex hormones and adiposity with plasma concentrations of fibrinogen and PAI-1 in postmenopausal women. *Am. J. Epidemiol.* 143:159–166.

Meredith, I.T., A.C. Yeung, and F.F. Weidinger (1993). Role of impaired endothelium-dependent vasodilation in ischemic manifestations of coronary artery disease. *Circulation* 87:56–66.

Messerli, F.H., and Ketelhut (1993). Left ventricular hypertrophy: a pressure-independent cardiovascular risk factor. *J. Cardiovas. Pharmacol.* 22:S7–S13.

Miller, W.C., A.K. Linderman, J. Wallace, and M. Niederpruem (1990). Diet composition, energy intake, and exercise in relation to body fat in men and women. *Am. J. Clin. Nutr.* 52:426–430.

Montoye, H., H. Kemper, W. Saris, and R. Washburn (1996). *Measuring Physical Activity and Energy Expenditure.* Champaign: Human Kinetics, pp. 17–25.

Moore, L.L., U.D.T. Nguyen, K.J. Rothman, L.A. Cupples, and R. C. Ellison (1995). Preschool physical activity level and change in body fatness in young children. *Am. J. Epidemiol.* 142:982–988.

Morrison, J.A., M.P. Alfaro, P. Khoury, B.B. Thornton, and S.R. Daniels (1996). Determinants of resting energy expenditure in young black girls and young white girls. *J. Pediatr.* 129:637–642.

Mo-suwan, L., and A.F. Geater (1996). Risk factors for childhood obesity in a transitional society in Thailand. *Int. J. Obes.* 20:697–703.

Muecke, L., B. Simons-Morton, I.W. Huang, and G. Parcel (1992). Is childhood obesity associated with high-fat foods and low physical activity. *J. Sch. Health* 62:19–23.

Nagy, T.M., B.A. Gower, C.A. Trowbridge, C. Dezenberg, R. M. Shewchuk, and M.I. Goran (1997). Effects of gender, ethnicity, body composition, and fat distribution on serum leptin concentrations in children. *J. Clin. Endocrinol. Metab.* 82:2148–2152.

Nguyen, V.T., D.E. Larson, R.K. Johnson, and M.I. Goran (1996). Fat intake and adiposity in children of lean and obese parents. *Am. J. Clin Nutr.* 63:507–513.

Obarzanek, E., G. Schrieber, P. Crawford, S. Goldman, P. Barrier, M. Frederick, and E. Lakatos (1994). Energy intake and physical activity in relation to indexes of body fat: the National Heart, Lung, and Blood Institute Growth and Health Study. *Am. J. Clin. Nutr.* 60:15–22.

Oscai, L (1989). Exercise and obesity: emphasis on animal models. In C. Gisolfi and D. Lamb (eds.) *Perspectives In Exercise Science and Sports Medicine Vol 2: Youth, Exercise and Sport.* Indianapolis: Benchmark Press, pp. 273–292.

Owens, S., B. Gutin, J. Allison, S. Riggs, M. Ferguson, M. Litaker, and W. Thompson (1998). Effect of physical training on total and visceral fat in obese children. *Med. Sci. Sports Exerc.* (in press).

Owens, S., B. Gutin, W. Karp, M. Ferguson, S. Moorhead, and J. Allison (1997). Relationship of total and visceral adipose tissue to cardiovascular health. In: N. Armstrong, B. Kirby, and J. Wellsman (eds.) *Children and Exercise XIX.* London: E&FN Spon, pp. 373–381.

Palgi, Y. B. Gutin, J. Young, and D. Alejandro (1984). Physiologic and anthropometric factors underlying endurance performance in children. *Int. J. Sports Med.* 5:67–73.

Panchenko E., A. Dobrovolsky, K. Davletov, E. Titaeva, A. Kravets, J. Podinovskaya, and Y. Karpov (1995). D-Dimer and fibrinolysis in patients with various degrees of atherosclerosis. *Eur. Heart J.* 16:38–42.

Pate, R., and D. Ward (1990). Endurance exercise trainability in children and youth. In: W. Grana (ed.) *Advances in Sports Medicine and Fitness Vol 3*. Chicago: Yearbook Medical, pp. 37–55.

Pate, R.R., B.J. Long, and G. Heath (1994). Descriptive epidemiology of physical activity in adolescents. *Pediatr. Exerc. Sci.* 6:434–447.

Payne, V.G., and J.R. Morrow (1993). The effect of physical training on prepubescent VO₂max: a meta-analysis. *Res. Q. Exerc. Sport* 64:305–313.

Payne, V.G., J.R. Morrow, L. Johnson, and S.N. Dalton (1997). Resistance training in children and youth: a meta-analysis. *Res. Quart. Exerc. Sport* 68:80–88.

Pi-Sunyer, F (1991). Health implications of obesity. *Am. J. Clin. Nutr.* 53:1595S-603S.

Pinhas-Hamiel, O., L.M. Dolan, S.R. Daniels, D. Standford, P.R. Khoury, and P. Zeitler (1996). Increased incidence of non-insulin-dependent diabetes mellitus among adolescents. *J. Pediatr.* 128:608–615.

Pivarnik, J.M., M.S. Bray, A.C. Hergenroeder, R.B. Hill, and W.W. Wong (1995). Ethnicity affects aerobic fitness in U.S. adolescent girls. *Med. Sci. Sports Exerc.* 27:1635–1638.

Poehlman, E.T., C.L. Melby, and M.I. Goran (1991). The impact of exercise and diet restriction on daily energy expenditure. *Sports Med.* 11:78–101.

Prentice, A.M., G.R. Goldberg, P.R. Murgatroyd, and T.J. Cole (1996). Physical activity and obesity:problems in correcting expenditure for body size. *Int. J. Obes.* 20:688–691.

Racette, S.B., D.A. Schoeller, R.F. Kushner, and K.M. Neil (1995a). Exercise enhances dietary compliance during moderate energy restriction in obese women. *Am. J. Clin. Nutr.* 62:345–349.

Racette, S.B., D.A. Schoeller, R.F. Kushner, K.M. Neil, and K. Herling-Iaffaldano (1995b). Effects of aerobic exercise and dietary carbohydrate on energy expenditure and body composition during weight reduction in obese women. *Am. J. Clin. Nutr.* 61:486–494.

Ravussin, E., and B.A. Swinburn (1992). Pathophysiology of obesity. *Lancet* 340:404–408.

Ravussin, E., S. Lillioja, W.C. Knowler, L. Christin, D. Freymond, W.G.H. Abbott, V. Boyce, B.V. Howard, and C. Bogardus (1988). Reduced rate of energy expenditure as a risk factor for body-weight gain. *New. Engl. J. Med.* 318:467–472.

Reaven, G. (1988). Role of insulin resistance in human disease. *Diabetes* 37:1595–1607.

Reaven, G.M., H. Ho, and B.B. Hoffman (1988). Attenuation of fructose-induced hypertension in rats by exercise training. *Hypertension* 12:129–132.

Reynolds, K., J. Killen, S. Beyson, D. Maron, C. Taylor, N. Maccoby, and J. Farquhar (1990). Psychosocial predictors of physical activity in adolescents. *Prev. Med.* 19:541–551.

Rice, S., C.J.R. Blimkie, C.E. Webber, D. Levy, J. Martin, D. Parker, and C.L. Gordon (1993). Correlates and determinants of bone mineral content and density in healthy adolescent girls. *Can. J. Physiol. Pharmacol.* 71:923:930.

Roberts, S., J. Savage, W. Coward, B. Chew, and A. Lucus (1988). Energy expenditure and intake in infants born to lean and overweight mothers. *N. Eng. J. Med.* 318:461–466.

Rocchini, A., V. Katch, A. Schork, and R. Kelch (1987). Insulin and blood pressure during weight loss in obese adolescents. *Hypertens.* 10:267–273.

Rollins, M., J. Jenkins, D. Carson, B. McClure, R. Mitchell, and S. Imam (1992). Power spectral analysis of the electrocardiogram in diabetic children. *Diabetologia* 35:452–455.

Ross, R., and J. Rissanen (1994). Mobilization of visceral and subcutaneous adipose tissue in response to energy restriction and exercise. *Am. J. Clin. Nutr.* 60:695–703.

Rowland, T. (1996). Is there a scientific rationale supporting the value of exercise for the present and future cardiovascular health of children? The con argument. *Ped. Exerc. Sci.* 8:303–309.

Rowland, T.W., V.B. Unnithan, N.G. MacFarlane, N.G. Gibson, and J.Y. Paton (1994). Clinical manifestations of the 'athletes heart' in prepubertal male runners. *Int. J. Sports Med.* 15:515–519.

Salbe, A.D., M. Nicolson, and E. Ravussin (1997). Total energy expenditure and the level of physical activity correlate with plasma leptin concentrations in five-year-old children. *J. Clin. Invest.* 99:592–595.

Sallis, J.F., B.G. Simons-Morton, E.J. Stone, C.B. Corbin, L.H. Epstein, N. Faucette, R.J. Iannotti, J.D. Killen, R.C. Klesges, C.K. Petray, T.W. Rowland, and W.C. Taylor (1996). Determinants of physical activity and interventions in youth. *Med. Sci. Sports Exerc.* 24:S248–S257.

Sallo, M., and R. Silla (1997). Physical activity with moderate to vigorous intensity in preschool and first-grade school children. *Ped. Exerc. Sci.* 9:44–54.

Saris, W. H. (1995). Effects of energy restriction and exercise on the sympathetic nervous system. *Int. J. Obes.* 19:S17–23.

Sasaki, J., M. Shindo, H. Tanaka, M. Ando, and K. Arakawa (1987). A long-term aerobic exercise program decreases the obesity index and increases the high density lipoprotein cholesterol concentration in obese children. *Int. J. Obes.* 11:339–345.

Sasson, Z., Y. Rasooly, T. Bhesania, and I. Rasooly (1993). Insulin resistance is an important determinant of left ventricular mass in the obese. *Circulation* 88:1431–1436.

Savage, M.P., M.M. Petratis, W.H. Thomson, K. Berg, J.L. Smith, and S.P. Sady (1986). Exercise training effects on serum lipids of prepubescent boys and adult men. *Med. Sci. Sports Exerc.* 18:197–204.

Schneider D.J., and B.E. Sobel (1991). Augmentation of synthesis of plasminogen activator inhibitor type-1 by insulin and insulin-like growth factor type-1: implications for vascular disease in hyperinsulinemic states. *Proc. Natl. Acad. Sci. USA* 88:9959–9963.

Schoeller, D., L. Bandini, and W. Dietz (1990). Inaccuracies in self-reported intake identified by comparison with the doubly labeled water method. *Can. J. Physiol. Pharmacol.* 68:941–949.

Schwartz, R.S., W.P. Shuman, V. Larson, K.C. Cain, G.W. Fellingham, J.C. Beard, S.E. Kahn, J.R. Stratton, M.D. Cerqueira, and I.B. Abrass (1991). The effect of intensive endurance exercise training on body fat distribution in young and older men. *Metabolism* 5:545–551.

Schwingshandl J., and M. Borkenstein (1995). Changes in lean body mass in obese children during a weight reduction program: effect on short term and long term outcome. *Int. J. Obes.* 19:752–755.

Segal, K., and B. Gutin (1983). Thermic effects of food and exercise in lean and obese women. *Metabolism* 32:581–589.

Segal, K., B. Gutin, J. Albu, and F. Pi-Sunyer (1987). Thermic effects of food and exercise in lean and obese men of similar lean body mass. *Am. J. Physiol.* 252:E110–E117.

Shea, S., C. Basch, B. Gutin, A. Stein, I. Contento, M. Irigoyen, and P. Zybert (1994). The rate of increase in blood pressure in children 5 years of age is related to changes in aerobic fitness and body mass index. *Pediatrics* 94:456–470.

Shimomura I., T. Funahashi, M. Takahashi, K. Maeda, K. Kotani, T. Nakamura, S. Yamashita, M. Miura, Y. Fukuda, K. Takemura K. Tokunaga, and Y. Matsuzawa (1996). Enhanced expression of PAI-1 in visceral fat: possible contributor to vascular disease in obesity. *Nat. Med.* 2:800–803.

deSimone, G., R.B. Devereux, G.F. Mureddu, M.J. Roman, A. Ganau, M.H. Alderman, F. Contaldo, and J.H. Laragh (1996). Influence of obesity on left ventricular midwall mechanics in arterial hypertension. *Hypertension* 28:276–283.

Sniderman, A., S. Shapiro, D. Marpole, B. Skinner, B. Teng, and P. Kwiterovich (1980). Association of coronary atherosclerosis with hyperapobetalipoproteinemia [increased protein but normal cholesterol levels in human plasma low density (beta) lipoproteins]. *Proc. National Acad. Sciences* 77:604–608.

Stampfer, M.J., R.M. Krauss, J. Ma, P.J. Blanche, L.G. Holl, F.M. Sacks, and C.H. Hennekens (1996). A prospective study of triglyceride level, low-density lipoprotein particle diameter, and risk of myocardial infarction. *JAMA* 276:882–888.

Stewart, K., and B. Gutin (1976). Effects of physical training on cardiorespiratory fitness in children. *Res. Quart.* 47:110–120.

Stubbs, R.J., P. Ritz, W.A. Coward, and A.M. Prentice (1995). Covert manipulation of the ratio of dietary fat to carbohydrate and energy density: effect of food intake and energy balance in free living men eating ad libitum. *Am. J. Clin. Nutr.* 62:330–337.

Suter, E., and Hawes, M. (1993). Relationship of physical activity, body fat, diet, and blood lipid profile in youths 10–15 yr. *Med. Sci. Sports Exerc.* 25:748–754.

Tracy, R.E., W.P. Newman, W.A. Wattigney, and G.S. Berenson (1995). Risk factors and atherosclerosis in youth autopsy findings of the Bogalusa Heart Study. *Am. J. Med. Sci.* 310:S37–S41.

Treiber, F., F. McCaffrey, K. Pflieger, W.R. Strong, and H. Davis (1993). Determinants of left ventricular mass in children. *Am. J. Hypertens.* 6:505–513.

Treiber, F., D. Papavassiliou, B. Gutin, D. Malpass, W. Yi, S. Islam, H. Davis, W. Strong (1997). Determinants of endothelium-dependent femoral artery vasodilation in youth. *Psychosom. Med.* 59:376–381.

Tremblay, A., N. Almeras, J. Boer, E.K. Kranenbarg, and J.P. Després (1994a). Diet composition and postexercise energy balance. *Am. J. Clin. Nutr.* 59:975–979.

Tremblay, A., J.P. Després, C. Leblanc, C.L. Craig, B. Ferris, T. Stephens, and C. Bouchard (1990). Effect of intensity of physical activity on body fatness and fat distribution. *Am. J. Clin. Nutr.* 51:153–157.

Tremblay, A., J. Simoneau, and C. Bouchard (1994b). Impact of exercise intensity on body fatness and skeletal muscle metabolism. *Metabolism* 3:814–818.

Troiano, R.P., K.M. Flegal, R.J. Kuczmarski, S.M. Campbell, and C.L. Johnson (1995). Overweight prevalence and trends for children and adolescents - The National Health and Nutrition Examination Surveys, 1963 to 1991. *Arch. Pediatr. Adolesc. Med.* 149:1085–1091.

Trost, S.G., R.R. Pate, M. Dowda, R. Saunders, D.S. Ward, and G. Felton (1996). Gender differences in physical activity and determinants of physical activity in rural fifth grade children. *J. Sch. Health.* 66:145–150.

Trowbridge, C.A., B.A. Gower, T.R. Nagy, G.R. Hunter, M.S. Treuth, and M.I. Goran (1997). Maximal aerobic capacity in African-American and Caucasian prepubertal children. *Am. J. Physiol.* 273:E809–E814.

U.S. Department of Health and Human Services (1996). Physical activity and health: a report from the surgeon general. Atlanta, GA: U.S. Department of Health and Human Services, Centers for Disease Control and Prevention, National Center for Chronic Disease Prevention and Health Promotion.

Vague P., I. Juhan-Vague, V. Chabert, M.C. Alessi, and C. Atlan (1989). Fat distribution and plasminogen activator inhibitor activity in nondiabetic obese women. *Metabolism* 9:913–915.

Webber, L.S., W.A. Wattigney, S.R. Srinivasan, and G.S. Berenson (1995). Obesity studies in Bogalusa. *Am. J. Med. Sci.* 310:S53–S61.

EXERCISE AND HEALTH IN CHILDREN **339**

Wei, M., S.P. Gaskill, S.M. Haffner, and M.P. Stern (1997). Waist circumference as the best predictor of noninsulin-dependent diabetes-mellitus (NIDDM) compared to body-mass index, waist/hip ratio and other anthropometric measurements in Mexican-Americans: a 7 year prospective-study. *Obes. Res.* 5:16–23.

Wells, J.C., M. Stanley, A.S. Laidlaw, J.M. Day, and P.S. Davies (1996). The relationship between components of infant energy expenditure and childhood body fatness. *Int. J. Obes.* 20:848–853.

Williams, B. (1994). Insulin resistance: the shape of things to come. *Lancet* 344:521–524.

Williamson, D.F., J. Madans, R.F. Anda, J.C. Kleinman, H.S. Kahn, and T. Byers (1993). Recreational physical activity and ten-year weight change in a US national cohort. *Int. J. Obes.* 17:279–286.

Woo, R., J. Garrow, and F. Pi-Sunyer (1982). Effects of exercise on spontaneous calorie intake in obesity. *Am. J. Clin. Nutr.* 36:470–477.

Woo, R., and F.X. Pi-Sunyer (1985). Effect of increased physical activity on voluntary intake in lean women. *Metabolism* 34:836–841.

Yanovski, J., S. Yanovski, K. Filmer, V. Hubbard, N. Avila, and B. Lewis (1996). Differences in body composition of black and white girls. *Am. J. Clin. Nutr.* 64:833–839.

Yoshizawa, S., H. Honda, N. Nakamura, K. Itoh, and N. Watanabe (1997). Effects of an 18–month endurance run training program on maximal aerobic power in 4– to 6–year-old girls. *Ped. Exerc. Sci.* 9:33–43.

Young, T., and D. Gelskey (1995). Is noncentral obesity metabolically benign? *JAMA* 274:1939–1941.

Zurlo, F., R.T. Ferraro, A.M. Fontvieille, R. Rising, C. Bogardus, and E. Ravussin (1992). Spontaneous physical activity and obesity: cross-sectional and longitudinal studies in Pima Indians. *Am. J. Physiol.* 263:E296–E300.

DISCUSSION

BAR-OR: Based on your efficacy studies, can you identify responders versus non-responders in children? What would be the characteristics of a child who does well in an activity program versus a child who does less well?

GUTIN: We have not done that but have plans to do so. I'm interested to hear that you think that's an important way to look at it.

BAR-OR: We don't have any clue either. We have seen about 2,000 obese children in the last 10 y, and we still don't know who will respond well and who will not.

GUTIN: We do have some indirect information about this matter. We did the analyses various ways, including using the baseline value as a covariate with change as the outcome variable; this would tell us, for example, whether those who were fattest at baseline were those who lost the most fat as a result of the training, but that wasn't so. We had lots of "good" hypotheses that turned out not to be correct.

BAR-OR: Another issue is the tracking of activity from childhood to adulthood. Bearing in mind that sedentarism has been recognized as a major risk factor in adulthood coronary artery disease, our major challenge is to induce a child to acquire active lifestyle habits that are sustained through adulthood. Can you comment on what approach one can take in order to enhance the likelihood that an active child will remain active in later years?

GUTIN: One of the main predictors of future increases in fatness is present fatness, so it would seem reasonable to reduce fatness as early in childhood as possible. We looked at one cohort starting at age three and four and followed them for 3 y; we found that even at that age the kids who were fattest at baseline were the ones who gained the most fat later on. So, when do you start with interventions? I don't know, but certainly it should be very early in childhood. One might argue that there is hereditary predisposition that leads these children to be fat at the beginning and continues to operate so they continue to get fatter afterward. But another possibility is that physical activity and fatness are inversely correlated. I'm not sure what the causal connection is.

I think the most parsimonious way to think about it is that it's cyclic. For some reason the kid is fat, which leads him to be less physically active because it's activity is more strenuous for fat children, and so on, or he's shunted aside in settings where there are lean as well as obese kids.

Let me digress for a moment on that matter. There's some evidence that when obese children were in a separate physical education class they were more active than when they were mixed together with non-obese kids. Now our obese kids were very active, and when I say active I should comment that 20 min of the program were devoted to work on machines, at least 5 min on at least four machines that they could chose, while the other 20 min involved games that were modified to keep them physically active and keep their heart rates up. But there were competitive games of various sorts, and these kids really went at it. So, the lesson we derived is that obese children will be active if you put them in the right environment; this was by no means a certainty when we started because we had heard so much about obese kids being inactive. So I would argue that having safe environments such as after-school programs where there's good supervision might help kids who are somewhat fatter to be more active, prevent their getting even fatter, and thereby encourage them to be even more active in the future. That would be one societal strategy I would suggest. Also, evidence is emerging that a low-fat diet makes very good sense. It looks like there's a synergism between inactivity and high-fat diets, such that the combination of the two is especially likely to lead to obesity.

BAR-OR: Our program lasts approximately 1 y. We usually find out that those who do not do well after 3 mo will not do well in the entire program, and that suggests that possibly one clue to success is a fast initial response. Do you have any thoughts about that? How can we induce a fast initial response? Obviously it should include a combination of exercise and diet.

GUTIN: Well, I wouldn't agree that it's so obvious that they should be done in combination. When you want people to change their behaviors, it's not necessarily a good idea to try to change more than one behavior at a time. On the other hand, it's possible that in the case of diet and exercise it's even better to focus on both at the same time. There was at least one study of adult women in a weight-control program that found out that those who were in the physical training program adhered to their diets more effectively. So there may be, at least with adults, a kind of healthy lifestyle where each behavior influences the other. Certainly, we know that diet can impose an energy deficit that's much greater than one can get from physical activity in a very short period of time. So you may have good reason to use diet initially to get that initial boost and reduce their fatness, which, as I said before, is more likely to make them more physically active. Then you may move them into a second phase where activity becomes important for long-term maintenance. Although that is a reasonable hypothesis, I don't know of any data that support it.

ROWLAND: I am concerned about how obesity in children affects aerobic fitness. If we take a group of obese children, we find that they have a lower maximal oxygen uptake per unit body weight. Is that simply because they have more fat in the denominator, or does obesity in children really have some negative impact on cardiovascular fitness? I think that's an important question to answer to address the dilemma of whether to use high intensity training or low intensity training; which of the two explanations for the low cardiovascular fitness would determine how you would construct the study.

GUTIN: Of course, this has to do with what you mean by the concept "cardiovascular fitness?" I am certainly willing to discuss what happens with absolute $\dot{V}O_2max$, but I would not call that cardiovascular fitness. Let me refer to a study we did some years ago where we had 11- and 12-year-old girls who varied quite a bit in fatness. We measured a variety of things to see what factors would predict their ability to run 2 km, including a $\dot{V}O_2max$ test expressed in mL/kg body weight and skin folds. The correlation between the sum of six skin folds and run time was 0.92. In other words, the fatter kids took a longer time to run the 2 km, and that correlation was so high there was no room for any other factor to come into the picture at all, including any way you looked at $\dot{V}O_2max$. So my answer is that there is a very tight relationship between body fatness and what I would consider a good index of cardiovascular fitness. Now, when you express $\dot{V}O_2max$ in L/min, then the fatter kid, who also has more fat-free mass (they go together to some degree), will have a higher $\dot{V}O_2max$, which is a bit counter-intuitive. If someone knows a way to solve this puzzle, then I welcome it.

DESPRES: I don't have the answer but just a suggestion. Select children in the cohort who have exactly the same amount of total body fat but different $\dot{V}O_2$max values and then observe the cardiovascular disease risk profile. If there is some difference, it's at least one indication that differences in $\dot{V}O_2$max may be involved.

GUTIN: That's a good suggestion with respect to whether one or the other is influencing the other cardiovascular risk factors. I'm not sure that's the question that Tom asked, however.

ROWLAND: Well, it's not a simple question and there's not a simple answer. What it boils down to is a choice between two possible goals of an exercise intervention for the obese child. Is the goal to improve cardiovascular fitness because each of these children has a low $\dot{V}O_2$max in mL/kg and should therefore be exercising three times a week for 35 min at a heart rate over 170? Or should one assume that the low $\dot{V}O_2$max simply reflects the fact that they have lots of fat to carry around, and that their true cardiovascular fitness is normal or above normal because they have increased fat-free mass? If the latter is correct, one should use low-intensity exercise designed to do volume work to burn off the fat; you don't need to worry about improving cardiovascular fitness. I think it comes down to a concrete question of how you're going to design your exercise program.

GUTIN: What you say is true, but it depends upon your outlook. From the point of view of optimal well being, which includes physiologic, psychological and social well being, moving that child from the midpoint on the continuum where risk factors are not an issue at all up to some higher level of function can be very important. This would include increasing the child's ability to run 1 km and keep up with the other kids without being ridiculed, and improving self-esteem and self-efficacy, which might predict future physical activity. If turns out that that a higher intensity of physical training is more efficacious, then I would argue for higher intensity physical training. I think there's no evidence whatsoever that a low intensity physical training is more efficacious at reducing fat mass. Am I wrong about that?

ROWLAND: You don't think that the obese child might better tolerate a lower intensity exercise program?

GUTIN: That's a reasonable hypothesis, but I asked if there were any data showing that low intensity physical training is more efficacious than higher intensity training at reducing fat mass?

ROWLAND: Well, from what we've heard before, the high intensity would be more efficacious in terms of energy expenditure, but in terms of the practical aspects of designing the program, I'm wondering if that's the best way to go.

GUTIN: The Surgeon General's report came down on the side of the public health message and suggested that relatively modest amounts of exercise would be desirable—not necessarily optimal. The thinking is that modest levels of exercise would reduce the chance that people would not want to even start because they could not aspire to high levels of activity and fitness. I think that's a reasonable public health message, but I'm a little concerned that we may stop there. It implies that small amounts of activity are also optimal, and I believe that this is not so. I believe that more is better, up to a much higher level than we typically advocate. When indirect calorimetry was first invented about 120 y ago and studies were done on factory workers and farmers, i.e., the typical men in that time, they had energy expenditures of 3500–3700 kcal/d, but typical values now are down around 2400. This is clearly not what we were evolutionarily designed to do; when we say people should do an extra 200 kcal/d, that's a drop in the bucket. I think we need to figure out ways to redress that balance somewhat. I'm not saying we can go back to a point where we add 1000 kcal/d; that would be quite a bit.

SATTERWHITE: You suggested that school-based interventions for the development of good habits or decreasing fatness have fared poorly. I have a question for Steve Johnson. Is this lack of adequate school-based physical activity a problem that's primarily financial, or is it based on concerns that we don't have enough time during the day to present the academic curriculum to students? Why is this trend going on with elimination of physical education programs from high school?

JOHNSON: We are experiencing total elimination of physical education programs, not just at the high-school level, but also in the elementary-schools. It is strictly a financial matter. In Nebraska, for example, our school systems are supported totally by property tax, and with property tax relief has come a significant decrease in support for physical education. Boards of education and school administrators need data on the importance of physical activity in adolescents and the long-term ramifications of eliminating the availability of these programs.

CLARKSON: One reason that obese children don't exercise, as you pointed out, is that they perform more poorly compared to their lean counterparts. A solution that you suggested was to have a separate class. If this is done in a school-based situation, it may be perceived as the remedial class, i.e., the "slow" class, and may become an embarrassment to attend. However, there is a form of exercise in which overweight children perform better than their lean counterparts, and that is strength and resistance training. Is anyone considering augmenting school programs so that more strength and resistance training is included?

GUTIN: There is good reason to believe that strength training would be a good modality for children in general. I'm not sure that they need more fat-free mass, but it may help them burn up calories and contribute to their self-esteem. The one psychological variable that has been shown to predict future physical activity is physical self-efficacy; strength training might influence the two major factors that predict future physical activity—physical self-efficacy and present body fatness. We plan to incorporate weight training into future studies.

HORSWILL: I was interested in how exercise seemed to enhance linear growth. Often for obese children, the recommendation is to use exercise to decrease their fat mass or slow their fat mass accretion. Exercise is suggested over dieting because of the potential negative effects of dieting on micronutrient intake, the loss of lean-body mass, and the slowing of linear growth. But the obese kids tend to have greater stature, greater linear growth rate, and a greater lean body-mass than do the non-obese kids. Do you think dieting alone really slows linear growth in obese kids, given that they are growing linearly faster than normal?

GUTIN: Studies done by pediatricians have failed to show that the typical kinds of weight control programs in children have any influence on linear growth. A study just reported from Thailand was quite interesting. They did a longitudinal prospective study to see what baseline characteristics would predict future development of fatness, and they found that children who were less physically active tended to get fatter. The question was, What kind of intervention might be called for? In Thailand there are still many nutritional deficiencies in wide areas of the country. If they were to have a community-wide effort to reduce energy intake, it probably would bump a lot of children even further down on the nutritional adequacy spectrum. So these authors concluded that they had to do something to increase physical activity. In our society, low-income people tend to have more obesity, but they probably have poorer nutrition as well. So if we work to emphasize reduction in total calories, it's quite conceivable we would bump a lot of those people into an even poorer nutritional state. That's another reason that it may not be a good idea to emphasize reduction in calories, except in clinical settings.

HORSWILL: Are there any data to show that exercise is of benefit to the child who has short stature or may suffer from cachexia and muscle wasting? Can exercise stimulate their growth and lean-body mass accretion?

GUTIN: I don't know of any information on that topic.

GISOLFI: Are children getting fatter because they're generating a larger population of fat cells, an increase in the size of the cell, or a combination of both? And when these kids engage in physical activity programs and training, are we decreasing the size of the cell, the number of cells or both? At what age does the population of fat cells become fixed?

GUTIN: In general, I can summarize by saying that when exercise, as opposed to dietary restriction, was used in growing animals, it was found that the total number of fat cells that resulted as they went into maturity was lower, so it looked like exercise was a better intervention than caloric restriction—at least if you extrapolate from the animal studies. In humans, the number of fat cells is probably established at the end of maturity for the most part, but there is some evidence that adults who continue to gain fat mass can increase the number of fat cells. And it looks like once you've gotten to a higher number and then you lose weight or lose fat, you still retain that greater number of cells, and presumably that makes it more difficult to ever go down in total fat mass again. I don't know of any studies with children that have looked at this.

GISOLFI: So, basically once a fat cell, always a fat cell?

GUTIN: Yes, I think that's true. However, there is also a kind of ratcheting effect in which you can increase the number of fat cells at any age if you get fat enough. Per Bjorntorp used to say that he never saw a fat cell that was a foot long. So, once you get big fat cells, they split, and then you have two fat cells.

DESPRES: We do a lot of adipose tissue biopsies in human subjects, and we have found a progressive increase in the number of adipose cells from birth to middle age; the stimulus for fat cell hyperplasia is fat cell hypertrophy. That's why it is so important during growth to minimize fat cell hypertrophy. If adipose cell size is reduced in children, and that's what happens if an exercise program induces mobilization of adipose tissue mass, the stimulus for adipose tissue hyperplasia may be reduced. Therefore, from birth to about 2 y of age there's an increase in adipose cell size, after which the adipose cell size remains fairly stable; it increases only slightly up to adulthood. There's a progressive increase in the number of adipose cells during that period. Hirsch and colleagues have done studies during growth indicating that the number of adipose cells increases if there are enlarged adipose cells present. It is therefore very important to keep adipose cell size within a certain range during growth.

GUTIN: Most of the hyperplasia takes place in childhood. It takes a sizable increase in the volume of fat to increase cell number later on in life, and that has tremendous implications for prevention. If we had to pick a time in life when intervention should be emphasized, it might well be childhood.

FIATARONE: Is there a prepubescent difference in visceral obesity?

GUTIN: We've only looked at 7- to 11-year olds so far, so I can't say anything about the role of puberty.

FIATARONE: Is there a gender difference in the amount of visceral obesity for similar amounts of total body fat at that age?

GUTIN: Keep in mind that our study was not designed to recruit a representative sample of all children, or even all obese children, so we would not feel comfortable making a statement about boys versus girls, blacks versus whites, except in-so-far-as their responses to the physical training might be different. I might comment that the study that we are about to begin will include 13- to 15-year olds, so we will have an opportunity to compare pre- and postpubescent children.

FIATARONE: Are the parents of these obese children also obese?

GUTIN: I can only tell you by the eyeball test; yes, many of the parents are obese.

8

Dietary Supplements and Pharmaceutical Agents for Weight Loss and Gain

Priscilla M. Clarkson, Ph.D.

INTRODUCTION

Degas' famous paintings of ballet dancers illustrate an ideal body type and weight consistent with the culture of the mid to late 19th century. Compared to today's ballet dancers, who strive to achieve a sylph-like image, Degas' dancers appear plump. Art reflects society such that now aesthetic standards for a pleasing body weight are quite a bit leaner than they were 100 y ago. Fat has become a disparaging characteristic for both men and women, albeit with different psychological and physiological consequences. In addition, men want to become more muscular, and women want a more toned body.

The concept of beauty has changed over the years (Brownell & Rodin, 1994), and along with this change has come challenges in how to obtain the ideal body. In Degas' day the challenge was to be sufficiently affluent to afford the amount of food needed to maintain a plump body. Today the challenge is to resist the overwhelming amount of food that can be purchased and ingested, and many seek miracle remedies to melt away fat and stack on muscle.

Weight loss and gain are also important concerns for athletes. Some athletes want to lose weight to comply with the aesthetic standards of their sport, as in the case of gymnastics and figure skating, or because they believe that lower weight will translate into improved performance. Strength and power athletes want to gain muscle mass either for aesthetic reasons (bodybuilding) or to increase force-generating capacity.

Treatments to reduce weight are always palliative and almost never curative, and for those who are initially successful, there is a significant percentage who regain the weight (Bray, 1996). Many "high-tech" nutritional supplements marketed to increase lean body mass may seem to be effective at first, but this is possibly due to a placebo effect. Ultimately, most nutritional supplements are ineffective, and some athletes then turn to pharmaceutical interventions.

Weight loss and weight gain are big business (Bray, 1996). Many products promise results such as "quick weight loss in 30 days and keep it off" and "gain 10 pounds of muscle in one week." Nutritional supplements receive little governmental oversight, and retailers have much freedom in making marketing claims, compared to prescription drugs, for which the Food and Drug Administration (FDA) carefully regulates clinical testing, advertising, and promotion. This chapter will review the various nutritional supplements and pharmacological interventions used to alter body composition and body weight. Among the nutritional supplements that will be discussed are chromium, creatine, protein, and amino acids. Pharmacological agents addressed are thermogenic drugs, anorectic (anorexiant) drugs, anabolic steroids, growth hormone, nicotine, diuretics, and β_2 agonists. In sections where a wealth of information exists, research findings will be summarized, pertinent examples provided, and recent or well-controlled studies highlighted.

WEIGHT LOSS

Most nutritional interventions center on ingesting diets with fewer calories and lower fat. Chromium and pyruvate are mononutrient supplements marketed as a means to lose fat (Nielsen, 1996); chromium is also purported to increase muscle mass. Pharmacological agents commonly used to decrease weight are thermogenic drugs, such as ephedrine or ephedrine/caffeine/aspirin combinations, and anorexiant drugs, such as fenfluramine and fluoxetine. Many individuals use nicotine in the form of tobacco smoking to control weight. Athletes who need to "cut weight" for competition often rely on quick weight loss from diuretics.

Nutritional Supplements for Weight Loss

Although products other than chromium and pyruvate are marketed to enhance weight loss, only these two agents will be discussed because preliminary studies of their effectiveness are available. Hydroxycitrate has become popular as a weight loss agent based upon results from animal research, yet no studies on its effectiveness in humans exist. Also, L-carnitine is marketed as a "fat burner" with no data to support its efficacy in humans.

Chromium. Chromium is an essential trace mineral that functions to potentiate the effects of insulin. Because of insulin's role in fat metabolism, it was theorized that chromium ingestion might enhance fat usage and loss. Chromium is marketed predominantly in the form of chromium picolinate, although chromium nicotinate and chromium chloride exist. Picolinic acid is an organic compound that serves as a chelator of chromium and is thought to enhance the absorption and transport of chromium, although how picolinate enhances chromium bioavailability is not clear (Evans, 1989).

Few studies have assessed the effects of chromium as a weight loss product (See Table 8-1). Evans (1989) reported results of two studies in which college students and football players ingested 200 µg/d of chromium picolinate for about 6 wk. During the supplementation period, the subjects participated in a weight training program. The study of untrained subjects showed no change in fat for the chromium supplemented group, but the placebo group significantly increased body fat by 1.1%. In the study using football players, the supplemented group lost 3.6% fat (3.4 kg), and the placebo group lost only about 1% fat (1 kg),

TABLE 8-1. *Effects of Chromium Supplementation on Body Composition.*

Study	Subjects	Length	Treatment	N	Initial BW (kg)	Control of diet or exercise	Primary Measurement	Change (kg) in LBM	Fat	BW	Effect of Chr on body composition significant?
Studies to Assess Weight Loss											
Lukaski et al. (1996)	Untrained	56 d	Placebo ChrCl 200µg ChrPic 200µg	12 12 12	79.9 79.3 79.2	Dietary intake assessed, Participated in strength training	DEXA	+1.4 +1.9 +1.9	-0.3 +0.4 -0.2	+0.6 +1.8 +1.3	No
Trent & Thieding-Cancel (1995)	Untrained ♂ & ♀ (17% ♀)	112 d	Placebo ChrPic 400µg	44 51	89.9 89.8	Diet and exercise logs kept	Circumference	-0.2 -0.3	-1.18 -0.62	-1.5 -1.0	No
Kaats et al. (1996)	Untrained ♂ & ♀ (~80% ♀)	72 d	Placebo ChrPic 200µg ChrPic 400µg	55 33 66	83.3 87.0 85.3	None	Underwater weighing	+0.09 +0.54 +0.68	-0.18 -1.62 -2.07	-0.14 -1.08 -1.40	Yes data analyzed only by BCI[1]
Studies to Assess Weight Gain											
Evans (1989) Study 1	Untrained ♂	40 d	Placebo ChrPic 200µg	5 5	NR	No diet control, participated in strength training	Skinfolds	+0.04 +1.6	NR NR	+1.25 +2.2	Yes
Study 2	Football Players	42 d	Placebo ChrPic 200µg	15 16	NR	No diet control, participated in strength training	Skinfolds	+1.8 +2.6	-1.0 -3.4	NR -1.2	Yes
Hasten et al. (1992)	Untrained	84 d	Placebo ♀ ChrPic 200µg ♀ Placebo ♂ ChrPic 200µg ♂	10 12 19 18	62.9 58.5 72.0 71.0	No diet control, participated in strength training	Skinfolds	NR NR NR NR	-5.6" -4.2 -3.3 -3.3	+0.6 +2.5 +1.3 +0.8	Only ChrPic ♀ BW change significant
Clancy et al. (1994)	Football Players	63 d	Placebo ChrPic 200µg	12 9	94.9 100.8	Diet assessed, urine Chr assessed, participated in strength training	Underwater weighing	<1 <1	NR NR	NR NR	No
Hallmark et al. (1996)	Untrained ♂	84 d	Placebo ChrPic 200µg	8 8	80.5 81.6	Diet assessed, urine Chr assessed, participated in strength training	Underwater weighing	+0.5 +1.0	+0.16 -0.78	+0.4 +0.4	No

" — These data are based on sum of skinfolds (mm) NR— Not Reported

BCI[1]-A body composition index (BCI) was calculated by adding the loss of body fat and gain in nonfat mass and subtracting the fat gained and lean tissue lost.

with the difference between groups being significant. However, percent body fat was only estimated from skinfolds, so differences could be attributed to the variability and low reliability of the measurement technique. Three other studies, in which subjects participated in weight training while taking the chromium supplements, did not substantiate these findings (Clancy et al., 1994; Hallmark et al., 1996; Lukaski et al., 1996). These studies did not use overweight individuals as subjects.

Two studies have assessed the effects of chromium picolinate specifically as a weight loss agent. Trent and Thieding-Cancel (1995) used a double-blind design to investigate the effects of a daily dose of 400 µg chromium picolinate or placebo for 16 wk in subjects who were participating in an aerobic exercise program three times per week, at least 30 min a session. The subjects consisted of navy personnel who were overweight and did not meet the body fat standards of 22% for men and 30% for women. Seventy-nine men and sixteen women completed the study. Percent fat was estimated by circumference measures. The results of the study showed only minimal changes in total body weight or percent fat over the course of the study, with no significant difference between groups. Sixty-two subjects lost some body fat, and of these, 32 were in the chromium-supplemented group, and 30 were in the placebo group. Thirty-one subjects gained body fat, and of these, 17 took the chromium supplement, and 14 took the placebo.

Trent and Thieding-Cancel (1995) concluded that chromium picolinate supplements used in conjunction with an aerobic exercise program did not enhance fat reduction. The authors further suggested that one explanation for the lack of effectiveness might be that subjects were not chromium deficient; chromium supplements may only be effective when compensating for a deficiency. However, establishing chromium status is difficult because few valid data are available for chromium content of foods (Kumpulainen, 1992), and there is no easy means to accurately determine status. Moreover, use of circumference measures to estimate body composition casts doubt on the reliability and validity of the findings.

Another study of chromium picolinate as a weight loss agent offered more promising results. Kaats et al. (1996) examined the effects of 200 µg and 400 µg of chromium per day or a placebo for 72 d in 154 subjects who responded to an advertisement. The body mass index (BMI; body weight (kg) divided by height (m) squared) was approximately 30 kg/m^2 for each of the three study groups. Body composition was assessed using underwater weighing. A body composition index (BCI) was calculated by adding the loss of body fat and gain in nonfat mass and subtracting the fat gained and lean tissue lost. Compared with the placebo, the chromium supplement resulted in significantly higher positive changes in BCI. The actual amount of total body weight loss and fat weight loss over the 72 d was 1.26 kg and 1.89 kg, respectively, for the chromium-supplemented group, compared with 0.14 kg and 0.18 kg, respectively, for the placebo. Statistical analyses were reported for only the BCI values, not for the actual changes.

At this time there is not valid scientific evidence to support the contention that chromium is an effective weight loss agent. Anderson and Kozlovsky (1985) raised the concern that many people are not ingesting the minimum of the recommended range of 50–200 μg per day. However, this range was established using less sophisticated equipment than is available today, so these recommended values may be too high (Stoecker, 1996). If this is correct, then the average diet could provide sufficient chromium. Furthermore, it has been suggested that too much chromium may be harmful. Stearns et al. (1995a) reported that chromium picolinate at high levels caused chromosome damage in cultured cells. The picolinate may facilitate chromium transport into cells, and once chromium is in the cell, it is slow to leave and accumulates. McCarty (1996) criticized the interpretation of the results for humans because the study used superphysiological doses in cell cultures.

In a second report, Stearns et al. (1995b) employed a pharmacokinetic model to predict chromium accumulation into cells in humans and estimated that chromium could accumulate to levels that would damage chromosomes. The authors also suggested that ingesting levels below the recommended range of 50–200 μg/d might be adequate. Because so little is known about chromium status, chromium balance, and chromium ingestion, a prudent course of action would be to ingest foods rich in chromium.

Pyruvate. Early animal studies found that supplementing diets with 3-carbon compounds (e.g., pyruvate or dihydroxyacetone) inhibited lipid accumulation in adipose tissue and inhibited fat gain and weight gain in growing animals (Cortez et al., 1991). It is thought that these 3-carbon compounds inhibit lipid synthesis and enhance energy expenditure, although the mechanism to explain these effects is unclear. Four studies examined the effects of these 3-carbon compounds on weight loss in human subjects. Stanko et al. (1992a) measured body composition and energy expenditure in 14 obese women housed in a metabolic ward for 21 d. The women were placed into groups that ingested diets with and without pyruvate substituted for glucose. The low-energy diet consisted of 4.24 MJ/d (about 1000 kcal/d) with either 30 g pyruvate or 22 g polyglucose (placebo). Subjects who ingested the pyruvate had a significantly greater weight loss (5.9 kg), compared with the placebo (4.0 kg). Bioelectrical impedance analysis showed a greater fat loss (4.0 kg) for pyruvate, compared with the placebo (2.7 kg). Nitrogen balance was comparable between groups.

Three additional studies of obese subjects were performed in the same laboratory using the same methodology. Stanko et al. (1992b) found that in obese women a combination of dihydroxyacetone (12 g) and pyruvate (16 g) resulted in a greater loss in body weight (6.5 kg) and fat weight (4.3 kg), compared to a placebo (26 g polyglucose) (5.6 and 3.5 kg, respectively). Nitrogen balance was similar between groups. Another study (Stanko et al., 1994) reported that despite the greater weight and fat loss with these 3-carbon compounds, compared to a placebo, there was no difference between groups in plasma concentrations of cholesterol, LDL cholesterol, HDL cholesterol, or triglycerides in hyperlipidemic overweight subjects. Thus, the supplements did not produce a lowering of these cardiovascular risk factors. In the latest study, Stanko and Arch (1996) examined the effects of the 3-carbon compounds on weight gain after weight loss. Subjects were energy restricted for 3 wk and were then re-fed with a hyperenergetic diet for 3 wks. Weight gain was significantly less in subjects receiving the diet containing pyruvate and dihydroxyacetone (0.8 kg weight gain) compared with the isoenergetically similar placebo (1.8 kg weight gain).

Three of the four studies described above (Stanko et al., 1992a, 1992b, Stanko & Arch, 1996) appear to be well-controlled; they took place in a controlled metabolic unit, the subjects were confined to bed except to walk to the lavatory or the metabolic kitchen, no medications were allowed during the study period, subjects were observed during meals to assure that they ingested the diets, and they were observed so that they did not perform any exercise. Although the weight-loss diets differed in 3-carbon compounds versus glucose, they were isoenergetic and set at a composition of 60% CHO, 40% protein, and < 1 g of fat. The 1994 study was an outpatient study in which subjects were given instruction on restricting physical activity and were provided with dietary guidelines and given a liquid supplement. Even with this lack of strict control, small differences in weight loss between the supplement and the placebo were found.

While these results are interesting, it should be noted that the weight loss in 21 d was less than a 1.7-kg difference between the supplemented and the placebo groups. Also, three of these studies used obese subjects, so effects on relatively lean individuals are not fully known. The study that used subjects who were not all classified as obese, but who were hyperlipidemic and overweight, found even smaller changes due to the supplement, although this is also the study that was less well-controlled (Stanko et al.,1994). The only adverse effects attributed to the supplement were that about 20% of the subjects experienced diarrhea and borborygmus.

Pharmacological Agents for Weight Loss

Weight reduction due to tissue loss occurs from two possible mechanisms: stimulating heat production or energy expenditure (thermogenic effects) or reducing food intake (anorectic effects). Pharmacological treatments act via these mechanisms to induce weight loss either by increasing thermogenesis or by suppressing appetite, or both. Nicotine (smoking) is commonly used to control weight and appears to increase thermogenesis in males but not in females, where its action may involve appetite suppression. Diuretics induce a quick weight reduction by facilitating water loss from the body.

Thermogenic/Anoretic Agents. The sympathetic nervous system is a primary regulator of thermogenesis (Landsberg & Young, 1993). Drugs have been identified or developed to act as agonists to receptors in the sympathetic nervous system (adrenergic receptors) or to prevent inhibition of sympathetic neural activity. Ephedrine and amphetamines are sympathomimetic, meaning that they stimulate (act as agonists to) adrenergic α and β receptors (Fitch, 1986; Hoffman & Lefkowitz, 1996; Hoffman et al., 1996; McKenry & Salerno, 1995; Morton & Fitch, 1992). Ephedrine has both thermogenic and anorectic effects, whereas newer drugs, β_3 agonists, have more thermogenic effects. Ephedrine effects are less pronounced than those of amphetamines. In the past, amphetamines were used as weight loss products, but their additional action as a central nervous system stimulant, their addictive properties, and their abuse potential have made them undesirable (Weintraub & Bray, 1989). Sympathomimetic compounds increase resting energy expenditure by about 10–20% and slightly increase the thermic effect of foods (Astrup et al., 1996). The extent to which these drugs influence energy expenditure during exercise for weight loss is not known.

There are two types of α receptors: α_1 and α_2. The α_1 receptors are found on effector organs such as heart and vascular smooth muscle, and the α_2 are found on presynaptic nerve terminals and on vascular and other smooth muscle cells where they mediate contraction. There are three types of β receptors: β_1, β_2, and β_3. The β_1 receptors are mainly located in the heart, where they mediate heart rate and force of contraction, and are also found in adipose tissue, where they mediate lipolysis. The β_2 receptors are located on pre-synaptic nerve terminals and post-synaptically in the heart, where they mediate contraction, and in smooth muscle, where they mediate relaxation. The β_3 receptors are located mainly in visceral fat and brown adipose tissue and have been proposed to function predominantly in thermogenesis (Hoffman et al., 1996; McKenry & Salerno, 1995; Stock, 1996).

Sympathomimetic drugs may effect thermogenesis by their action on skeletal muscle and adipose tissue. Skeletal muscle, which plays an important role in resting energy expenditure and thermogenesis, contains β_2 receptors and possibly β_3 receptors (although this has not been proven). Adipose tissue contains α_2, β_1, and β_2 receptors that appear to be involved in lipolysis and mobilization of lipids (Kempen et al., 1994).

Sympathomimetic drugs exert their effect as appetite suppressors via activation of β-adrenergic and/or dopaminergic receptors within the perifornical hypothalamus (Wellman, 1992). Anorexiant drugs also appear to bind to the paraventricular nucleus, and neurochemical activity in this area may play a role in integration of behavioral, metabolic, and neuroendocrine responses to control appetite (Blundell & Greenough, 1994). Serotonin and norepinephrine are found in high concentrations in the paraventricular nucleus and, when released, function to control appetite. Anorexiant drugs can also prolong the effect of serotonin or norepinephrine by inhibiting their reuptake into presynaptic neurons (Norton et al., 1993).

Ephedrine. Ephedrine occurs naturally in several plants and is structurally related to the amphetamines (Wagner, 1991). It both suppresses appetite and increases thermogenesis (Astrup et al., 1992c; Daly et al., 1993) and may act as a β_3 agonist (Dulloo, 1993), but this is still unclear.

Therapeutic uses of ephedrine to control asthma (by stimulating β receptors in lungs to induce brochodilation) and urinary incontinence (by stimulating α receptors in smooth muscle of the bladder) have dwindled over the years as drugs with less central nervous system action have been developed (Hoffman & Lefkowitz, 1996). However, ephedrine is a very popular drug with athletes, and there is considerable information available to athletes over the Internet regarding purported benefits of ephedrine, and combinations of ephedrine, caffeine, and aspirin, in improving body composition. Although regulation of ephedrine is tightening, it is still available in some states over-the-counter and is easier to obtain than other prescription drugs. Ephedrine is not approved by the FDA for weight control.

Pasquali and Casimirri (1993) reported that obese patients who ingested 150 mg of ephedrine or a placebo daily for 3 mo showed a significantly greater weight loss with ephedrine. Several other studies showed that ephedrine significantly promotes weight reduction in adult obese subjects (Astrup et al., 19920a; Dulloo et al., 1986) and reduces nitrogen loss (Pasquali et al., 1987). The reduction in nitrogen loss could be due to protein sparing caused by stimulation of β_2 receptors affecting protein synthesis and counteracting lean tissue loss (Dulloo, 1993). Moreover, ephedrine prevented the fall in resting metabolic rate associated with low calorie diets (Pasquali et al., 1992).

Ephedrine produces side effects because stimulation of β_2 receptors can cause tremor and nervousness (Atkinson & Hubbard, 1994), while stimulation of α and β_1 receptors causes increases in blood pressure (vasoconstriction) and heart rate. In long-term treatment of obesity with ephedrine there appears to be a down-regulation of adrenoreceptor types associated with undesirable cardiac and pressor effects but a continued stimulation of adrenoreceptors mediating thermogenesis, fat loss, and protein sparing (Dulloo, 1993). More severe adverse reactions to ephedrine misuse include myocardial infarction, stroke, seizures, psychosis, and death. The death of a Tufts University Graduate student due to myocardial necrosis raised concern over ephedrine (Goldberg, 1996). Several empty bottles of a sports product containing ephedrine designed to enhance muscle mass and burn fat were found in the student's room although no direct link has been established between the student's death and ephedrine use. Risks of ephedrine also include cardiac arrhythmia and hypertension (Hoffman & Lefkowitz, 1996). Use of ephedrine for those with diabetes mellitus, hypertension, and hyperthyroidism is dangerous, and there are significant drug interactions with antidepressants, anesthetics, cocaine, and β blockers (McKenry & Salerno, 1995). A nationwide movement to restrict the availability of ephedrine is currently underway. This is a prudent course of action given the possibility of death from use of ephedrine and given the fact that there is no valid research to support the suggestion that ephedrine is an effective weight loss agent in non-obese individuals.

Ephedrine/Caffeine. To enhance effectiveness as a weight loss agent, ephedrine has been combined with caffeine. Although caffeine is commonly used for weight loss, data do not support its effectiveness by itself (Astrup et al., 1992c). Ephedrine stimulates the release of norepinephrine, which in turn stimulates the release of adenosine. Adenosine serves as a prejunctional inhibitor of norepinephrine. Caffeine exerts an antagonistic effect to adenosine and thus potentiates the release of norepinephrine. Caffeine may act in other ways to enhance the effects of ephedrine, but these are not well established (Dulloo et al., 1994). For example, ephedrine may suppress food intake via adrenergic pathways in the hypothalamus, and this effect could be potentiated by caffeine (Astrup et al., 1992c).

A combination of ephedrine and caffeine has been found to increase energy expenditure and enhance weight loss in obese subjects (Astrup et al., 1991, 1992a, 1992b; Dulloo & Miller, 1986). A double-blind placebo-controlled study of three doses of ephedrine and caffeine (10mg/200mg,

20mg/100mg, and 20mg/200mg) (Astrup & Toubro, 1993; Astrup et al., 1991) found that the combination of 20 mg ephedrine and 200 mg caffeine was significantly more effective than the other treatments. The 20 mg/200 mg combination was also found to be effective in promoting a dietary-induced weight loss over 24 wk (Breum et al., 1994). After 8 wk of ephedrine/caffeine (20mg/200mg) there was a significantly greater fat loss despite similar losses in total body weight compared to a placebo (Astrup & Toubro, 1993; Astrup et al., 1992b). The greater energy expenditure for the ephedrine/caffeine group was due to fat oxidation (Astrup et al., 1992b).

Although not all studies found ephedrine/caffeine combinations to be as efficacious as those reported previously (Molnár, 1993; Pasquali & Casimirri, 1993), most of the evidence suggests that the combination of ephedrine and caffeine is more effective than ephedrine alone in promoting weight loss in adults. Based on results of their studies, Astrup and Toubro (1993) estimated that about 80% of weight loss was due to an anorectic effect and 20% was due to a thermogenic effect.

Ephedrine/Caffeine/Aspirin. Ephedrine has also been combined with both caffeine and aspirin to further enhance its effectiveness. Aspirin has been used in this combination because aspirin inhibits the synthesis of prostaglandins. Ephedrine stimulates release of norepinephrine, which stimulates the synthesis of prostaglandins by the activated tissue. Prostaglandins act as prejunctional inhibitors. Aspirin is a prostaglandin blocker and may prevent inhibition of norepinephrine release induced by the prostaglandins. This would enhance the action of ephedrine on sympathetically mediated thermogenesis (Geissler, 1993).

Daly et al. (1993) had obese individuals ingest either a combination of ephedrine (75 mg), caffeine (150 mg) and aspirin (330 mg) (ECA) or a placebo for 4 wk, and then the dose of ephedrine was increased to 150 mg/d for another 4 wk (Figure 8-1a). In the second part of the study, the placebo group (non-blinded) took the ECA combination for 8 wk (the increase in ephedrine dose occurred after the first week) (Figure 8-1b). In part three, subjects taking the ECA combination continued for 7–26 mo. The mean weight loss over the 8 wk in part one of the study was 2.2 kg for the ECA group (p < .05) and 0.7 for the placebo. In part two, the mean weight loss was 3.3 kg (p < .05), compared to only 1.3 kg during the 8 wk the subjects were taking the placebo. In part three, the average weight loss in five subjects after 5 mo was 5.2 kg, compared to 0.03 kg gained during 5 mo with no intervention (p < .05). The ECA was well tolerated with only minor occasional side effects of dry mouth, transient nervousness, or constipation in a few subjects.

Geissler (1993) examined energy expenditure in formerly obese women and in women with no history of obesity who were matched by

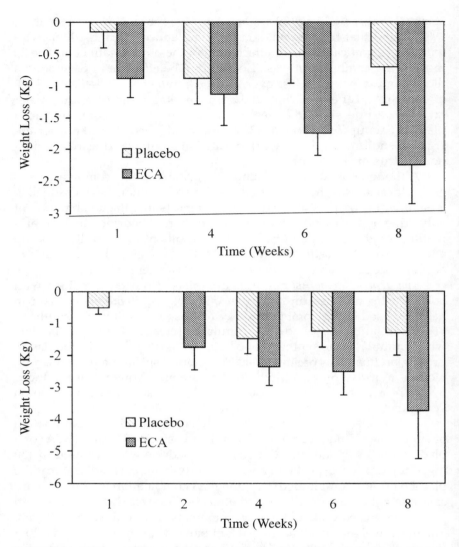

FIGURE 8-1. *Mean cumulative weight loss over 8 wk in: (a) subjects taking a placebo and subjects (ECA) taking a combination of ephedrine, caffeine, and aspirin, and (b) subjects who were the placebo group in part a returned 5 mo later and were assigned either to a placebo or ECA. Data from Daly et al. (1993).*

age, height, and weight. A 15% lower energy expenditure was found for the previously obese subjects, compared with the lean subjects. The authors suggested that the propensity to gain weight may result from a lower metabolic rate due to a dysfunction of the sympathetic nervous system. Ephedrine could correct the dysfunction by increasing thermo-genesis, which would then have the effect of regulating weight better. Horton and Geissler (1991) tested the effects of 30 mg ephedrine and 300 mg of aspirin, alone and combined, on the acute thermogenic response to a liquid meal in 10 lean and 10 obese women. The combination was significantly more effective in increasing the thermic response in the obese group only.

Ephedrine Combinations, Diet, and Exercise. When these drugs are coupled to a diet-and-exercise regimen, they can be a more effective tool for weight reduction. Astrup et al. (1992a) and Toubro et al. (1993) reported on the effects of diet restriction (total amount of energy ingested was 4.2 MJ/d) with either ephedrine (20 mg), ephedrine/caffeine (20 mg/200 mg), caffeine (200 mg), or placebo, three times per day for 24 wk. All groups demonstrated a decrease in body weight. The ephedrine/caffeine combination resulted in significantly more weight loss than oc-curred with the placebo (16.6 kg and 13.2 kg, respectively), and there was no significant difference among ephedrine, caffeine, and placebo groups (Figure 8-2). Differences between ephedrine and ephedrine/caf-feine did not reach statistical significance. When the weight losses were adjusted for differences in initial body weight, the ephedrine/caffeine group lost 3.8 kg more than the placebo group, whereas the ephedrine-without-caffeine group lost only 1.7 kg more than the placebo group.

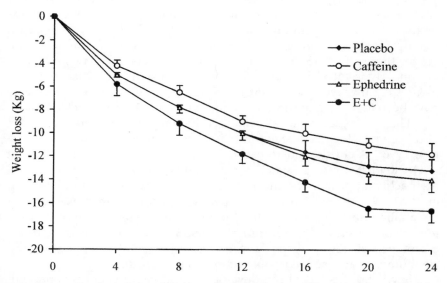

FIGURE 8-2. *Changes in body weight in groups taking placebo, caffeine, ephedrine, or ephedrine plus caffeine (E + C). All subjects maintained a diet of 4.2 MJ/day.* Data from Toubro et al. (1993).

Although the amount of weight loss was not dramatic relative to the amount of weight that obese individuals would be recommended to lose, there seems to be some benefit from ephedrine when combined with caffeine and/or aspirin ingestion, even without caloric restriction. In the treatment of obesity, small weight losses can improve health. Ephedrine alone or when coupled with aspirin and/or caffeine appears to be a promising treatment for obesity, and these drugs combined with exercise and diet intervention warrant further study. Most studies have neither controlled for nor assessed physical activity levels of the subjects.

Because studies on the effects of these drugs have used obese individuals as subjects, their effectiveness for those who may want to lose only a few pounds is not known. Dulloo and Miller (1986) did find that lean subjects showed an increased diet-induced thermogenesis (50%) with a combination of ephedrine, caffeine, and theophylline, albeit significantly smaller than for post-obese subjects (those who have been obese and were considered predisposed to gaining weight) (200%). However, overall, the lean subjects had significantly greater increases in energy expenditure than did the post-obese. Because cessation of the drugs commonly results in weight gain, drugs may not be the best tool for weight loss in mildly overweight individuals who, perhaps, would benefit more from behavior modification leading to an adjustment in diet.

β_3 *Agonists.* β_3 adrenergic receptors may play a role in lipolysis and release of free fatty acids into circulation and in regulation of energy expenditure and fat accumulation (Lönnqvist et al., 1995). It is thought that β_3 receptors on brown adipose tissue or in visceral fat are responsible for these effects (Stock, 1996). In studies of rats, the drugs may predominantly involve the action of brown adipose tissue, whereas in humans they involve visceral fat (although β_3 adrenergic receptors also have been identified in the gall bladder and colon) (Lipworth, 1996).

The β_3 receptor gene has been identified in humans, and a mutation of this gene, which had been found in obese individuals (Napoli & Horton, 1996), is considered to cause a reduced ability to metabolize fat (ADA Report, 1997). β_3 agonists have little or no anorectic effects, and their action appears to be entirely peripheral rather than central (Astrup et al., 1992c). Administration of specific β_3 agonists increases resting metabolic rate and increases the thermic effect of food (Napoli & Horton, 1996), presumably by stimulating visceral and brown adipose tissue thermogenesis (Stock, 1996). It is interesting to note that ephedrine and clenbuterol may also have some action on β_3 receptors.

Several drugs have been developed to serve as β agonists, particularly acting on the β_3 receptors (BRL35135, ZD2079, CL316243, Ro49-2148, and BRL26830A). Most of these compounds, with the exception of

BRL 26830A, have not proven effective in weight reduction in humans (Stock, 1996). However, BRL 26830A was found to increase metabolic rate and improve weight loss, compared to a placebo, when given with an energy-restricted diet (Astrup et al., 1992c; Connacher et al., 1992; MacLachlan et al., 1991). Connacher et al. (1992) had obese subjects take either BRL 26830A or placebo for 18 wk while they followed a prescribed diet. The drug produced a significantly greater weight loss (15.4 kg), compared with the placebo (10 kg). Twelve of the 16 subjects reported tremor that was mild, occurred within 1 h of dosing, but diminished with time on the treatment.

It has been disappointing that the β_3 drugs have not been more successful in humans because they have been proven quite effective in enhancing weight loss in the rat (Arch & Wilson, 1996). There appears to be a lower number of β_3 receptors relative to β_1 and β_2 receptors in those tissues that mediate thermogenesis in humans versus rats. The significant side effects of the β_3 agonists in humans, such as an increase in tremor, show that they also have some effects as β_2 agonists on skeletal muscle β_2 receptors. Research is underway to develop a version of β_3 agonists that can increase lipolysis and thermogenesis without any side effects. Whether the weight loss is maintained upon cessation of the drug is not known. Until a compound is developed that has good selectivity and efficacy at the human β_3 adrenergic receptor, the true potential of the β_3 agonists as weight loss agents cannot be evaluated (Arch & Wilson, 1996).

Anoretic Agents. There are two general categories of anoretic agents: the amphetamine and amphetamine-related drugs and the serotonergic drugs. The first category includes amphetamine, methamphetamine, and dextroamphetamine, which are all potent central nervous system stimulants. Amphetamines have had a long history of use as anorexiant drugs and work as catecholaminergic agents. Because of their side effects, potential for abuse, and addiction, other drugs were developed.

Catecholaminergic Agents. Amphetamine-related anorexiant drugs include benzphetamine, diethylpropion, phentermine, phendimetrazine, and mazindol. These agents are structurally related to amphetamines, but their potential for abuse and addictive properties are less. However, they are recommended for only short-term use. These drugs have been shown to reduce hunger and food intake in normal and obese subjects (Atkinson & Hubbard, 1994). The use of phentermine in conjunction with fenfluramine will be discussed in the next section.

Phenylpropanolamine is chemically related both to ephedrine and amphetamines. It is commonly found as the active ingredient in commercially available diet pills as an appetite suppressor (Greenway, 1992) and is the only appetite suppressant approved by the FDA to be available without prescription. Phenylpropanolamine is also a nasal decongestant and is found as the active ingredient in many over-the-counter cold medications. In a meta-analysis, Greenway (1992) reported that phenylpropanolamine was a safe and effective weight loss agent, especially in the first 4 wk of use, but its effectiveness is still controversial. Whereas the abuse potential of phenylpropanolamine is much less than that for amphetamines, it should not be used indiscriminately and should be used with caution by those with hypertension and by men with enlarged prostates (Hoffman & Lefkowitz, 1996). Although side effects are less for phenylpropanolamine compared with amphetamines, it does act as a central nervous system stimulant and produces cardiovascular side effects. Because of this health hazard, over-the-counter compounds containing phenylpropanolamine should not be indiscriminately used.

   Serotonergic Agents. Recently, the drugs, fenfluramine, dexfenfluramine, and fluoxetine, which act as serotonergic agents, have proven successful as anorexiants (Silverstone & Goodall, 1992) and may be less dangerous than the amphetamines. Although they are structurally related to the amphetamines, they are pharmacologically different. The racemic compound, d,l-fenfluramine, and the dextro isomer, d-fenfluramine (dexfenfluramine), both result in weight loss, but dexfenfluramine seems to be the more effective (Atkinson & Hubbard, 1994). Fenfluramine has a selective effect on carbohydrate intake; it reduces carbohydrate snacking in obese subjects who have a tendency toward frequent snacking (Silverstone & Goodall, 1992). Fenfluramine is thought to release serotonin from nerve endings and block its reuptake. Prescribed together, phentermine (a catecholaminergic agent) and fenfluramine ("Fen-phen") have been used to facilitate adherence to a restrictive diet (ADA Report, 1997).

   Several long-term studies demonstrated the effectiveness of fenfluramine as a weight loss agent (Guy-Grand, 1992; Guy-Grand et al., 1989). In one study, obese subjects took 30 mg/d dexfenfluramine or placebo for 1 y while being prescribed a control low-calorie diet. Significantly greater weight loss was found for the group taking the drug (10.26%), compared with the group taking the placebo (7.18%). Ten percent of the obese subjects maintained a significant weight loss over the year, whereas most patients did not continue to lose weight after 6 mo (Guy-Grand et al., 1989).

   Breum et al. (1994) compared an ephedrine/caffeine (60mg/600mg) combination to dexfenfluramine (30 mg) for 15 wk in obese subjects who were provided instruction to maintain a 5.0 MJ daily energy intake and participate in a recommended exercise program. There was a significant weight loss for both groups, but the weight loss for the ephedrine/caffeine group (8.3 kg) was not significantly different than that for the dexfenfluramine group (6.9 kg). The ephedrine/caffeine combination resulted in a significantly greater weight loss for subjects who had body mass indexes (BMIs) equal to or over 30 kg/m² (9.0 kg), but the amount of difference was not large (2 kg) between treatments. O'Connor et al. (1995) had obese subjects who were participating in a lifestyle weight loss program (1500 kcal diet for men and 1200 kcal for women and prescribed exercise) take 30 mg dexfenfluramine or placebo daily for 6 mo. The drug caused a significant weight loss of 9.7 kg greater than that of the placebo (Figure 8-3). After 5 mo discontinuation of the drug, weight was regained to pre-treatment levels.

Levitsky and Troiano (1992) reported that, in addition to the primary anorectic effects, fenfluramine potentiates the expenditure of energy whenever an increase in energy expenditure occurs. It increases the thermic effect of food in human studies and the energy cost of exercise in animal studies. However, thermogenic properties of fenfluramine are still controversial (Schutz et al., 1992). Stunkard (1982) suggested that fenfluramine may lower the body weight set point.

Stahl and Imperiale (1993) examined results of 36 studies of mazindol and fenfluramine in the treatment of obesity. The amount of weight lost over a median duration of 12 wk for the drug-treated groups (5.15 kg

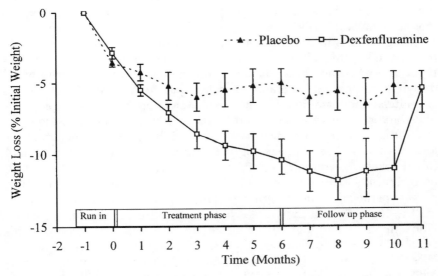

FIGURE 8-3. *Changes in weight loss expressed as a percentage of initial weight for subjects taking placebo or dexfenfluramine (treatment phase) and after stopping the treatment (follow up phase). Data from O'Connor et al. (1995).*

loss) was about 3 kg greater than that of the placebo group (1.91 kg loss). No difference was found between the mazindol-treated and the fenfluramine-treated groups. However, dropouts due to adverse drug effects were higher for fenfluramine trials (9% of subjects) compared with mazindol trials (4% of subjects). Dropout rates due to perceived lack of effect were also higher with fenfluramine (3%) compared with mazindol (1%). On the whole, dropout rates were fairly low, and modest weight loss was found.

A comprehensive, well-controlled series of studies that led to the popularity of the combination or fenfluramine and phentermine (Fenphen) found that this combination resulted in a weight loss of 14.2 kg (4.6 kg for the placebo group) after 34 wk, and the weight loss was maintained for 190 wk (Weintraub et al., 1992a-d). Subjects stopped taking the drug and were followed for an additional 20 wk (Weintraub et al., 1992e). The Fen-phen group gained back about half of the weight while the placebo group gained back most of the weight. In November 1997 a new drug (Sibutramine) was approved by the FDA that combines fenfluramine and phentermine like drugs in one pill. Although it appears that this combination of drugs is more successful than single-drug treatments, no direct comparisons have been made (National Task Force on the Prevention and Treatment of Obesity, 1996).

Eighteen million prescriptions for Fen-phen were written in 1996 (Miller, 1997). Although these weight loss drugs were approved only for the treatment of obesity, it is suspected that they are being prescribed for women who want to lose only a few pounds for cosmetic reasons. The FDA regulations initially did not restrict a physician from prescribing these drugs in other situations. However, on September 15, 1997, the FDA reported that dexfenfluramine and fenfluramine were voluntarily withdrawn from the market because of their linkage to heart valve defects.

Fluoxetine (commonly known as Prozac) appears to block reuptake of serotonin in nerve endings and thereby potentiates the action of serotonin in serotonergic synapses (Weintraub & Bray, 1989). Fluoxetine belongs to a new class of drugs (e.g., fluoxetine, paroxetine, and sertraline) called selective serotonin reuptake inhibitors (SSRIs) that are currently used clinically to treat depression. The SSRIs have also been shown to suppress appetite and cause weight loss. Fluoxetine was the first widely used SSRI in the U.S., and thus research has focused primarily on this drug. Fluoxetine may suppress intake of fat and carbohydrate more than protein intake (Silverstone & Goodall, 1992). In studies of a large number of obese subjects, fluoxetine has been found to be more effective than a placebo in inducing weight loss (Wise, 1992). Stinson et al. (1992) had obese subjects ingest a placebo or 60 mg fluoxetine for 14 d. The drug did not alter metabolism or thermogenesis but did produce a significant weight loss (1.16 kg), whereas the placebo did not alter weight. The weight loss was primarily due to the anorectic effect of the drug. Compared to amphetamines, the potential for abuse is less, as are the side effects.

The exact mechanisms to explain the action of anorexiant agents on weight loss in obesity are still unclear. However, weight loss is generally regained when these drugs are discontinued (Munro et al., 1992). Pfohl et al. (1994) found that patients taking dexfenfluramine for 1 y lost 11.2% of their initial body weight. They were then followed for 3 y and had regained slightly more than the lost body weight. Moreover, the weight rebound was associated with marked increase in cardiovascular risk factors (increases in serum total cholesterol, triglyceride, blood glucose, and systolic blood pressure). Aging, diet, or increased visceral fat could not explain this increase totally. The authors concluded that weight cycling itself may increase cardiovascular risk factors and that the prevention of weight gain should be the focus of future efforts

For both fenfluramine and fluoxetine there is some small potential for drug abuse and habituation (Hoffman & Lefkowitz, 1996; McKenry & Salerno, 1995; Sanders-Bush & Mayer, 1996). Side effects of fenfluramine include ataxia, sleep disturbances, and increased weakness, and this drug is contraindicated for those with cardiovascular disease, particularly dysrhythmias, hypertension, and hyperthyroidism. Although most of the side effects are mild and self limiting, serious conditions such as primary pulmonary hypertension, heart value, and heart valve defects have been reported with the use of Fen-phen (Abenhaim et al., 1996). Side effects of fluoxetine include insomnia, increased sweating, anxiety, tremor, and dry mouth. With use of these drugs there is a tendency for reliance on medication at the expense of improvement in diet and exercise behavior. Anorexiant agents are recommended to be used with other weight reduction methods, such as diet, exercise, and behavior modification.

Nicotine. Tobacco contains nicotine, which is a natural alkaloid with the primary action of stimulating autonomic ganglia but also affects the neuromuscular junction (Taylor, 1996). Nicotine has no therapeutic use (McKenry & Salerno, 1995). The effects of nicotine on the body are complex and often unpredictable because of its action on a variety of neuroeffector and chemosensitive sites as well as on stimulating and desensitizing receptors (Taylor, 1996). Smoking has long been used as a means to control weight; the mechanisms responsible for this effect are unclear but likely are due to an increase in thermogenesis and decrease in appetite. Nicotine increases catecholamines, particularly noradrenalin, which may be responsible for increasing energy expenditure (Perkins, 1997). Because tobacco smoking can impair performance, most athletes in the United States do not smoke.

Rásky et al. (1996) reported that the incidence of smoking significantly correlated with lower body mass index. Heavy smoking and the cessation of smoking were related to a higher relative weight. From analysis of data obtained from the third National Health and Nutrition Examination Survey (1988–1991), weight change over a 10 y period for subjects who stopped smoking was found to be 4.4 kg for men and 5.0 kg for women over that for those who kept smoking in that same time period (Flegal et al., 1995). Smokers who had ceased smoking within the past 10 y were significantly more likely to become overweight, compared with those who had never smoked (Flegal et al., 1995). Post-cessation weight gain is considered to be due to a decrease in metabolic activity by reduction in nicotine intake (Gray et al., 1995), but its effects on appetite are less clear (Perkins, 1992).

Audrain et al. (1995) examined the effects of smoking on resting energy expenditure (REE) and found that REE was increased in the 30 min post-smoking assessment period. Increases were greatest for normal weight subjects. Obese subjects had less of an increase in the 20 min after smoking, and this was followed by a decreased REE. Thus, obese subjects show an attenuated effect of smoking on energy expenditure, suggesting that smoking is a less effective weight control strategy for obese individuals. Exposure to nicotine significantly increased energy expenditure in males, and the effect was greatest in physically active men with longer smoking exposure histories (Perkins et al., 1995; Perkins et al., 1996). Jensen et al.(1995) found that fat oxidation increased with increasing nicotine uptake in male subjects. Women appear to have a reduced responsiveness regarding energy expenditure, and it was suggested that nicotine may control weight in women by affecting appetite (Perkins et al., 1996).

The effects of nicotine on hunger and appetite are less well understood. In 1991, Perkins et al. found that male smokers reported greater satiation following a meal than did non-smokers, and a nasal spray of nicotine every 20 min for 2 h reduced caloric intake during a meal. However, in a 1992 study from this laboratory (Perkins et al., 1992), male and female smokers after an overnight fast and abstinence from smoking received a nasal spray of nicotine or placebo every 30 min for 2 h. There was no difference in self reports of hunger, and, when given food ad lib, the subjects who received the nicotine spray had greater caloric intake. In a similarly designed study, but using actual cigarette smoking rather than nasal spray, there was no effect of acute cigarette smoking on hunger (Perkins et al., 1994). The authors therefore questioned the notion that nicotine or smoking has an acute anorectic action.

Nicotine must affect food intake and/or appetite in some way over time. Jorenby et al. (1996) reported that a transdermal nicotine patch given for 5 wk to subjects who ceased smoking resulted in a reduced appetite and weight gain, compared to a placebo transdermal patch. In a study of satiety following meal consumption, Perkins et al. (1995) found that smoking had no effect on initial hunger ratings after fasting, but after food intake, the hunger rating declined significantly more in the smoking condition. Perkins (1997) recently suggested that the smaller metabolic effect of nicotine in females must indicate that its action regarding body weight involves a change in food intake.

Several strategies have been used to counteract the weight gain after smoking cessation. Talcott et al. (1995) reported that an intensive program that limits alcohol and high-fat foods and encourages increased physical activity can prevent weight gain after cessation of smoking. A prospective examination of data from the Nurse's Health Study found that smoking cessation was associated with a gain of about 2.4 kg in middle-aged women and that moderate increases in physical activity minimized the weight gain (Kawachi et al., 1996). Other studies have examined drug interventions. Norregaard et al. (1996) found that a combination of ephedrine and caffeine was useful in attenuating weight gain in the 12 wk after smoking, but after 1 y there was no effect. Dexfenfluramine and fluoxetine were effective in reducing weight gain in the 4 wk after smoking cessation, and dexfenfluramine was still effective after 3 mo. However, when the drug was discontinued, similar weight gains to the placebo condition were found in the next 3 mo. Use of drugs to counteract weight gain with smoking cessation are only minimally effective, and substitution of one drug for another seems inappropriate, at best. Diet and exercise strategies are a more sensible choice (Winslow et al., 1996).

Diuretics. Diuretics are used for rapid weight loss. Most commonly used diuretics act by blocking the reabsorption of electrolytes in the kidneys, thus facilitating water loss from the body. Diuretics are used therapeutically for the treatment of edema due to congestive heart failure (Jackson, 1996) and to treat hypertension (McKenry & Salerno, 1995). Continued use of diuretics can result in electrolyte imbalance, which in turn can affect cardiac function and produce muscle cramps. Athletes, such as wrestlers, lightweight crew, bodybuilders and jockeys, who must make a particular weight classification or for whom a low body weight during competition is advantageous have abused diuretics.

The three major categories of diuretics (thiazide diuretics, loop diuretics, and potassium sparing diuretics) differ in their mechanisms of action (Jackson, 1996; McKenry & Salerno, 1995). The thiazide diuretics act on the distal tubules of the kidneys to prevent active sodium reabsorption. The loop diuretics are the most powerful diuretics and act by blocking reabsorption of sodium and chloride ions from the ascending limb of the loop of Henle. The potassium sparing diuretics block sodium/potassium exchange in the late distal tubule and the collecting duct, resulting in excretion of sodium and chloride and retention of potassium. The thiazide and loop diuretics result in a potassium loss from the body, and potassium supplements are often recommended. On the other hand, the potassium-sparing diuretics can cause excessive potassium retention. The action of these drugs is important to take into account because diet and other drugs can have interactive effects. For example, high-potassium diets or potassium supplements would benefit those taking thiazide or loop diuretics but would be dangerous for those taking potassium-sparing diuretics. Disturbances in electrolyte balance can adversely affect many systems, especially cardiac function. Severe disturbances in cardiac electrolyte balance can be life threatening. To increase drug efficacy, some diuretics now include one or more antihypertensive agents (e.g., ACE inhibitors, α-blockers, and β-blockers), and diuretic types are combined (e.g., a potassium-sparing diuretic with a thiazide diuretic).

Diuretics result in weight loss of about 3–4% over a 24 h period (Caldwell et al., 1984; Claremont et al., 1976; Wagner, 1991). For example, 3.4 mg of furosemide (loop diuretic) per kg of body weight given to subjects who were instructed to follow a low calorie/low fluid diet resulted in a significant mean 4.2% weight loss in 24 h (Caldwell et al., 1984). Using a lower dose (40 mg furosemide), Armstrong et al. (1985) reported a 1.6–2.1% weight loss in 5 h.

Diuretic-induced weight loss has been found to impair exercise performance (for review see: Murray, 1995; Sawka & Pandolf, 1990). Nielsen et al. (1981) examined the effect of diuretic-induced dehydration (80 mg furosemide) on cycle ergometry performance; the 18% decrease in physical work capacity was attributed to dehydration, electrolyte shifts, and hyperthermia. Claremont et al. (1976) reported that 40-80 mg furosemide caused an increased heart rate during subsequent exercise and significant increases in muscle and rectal temperatures during exercise in the heat. Likewise, Caldwell et al. (1984) reported that 1.7 mg/kg furosemide significantly reduced maximal work capacity, and Armstrong et al. (1985) found that 40 mg furosemide significantly increased running time in 5,000 and 10,000 m trials. Although laboratory data suggest that diuretics can limit performance, whether or not they actually affect performance during competition is less certain (Horswill, 1994; Steen, 1991).

Although athletes who use them consider diuretics safe, the consequences of diuretic use are of concern. However, the information concerning diuretic abuse in athletes is currently limited to anecdotal evidence and case studies. Bodybuilders find diuretics essential for reducing bloating before competition (Sturmi & Rutecki, 1995). A 27-y-old bodybuilder collapsed shortly after a professional competition and presented with hyperkalemia (Sturmi & Rutecki, 1995). This bodybuilder was using two potassium-sparing diuretics and potassium supplements, which led to excessive potassium retention. In another case report, a 24-y-old professional bodybuilder was taken to the hospital and presented with hyperkalemia and abnormal EKG. He was taking multiple diuretics in a 36 h period before competition (Al-Zaki & Talbot-Stern, 1996). He denied current use of anabolic steroids, alcohol, or other drugs, but it is unclear whether he was taking any of these drugs.

Diuretics represent about 6% of drug abuse by athletes (Al-Zaki & Talbot-Stern, 1996). They can lead to electrolyte imbalance, and because the loss of electrolytes principally involves sodium, a sustained imbalance between sodium intake and sodium loss can be life threatening. In case studies cited above, the patients described symptoms of muscle cramps, spasms and paralysis, conditions associated with hyperkalemia induced by use of potassium-sparing diuretics complicated by use of potassium supplements. Because of the dangers associated with diuretic use, most diuretics are available only by prescription to treat medical conditions such as reducing fluid load with congestive heart failure. To prescribe these to athletes for weight-reduction purposes would be considered a breach of medical ethics.

WEIGHT GAIN

Individuals who desire to gain weight want to do so by increasing muscle mass. Not only is this important for bodybuilders and strength-training athletes, but the ideal for all young men is to be muscular, and today that image is more muscular than ever. Even women want to obtain a more toned or muscular body, as titles of exercise videos such as Buns of Steel© attest. Nutritional supplements to increase muscle mass abound. When these fail to achieve the desired outcome, many athletes have turned to pharmaceutical interventions.

Nutritional Supplements for Weight Gain

The four most popular supplements to enhance muscle mass are chromium, creatine, protein, and amino acids. These supplements are often promoted and even available for purchase in weight training centers. The efficacy of other supplements marketed for weight gain, such as protein formulations that include such ingredients as "special" enzymes, spirulina, or brewer's yeast, have not been scientifically tested.

Chromium. Chromium supplements have been shown to increase muscle mass and growth in animals (Stoecker, 1996), but data on humans are scant (Table 8-1). Evans (1989) was the first to report that chromium increased lean tissue in exercising humans. The theoretical basis to suggest that chromium may exert such an effect is that chromium potentiates insulin action, and insulin stimulates amino acid uptake by cells (Lefavi et al., 1992; Mertz, 1992). In the Evans' studies, untrained college students and trained football players were given 200 μg of chromium picolinate or a placebo each day for 40–42 d while they were on a resistance exercise program. The authors reported that untrained subjects and the football players on chromium supplements gained significantly more lean body mass, compared to the placebo group. However, lean body mass was only estimated from circumference measures, and the changes observed were small so that it is possible that measurement error influenced the results.

Four studies have since tried to confirm the results of the Evans' studies. Hasten et al. (1992) gave students participating in a weight training program either 200 μg of chromium picolinate or a placebo for 12 wk. Only small increases in body weight were found for males either on the placebo or the chromium supplements or for females on the placebo. However, the treatment effect was significant due to the females who took the chromium supplements and gained 2.5 kg of body weight (Figure 8-4). The authors offered several speculations for the in-

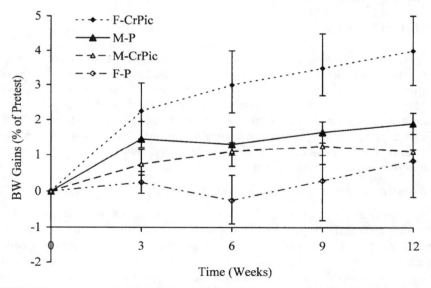

FIGURE 8-4. *Body weight gains over 12 wk expressed as a percentage of initial weight. F-CrPic = women taking chromium picolinate supplements; M-P = men taking the placebo; M-CrPic = men taking chromium picolinate supplements; and F-P = women taking the placebo.* Data from Hasten et al. (1992).

crease in body weight for only the females taking chromium: 1) females may have a chromium deficient diet (diet was not assessed); 2) the dose per body weight was greater for females; 3) females may be less insulin resistant than are males, and 4) the relatively large gain found for untrained subjects just beginning a weight training program may mask any effect of the supplement for the males. However, it is not known from this study if the increase in body weight for the females was due to muscle mass.

To further examine the effects of chromium on lean body weight in athletes, Clancy et al. (1994) gave chromium picolinate (200 µg/d) supplements or placebo for 9 wk to college football players participating in a resistance-training program. Underwater weighing and anthropometric measurements were used to assess changes in body composition, food diaries were kept, and urinary chromium excretion was assessed. Changes in skinfold measures, percent body fat, lean body mass, and circumference measures were not significantly different between groups. Urinary chromium excretion before supplementation was low and undetectable in many subjects, and this was also found for the subjects on the placebo group at weeks 4 and 9. However, for the chromium-supplemented group, urinary chromium excretion significantly increased at 4 wk and remained elevated through 9 wk. These data could suggest that chromium stores were adequate and extra ingested chromium was excreted. Another study (Hallmark et al., 1996), using virtually the same study design as the Clancy et al. (1994) study but with untrained males, also found no benefit to lean body mass with chromium supplements.

In a well-controlled study, Lukaski et al. (1996) examined the effect of 8 wk of chromium chloride, chromium picolinate, or a placebo in untrained men who started a resistance-training program. Body composition was carefully assessed by skinfolds, circumferences, and dual X-ray absortiometry. Compliance and dietary intake were also assessed. The subjects were matched for specific physical and nutritional characteristics before assigning them to groups. The two types of chromium supplements similarly increased urinary chromium excretion significantly (Figure 8-5). No effect of the supplements was found on any measure of body composition.

Thus, it appears that chromium supplements are not effective in increasing lean body mass. They may be effective in subjects who are chromium deficient, but this has not been established. Further studies are needed to determine the relationship between chromium status and muscular adaptations to resistance training.

Creatine. Creatine has received widespread attention as an ergogenic aid (Balsom et al., 1994; Volek & Kraemer, 1996). Several studies

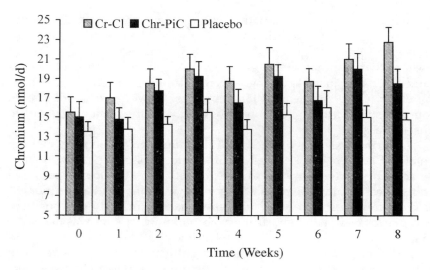

FIGURE 8-5. *Urinary chromium excretion in 3-d pooled samples taken prior to (0) and during 8 wk of resistance training while taking either chromium chloride (light shaded bar), chromium picolinate (dark shaded bar) and placebo (open bar).* Data from Lukaski et al. (1996).

also reported that creatine supplementation (20–30 g/d for about 5 d) caused a significant increase in body weight of about 1–3 kg (See Table 8-2). In the one study to assess body composition by underwater weighing, Earnest et al. (1995) gave subjects 20 g creatine per day for 28 d and found a 1.7 kg increase in body weight, but there was no significant increase in fat free mass. It was interesting to note that the increase in body weight occurred despite a lower daily energy intake for the creatine-supplemented group.

Balsom et al. (1993a) reported that eight subjects gained from 0.3–2.5 kg of body weight after ingesting 30 g of creatine for 6 d. The subject who gained 2.5 kg was a vegetarian. Harris et al. (1992) found that creatine uptake was greatest in two vegetarian subjects, which is consistent with other findings that creatine stores are lower in vegetarians (Delanghe et al., 1989). The variability in response to creatine may reflect an individual's creatine status before supplementation.

The mechanism to explain the increase in body weight is not known. Ingestion of 20 g of creatine markedly increases muscle creatine levels in 4–5 d (Harris et al., 1992). Creatine could act as an osmotic agent in skeletal muscle and increase water retention in cells (Volek & Kraemer, 1996). Hultman et al. (1996) found a 0.6 L decline in urinary volume that occurred at the onset of creatine ingestion, suggesting that increases in body weight could be due to body water retention. The au-

TABLE 8-2. *Effects of Creatine Supplementation on Body Weight.*

Study	Subjects	Length	Treatment Creatine g/d	N	Initial BW (kg)	Change (kg) in body weight	Effect of Cr significant?
Earnest et al. (1995) *	Weight trained ♂	28 d	Placebo 20	4 4	86.5	-0.1 +1.7	Yes
Viru et al. (1993)	Middle distance runners	6 d	Placebo 30	5 5	NR NR	NR +1.8	NR
Balsom et al. (1993a)	♂ PE students	6 d	Placebo 25	8 8	NR 84.2	NR +1.1	Yes
Balsom et al. (1995)	Active ♂	6 d	20	7	78.3	+1.1	Yes
Balsom et al. (1993b)	Active ♂	6 d	Placebo 20	9 9	73.6 73.5	-0.5 +0.9	Yes
Greenhaff et al. (1994)	Recreational	5 d	20 g	8	80.0	+1.6	Yes
Redondo et al. (1996)	College athletes	7 d	Placebo 25 g	9 9	69.7 63.5	0.0 -0.8	NR
Mujika et al. (1996)	Elite swimmers	5 d	Placebo 20 g	10 10	70.4 71.7	-0.3 +0.7	Yes
Stroud et al. (1994)	Active ♂	5 d	20 g	8	75.9	+1.0	Yes
Green et al. (1996)	Healthy ♂	5 d	20 g (no sugar) 20 g (with sugar)	12 9	79.0 (mean for both groups)	+0.9 +1.6	Yes
Söderlund et al. (1994)	♂	6 d	20 g	6	NR	+1.5	Yes
Dawson et al. (1995) 2 studies	Active ♂	5 d	Placebo 20 g	9 9	76.8 77.4	-0.1 +0.7	Yes
	Active ♂	5 d	Placebo 20 g	11 11	74.5 75.7	+0.4 +0.5	No

* This study also assessed lean body mass by underwater weighing and found a −0.5 change for the supplemented group and a +1.6 kg change for the placebo group. In all the other studies only body weight was measured, and diet was neither controlled nor assessed. Dietary intake was assessed in one study (NS). Dietary intake was assessed (NS). In all the other studies only body weight was measured, and diet was neither controlled nor assessed, other than instructing subjects to maintain normal diet and exercise patterns.

NR—Not Reported

thors noted that the time course of changes in urinary volume paralleled the time course of muscle creatine uptake found in a previous study (Harris et al., 1992). Flisińska-Bojanowska (1996) reported that creatine ingestion (100 mg/kg body weight) for 6–9 d in rats increased soluble and myofibrillar protein in skeletal muscle, especially red muscle. However, Ööpik et al. (1995) did not find an increase in protein synthesis in rats ingesting a larger dose of creatine (400 mg/kg body weight) for 7 d, nor did they find an increase in water content of muscle or in relative muscle weight. Further research is needed to explain what causes the rapid increase in body weight in humans after creatine ingestion.

Protein. Many supplements containing protein and various amino acid combinations are marketed to those who wish to increase lean muscle mass. Weight lifters and bodybuilders believe they need this extra protein. The recommended dietary allowance for protein intake is 0.8 g · kg^{-1} · d^{-1} (Food and Nutrition Board, 1989), but several studies have indicated that athletes require greater amounts. Other detailed reviews are available for additional information concerning protein requirements in athletes (Lemon, 1991, 1992, 1994).

Exercise increases protein use or protein degradation. Muscle protein synthesis was significantly increased for up to 24 h after strength-trained subjects performed a bout of heavy resistance exercise (Chesley et al., 1992). Subjects were infused with ^{13}C-leucine, and muscle biopsy samples were taken before, 4 h, and 24 h after exercise to determine the amount of ^{13}C-leucine isotope in the sample. An incorporation of this isotope into muscle indicated that leucine was being assimilated into protein. In another study using a similar technique, protein synthesis was elevated for 2 wk during the beginning of a resistance training program in previously untrained individuals (Yarasheski et al., 1993). Thus, resistance training increases protein synthesis in skeletal muscle, and this may, in a large part, serve to explain the increased protein requirement for strength-training athletes.

Protein needs during strength training have been assessed by several nitrogen balance studies. Tarnopolsky et al. (1988) examined nitrogen balance and body composition in six male bodybuilders who had been training for at least 3 y and not using anabolic steroids. The bodybuilders consumed two diets for 10 d each, one consisting of 1.05 g of protein · kg^{-1} · d^{-1} and the other consisting of 2.77 g of protein · kg^{-1} · d^{-1}. Both protein intakes caused a positive nitrogen balance, but the values were significantly greater on the high protein diet. However, there was no decrease in any of the anthropometric measures on the low protein diet, nor was there an increase on the high protein diet. Thus, it appears that lean body mass was not altered in response to higher nitrogen retention, at least in this short period of time.

Marable et al. (1979) studied college men who consumed either 0.8 g or 2.4 g of protein/kg body weight for 28 d, with some subjects participating in a resistance exercise program and others serving as controls. The authors concluded that the lower protein diet was marginal in maintaining nitrogen balance, whereas the diet with more protein did maintain balance. Other studies reported that a protein intake of about 2.0 g of protein $\cdot$ kg^{-1} $\cdot$ d^{-1} was required to maintain a positive nitrogen balance in strength-training athletes (Celejowa et al., 1970; Laritcheva et al., 1978). However, when 2 g of protein $\cdot$ kg^{-1} $\cdot$ d^{-1} was consumed by strength athletes to supplement their dietary intakes of 1.3 g of protein $\cdot$ kg^{-1} $\cdot$ d^{-1} for 4 wk, whole body protein synthesis increased, and significantly more lean body mass was achieved (Fern et al., 1991) (Figure 8-6). This study also found an increase in amino acid oxidation, which suggests that protein intake exceeded what was needed for muscle growth (Lemon, 1994). Tarnopolsky et al. (1992) found that increasing protein intake to 2.4 g of protein $\cdot$ kg^{-1} $\cdot$ d^{-1} did not increase protein synthesis more than 1.4 g $\cdot$ kg^{-1} $\cdot$ d^{-1} but did increase amino acid oxidation.

Protein and other nutrient intake could affect hormonal status. Volek et al. (1997) found that resting blood testosterone concentrations in 12 men were negatively correlated with percent energy from protein ($r = -0.71$) and with the protein to carbohydrate ratio ($r = -0.63$) but were correlated positively with percent fat, saturated fatty acids, and

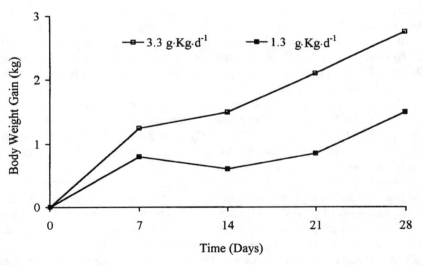

FIGURE 8-6. *Changes in body weight over 28 d while subjects ingested a diet of either 1.3 g of protein/kg of body weight or 3.3 g of protein/kg body weight. All subjects participated in a heavy resistance-training program during the 28 d. Data from Fern et al. (1991).*

mono-unsaturated fatty acids. These data suggest that dietary nutrients may modulate resting concentrations of testosterone. Further studies are needed to confirm and explain these findings.

Lemon (1995) suggested that a range of 1.4–1.8 g of protein $\cdot$ kg$^{-1} \cdot$ d^{-1} is needed for most strength-training individuals. A beginning athlete in the first 2–3 wk of training may need more protein than an experienced athlete would (Lemon, 1992). However, once adapted to the training, a positive nitrogen balance returns. Ingestion of protein at the low end of the range is suggested for experienced athletes, and ingestion of the high end is suggested for beginners. At this point there is not sufficient information to definitively state that protein intake above 2.0 g of protein $\cdot$ kg$^{-1} \cdot$ d^{-1} will enhance muscle mass.

If athletes require more protein than non-athletes, should they then consider taking protein supplements? Most athletes ingest a large amount of energy, and their protein intake generally meets or exceeds the recommended range for strength-trained athletes. Athletes ingesting energy-restricted diets, athletes who make poor food choices, and vegetarians may not meet their protein needs. Adequate energy intake as well as adequate protein is needed to promote muscle mass gains. In fact, protein needs can be greater when energy intake is low (Butterfield et al., 1992). Also, inadequate ingestion of carbohydrate causes more rapid depletion of glycogen during exercise, which would contribute to increased use of protein for energy (Lemon, 1992).

Amino Acids. Arginine and ornithine and even histidine, lysine, methionine, and phenylalanine are purported to have an anabolic effect. Two studies (Elam, 1988; Elam et al., 1989) reported that ingestion of arginine and ornithine in conjunction with resistance training significantly increased body mass and decreased body fat compared to placebo. However, body composition was only estimated from skinfold measures, and diet was not controlled.

It is claimed that these amino acids stimulate growth hormone and insulin release, which will increase muscle mass (Jacobson, 1990; Kreider et al., 1993). Bucci et al. (1990,1992) were among the first to investigate this possibility in athletes. Bodybuilders were given 40, 100, or 170 mg/kg of L-ornithine on three occasions. No increase in serum insulin was found, but there was a significant increase in growth hormone after 170 mg ornithine/kg body weight (about 12 g). In the only study to use lower amino acid doses and find a significant positive response, Isidori et al. (1981) reported that 1.2 g l-lysine and 1.2 g l-arginine, together but not alone, produced an increase in growth hormone and insulin.

In contrast, Fogelholm et al. (1993) examined the effect of 4 d of combined L-arginine, L-ornithine, and L-lysine supplements (2 g/d each) on serum growth hormone and insulin and found no effect. Lambert et al. (1993) had male bodybuilders ingest 2.4 g arginine/lysine supplement, a 1.85 g ornithine/tyrosine supplement, or a protein drink and found no enhancement of growth hormone release. When elite junior weight lifters were given an amino acid supplement containing most amino acids during 1 wk of high volume training, the supplement did not increase blood levels of growth hormone, testosterone, or cortisol at rest or during exercise (Fry et al., 1993). Although Suminski et al. (1997) found that 1.5 g L-arginine and 1.5 g L-lysine increased growth hormone at rest, the increase was small (7.5 μg/L), transient, and highly variable among subjects. Furthermore, ingestion of these amino acids prior to a bout of resistance exercise did not affect the growth hormone response to exercise. Walberg-Rankin et al. (1994) found that 200 mg arginine/kg neither increased serum growth hormone after supplementation nor influenced weight loss, fat, lean tissue, or strength over 10 days. The latter study was the only one to assess body composition and muscle function.

The weight of the evidence suggests that amino acid supplementation is unlikely to increase growth hormone release and alter body weight. Commercially available amino acid supplements contain less than 4 g per serving. Higher levels of amino acids can cause mild to severe stomach cramping and diarrhea. When the manufacturer-recommended doses were ingested, the purported increases in growth hormone and insulin did not occur. Thus, there is little reason to believe that amino acid supplements will promote gains in muscle mass.

Pharmacological Agents for Weight Gain

Pharmacological agents for weight gain are among the most abused drugs in sport (Wadler, 1994). In the 1996 Atlanta Games, two Olympic athletes were disqualified for positive steroid tests. Some commercial publications openly discuss drug use, effectiveness, and testing. Articles abound on the latest high-tech drugs, such as clenbuterol, as well as the old stand-bys, the anabolic steroids.

β_2 **Agonists.** Clenbuterol, salbutamol (albuterol), and metaproterenol are β_2 agonists that purportedly enhance muscle mass. Animal studies have shown that clenbuterol causes muscle hypertrophy, a decrease in fat deposition, and a conversion of slow-twitch fibers to fast-twitch fibers (Dodd et al., 1996; Prather et al., 1995; Spann & Winter, 1995), although not all studies have reported a fiber-type conversion (Ingalls et al., 1996). Criswell et al. (1996) found that 6 wk of clenbuterol treatment in rats increased type II fiber area due to hypertrophy of the type II fibers as well as an increase in fiber frequency, which suggests an increase in number. The mechanisms underlying these effects are not clear, but it is thought that clenbuterol exerts a suppressive effect on the balance of protein synthesis and protein degradation and reduces fat stores (Astrup et al., 1992c; Prather et al., 1995). β_2 agonists also have thermogenic properties, as discussed in a previous section (Astrup et al., 1992c). It should be noted that β_2 agonists are not completely selective for β_2 receptors but also have some activity on β_1 receptors (Hoffman & Lefkowitz, 1996; McKenry & Salerno, 1995). This latter action may not be evident with therapeutic levels of the drugs; however, if these drugs are abused, then blood levels could be reached that activate β_1 receptors and lead to serious cardiac-related problems.

Although clenbuterol is widely accepted in the athletic arena as a drug to enhance muscle mass, there are no studies of the effects of clenbuterol on muscle mass in athletes. In one animal study (Murphy et al., 1996) it was noted that clenbuterol increased muscle mass in animals that were untrained but not in animals that were trained. Salbutamol is commonly used to treat asthma, and preliminary results of animal studies suggest it may be anabolic as well (Martineau et al., 1992). A few studies have found positive effects on muscle strength but not on muscle mass.

Maltin et al. (1993) studied the effect of 20 µg of clenbuterol given twice daily for 4 wk to patients recovering from open medial meniscectomy. Drug or placebo treatment was started 12 h after the surgery. Knee extension isometric strength and cross sectional area of the knee extensors—assessed by computed tomography (CT)—were determined before and after surgery. The subjects taking clenbuterol showed a significantly faster recovery of strength when compared with the placebo group. There was about a 50% loss in isometric strength at 1 wk post-surgery for both groups; however, at 3 wk post-surgery the strength of patients in the clenbuterol group had returned to baseline, but there was still a significant strength loss for the placebo group. For the unoperated leg, there was no change in strength over the 4 wk of recovery. The change in cross sectional area was small for both groups, with no difference between the groups. The mechanism to explain the faster strength recovery rate with clenbuterol is not known, but the authors suggested that β_2 agonists could affect muscle excitability, which may contribute to improved strength. Clenbuterol also has an antidepressant action and may serve as an analgesic, although the authors consider this an unlikely explanation for the faster recovery (Maltin et al., 1993).

Signorile et al. (1995) tested the effect of 80 mg/d metaproterenol or placebo for 4 wk on isometric strength and cross sectional area of the elbow and wrist flexors and extensors of 10 males with spinal cord injuries; they found that the drug improved strength but did not affect cross-sectional area. Elbow flexion isometric strength for the drug and placebo groups significantly increased 4.7 kg and 2.6 kg, respectively. Corresponding values for wrist flexion isometric strength were 5.7 kg and 2.6 kg and for wrist extension isometric strength were 2.9 kg and −0.1 kg, respectively. There was no significant change for elbow extension strength, but only four subjects had measurable triceps function.

In a study of 12 healthy men, Martineau et al. (1992) examined the effect of a slow-release formulation of salbutamol (8 mg Volmax® twice daily) or placebo after 14 and 21 d of treatment. Isometric strength of the quadriceps and hamstring muscles of both legs and grip strength were assessed weekly. For the drug-treated group but not the placebo group, there was an improvement in strength for both quadriceps muscles (13.5%; ranging from 10–27% in five of the six subjects—no change for one subject) and non-dominant hamstrings muscles (18.0%; ranging from 13–48%) but no improvement for hand grip muscles. No changes in body weight, skinfold thickness, or limb circumferences were found.

The effects of 16 mg/d of albuterol or placebo were assessed in healthy men for 6 wk while they participated in an isokinetic strength training program for the knee extensors (Caruso et al., 1995). Before and after training, both concentric and eccentric strength were assessed as mean peak torque, total work, and average power for 10 repetitions at 45°/s. There was no difference between treatments in the change in thigh cross-sectional area estimated by circumference measures. Although the authors stated that most measures of strength showed a greater increase with the drug, compared with the placebo, scrutiny of the strength data and examination of the reported statistical analysis show that only eccentric total work and average power demonstrated significant interaction terms in the analysis of variance. Eccentric total work for the placebo and albuterol conditions increased 13.2% and 45.0%, respectively. Eccentric average power increased 15.9% and 41.0%, respectively, for the placebo and albuterol groups. However, the amount of absolute and relative change in concentric average power from before to after treatment for the placebo group was 11.9 N·m and 49.5%, respectively, compared with 12.7 N·m and 36.4% for the albuterol group.

Although these studies did not find an increase in muscle size with β_2 agonist treatments, the doses used in clinical studies may be much smaller than those used by athletes. The doses used were greater than doses recommended for the treatment of asthma but still below those used in animal models in which the drugs were shown to increase muscle mass (Prather et al, 1995). Due to other activities of the drug when used in excess, use of β_2 agonists may cause serious problems for individuals with cardiac problems, diabetes mellitus, hyperthyroidism, and hypertension. Significant drug interaction occurs with monamine oxidase inhibitors and tricyclic antidepressants. The most prominent side effect is skeletal muscle tremor, but tachycardia, nausea, and anxiety are also reported (Hoffman & Lefkowitz, 1996; McKenry & Salerno, 1995).

Clenbuterol is often used in combination with other drugs such as growth hormone, ephedrine, and anabolic steroids (Prather et al., 1995). Also, it should be noted that most studies assessed muscle mass by circumference measures, and because these measures are quite variable, it may be impossible to detect small differences. At present there are no data showing that clenbuterol or other β_2 agonists have anabolic effects in humans.

Anabolic-Androgenic Steroids. Anabolic-androgenic steroids are synthetic derivatives of testosterone that are widely used to increase muscle mass in athletes (Lamb, 1984; Wade, 1972). Testosterone is the most abundant of the male sex hormones called androgens, which are secreted by the testes. Secretion of testosterone after puberty results in male secondary sex characteristics, including anabolic effects on muscle. The synthetic derivatives of testosterone increase protein synthesis in muscle and hence are commonly called anabolic steroids, but a pure anabolic steroid with no androgenic effects has not been developed (Bahrke et al., 1996).

Not only do anabolic steroids stimulate protein synthesis, they also have anti-catabolic effects by competing with glucocorticoids for receptor sites (Haupt & Rovere, 1984). These drugs were introduced in the 1950s to treat victims of muscle wasting diseases (Marieb, 1992) and are used to reverse protein loss after trauma, surgery, or prolonged immobilization, and to treat delayed male puberty (McKenry & Salerno, 1995; Wilson, 1996). They are also used to maintain muscle mass in the elderly. It was not long after these steroids were developed that they began to be used by athletes. Numerous reviews are available on anabolic steroids and their impact in sport (e.g., Bahrke et al., 1996; Bahrke & Yesalis, 1994; Haupt & Rovere, 1984; Hough, 1990; Lombardo et al., 1991).

Several studies have reported increases in body weight or muscle mass with anabolic steroid use. Hervey et al. (1981) found that experienced weight lifters taking 100 mg/d of methandienone (Dianabol®) for 6 wk with no dietary controls showed a significant increase in lean body mass that amounted to only 3.13 kg. Loughton and Ruhling (1977) reported 5.6 kg and 5.0 kg increases in body weight in trained and untrained subjects, respectively, when they ingested anabolic steroids (10 mg/d of Dianabol® for 3 wk and then 5 mg/d for 3 wk) while participating in a training program, compared with 3.0 and 1.2 kg, respectively, for the placebo groups. Griggs et al. (1989) reported that testosterone enanthate (3 mg $\cdot$ kg^{-1} $\cdot$ wk^{-1}) for 12 wk significantly increased body weight by 5 kg and also increased muscle protein synthesis. In a longer term study, Alén et al. (1984) found that 24 wk of steroid self administration (an average of 31 mg/d each of methandienone, stanozolol, and nandrolone, and an average of 178 mg/wk of testosterone) during strength training produced a 5.1 kg increase in body weight, compared to a −0.6 kg change for the control group. It is interesting to note that when the treatment was discontinued, within the following 6 wk subjects lost more than half of the weight gained.

The American College of Sports Medicine (1987) in a position statement concluded that steroid use in the presence of an adequate diet will increase fat free mass, but the amount of weight gain is relatively small (3–6 kg). However, most studies of steroid effects used doses much smaller than those reportedly used by athletes. Moreover, athletes use multiple hormones in various combinations and may take 10–100 times the therapeutic dose of a given drug (Thein et al., 1994; Wadler et al., 1994). Other problems with many of the studies are that diet, exercise, or the subjects' levels of training were not well controlled.

In a well-controlled study, Bhasin et al.(1996) examined the effects of supraphysiologic doses of testosterone in four groups of men who had weight training experience: placebo with no exercise, testosterone with no exercise, placebo with resistance training, and testosterone with resistance training. The dose was 600 mg testosterone enanthate or placebo injected intramuscularly weekly for 10 wk. Subjects in the exercise group received controlled, supervised strength training 3 d/wk. Intake of energy and protein was controlled; subjects followed a standardized diet containing 36 kcal $\cdot$ kg^{-1} $\cdot$ d^{-1} with 1.5 g $\cdot$ kg^{-1} $\cdot$ d^{-1} protein. Muscle size was assessed by magnetic resonance imaging (MRI) of the arms and legs, and body composition was determined by underwater weighing. Strength was assessed by one-repetition maximums (1 RM) of the bench press and the squat. There were no changes in body weight or muscle size for the placebo group. Both groups that received testosterone showed significant increases in body weight and in triceps and quadriceps cross-sectional areas. The testosterone/exercise group demonstrated the greatest increase in body weight (6.1 kg), which was entirely accounted for by the change in fat free mass. The testosterone-only group showed an increase of 3.5 kg (Figure 8-7). Both groups who received testosterone showed a significant increase in bench-press and squatting strength. However, the testosterone/exercise group demonstrated the greatest increase in squatting and bench-press strength, compared with the testosterone/no exercise group. These data clearly show that supraphysiologic doses of testosterone, especially when combined with resistance exercise, increased muscle mass.

There are many known side effects of using anabolic-androgenic steroids (Haupt & Rovere, 1984; McKenry & Salerno, 1995; Wilson, 1996). Side effects reported by athletes include changes in libido, increased aggressiveness, muscle spasms, and gynecomastia, which were reversible upon discontinuance of the drugs. Use of anabolic steroids

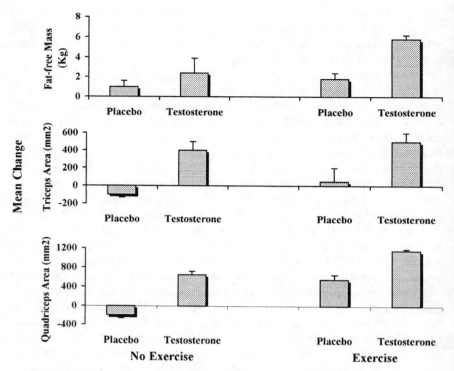

FIGURE 8-7. *Changes in fat-free mass, triceps area, and quadriceps area in subjects receiving placebo or testosterone for 10 wk. Subjects in each group were assigned to either a resistance-training regimen or no exercise for the 10 wk.* Data from Bhasin et al. (1996).

has also been linked to liver damage, cardiomyopathy, cancer, and testicular atrophy (Thein et al., 1995). Many of the anabolic steroids that are being used by athletes are either veterinary drugs or other unapproved derivatives for which safety data for humans is incomplete (Wilson, 1996).

   Human Growth Hormone. Administration of growth hormone (GH) is currently used in replacement therapy to treat growth hormone deficiency in children (Ascoli & Segaloff, 1996). Also, GH is being investigated as an adjunct treatment for several catabolic conditions such as burn injures, surgery, and malabsorption and may prove useful in the treatment of osteoporosis because of its role in calcium retention and osteogenesis (Ascoli & Segaloff, 1996). However, in the 1980's it grew in favor among athletes as a rival or complementary hormone to anabolic steroids (Wadler, 1994). GH may be popular because its use is more difficult to detect than anabolic steroid use. Sensitive tests for GH use by athletes are being developed, and it is expected that they will be available for the 2000 Olympic Games in Australia (David Cowan, 1997, personal communication).

Growth hormone increases protein deposition by facilitating amino acid uptake and protein synthesis and reducing protein catabolism (Thein et al., 1995; Wadler et al., 1994). Studies have found that patients with GH deficiency who received GH injections showed increases in lean body mass (Wirth & Gieck, 1996). How GH exerts an effect on target cells is not completely understood, but some of its action appears to involve the somatomedin peptides, specifically insulin-like growth factor (IGF-1). GH stimulates the liver to produce somatomedins, which have potent growth-promoting effects. IGF-1 may mediate many of the actions of growth hormone, and it is being investigated as a therapeutic agent (Ascoli & Segaloff, 1996).

Few studies have assessed the effects of growth hormone on muscle mass in healthy men. Yarasheski et al. (1992) examined GH administration (40 $\mu g \cdot kg^{-1} \cdot d^{-1}$) for 12 wk in untrained men (21–34 y) who were participating in a resistance exercise program. They found a greater increase in fat-free body mass and whole-body protein synthesis in the group receiving GH, compared with the placebo. However, muscle protein synthesis and muscle size (assessed by circumference measures) for the quadriceps were similar in both groups. The authors suggested that the increase in fat-free mass might be due to increases in lean tissue other than skeletal muscle. Prolonged GH administration may induce a down-regulation of the muscle GH receptors, thus exerting no effect on muscle mass (Yarasheski et al., 1992).

A study of resistance trained men (22–33 y) who were administered 30–50 $\mu g /$ kg of GH (3 times per wk) or placebo for 6 wk while continuing to participate in resistance exercise showed that those who received GH had a significant increase in fat-free weight and a decrease in fat mass, compared to the placebo group, but the changes were small (Christ et al., 1988). Moreover, this study reported that exogenous GH suppressed endogenous GH release. In contrast, Deyssig et al. (1993) evaluated the effects of placebo vs. GH therapy (0.09 U $\cdot$ kg^{-1} d^{-1}, i.e., about 35 $\mu g \cdot$ kg$^{-1} \cdot$ d^{-1}) for 6 wk in experienced male power athletes and reported no significant change in body weight or body fat as a result of GH treatment. Yarasheski et al. (1993) examined the effect of short-term GH injections (40 $\mu g \cdot$ kg^{-1} d^{-1} for 14 d) in experienced weight lifters and found that the GH treatment did not increase the rate of muscle protein synthesis or reduce the rate of protein breakdown.

In a study of older men (61–81 y), Rudman et al. (1990) found that 6 mo of GH injections resulted in a significant 8.8% increase in fat-free mass and a significant 14.4% decrease in fat mass while the placebo group showed no change. Likewise, Taaffe et al. (1994) found that older subjects (65–82 y) who participated in a weight training program for 14 wk and were then given injections of GH showed a significant increase in lean body mass and a decrease in fat mass, compared with the placebo. Welle et al. (1996) reported that older subjects given GH injections for 3 mo significantly increased both lean body mass and muscle mass evaluated by urinary creatinine excretion, but the rates of myofibrillar protein synthesis or whole body protein synthesis were not affected. Also, Yarasheski et al. (1995) found that compared to the placebo group, there was no increase in muscle protein synthesis and urinary creatinine excretion, despite a significant increase in fat free mass, in older men who were treated with GH for 16 wk while participating in a resistance exercise program. Also, Papadakis et al. (1996) found that 6 mo of GH treatment in older men did not improve muscular strength, $\dot{V}O_2$max, or performance on motor control tests. These studies used GH doses of about 20–40 µg/kg body weight.

Thus, it appears that GH may increase lean body mass and decrease fat mass, but the increase in lean tissue is not due to an increase in muscle protein synthesis. However, Welle et al. (1996) pointed out that only a small increase in protein synthesis may be needed to increase muscle mass, and a small increase may not be detectable statistically, considering the variability in the measures. The increase in lean tissue also could be due to an increase in fluid retention or an increase in connective tissue or organ mass (Wirth & Gieck, 1996).

Use of GH has several side effects. It can cause a thickening of bones leading to disfigurement, a condition known as acromegaly. GH also can also cause glucose intolerance, impaired thyroid function, peripheral neuropathy, increased plasma cholesterol and triglyceride concentrations, coronary artery disease, cardiomyopathy, and muscle and joint weakness (Thein et al., 1995). Use of GH in diabetes mellitus is especially risky because GH induces insulin resistance (Ascoli & Segaloff, 1996). Also, concomitant glucocorticoid therapy, as is used in the treatment of asthma, allergy and rheumatoid disorders, may interfere with the growth promoting effects of GH.

PRACTICAL IMPLICATIONS

Losing weight is a preoccupation not only of many overweight individuals in the general population but also of numerous athletes who are already relatively lean. These athletes want to lose weight for a number of reasons. In sports such as gymnastics and dance, where aesthetics matter, athletes strive to achieve a certain slender image. Distance runners and other athletes who need to move a given mass are convinced that a lower body weight will translate into improved performance, although inappropriate weight loss could actually impair performance and may precipitate an eating disorder (Clarkson & Going, 1996). Another reason athletes want to lose weight is to "cut weight" prior to a weigh-in, such as in wrestling, or prior to competition, such as in bodybuilding. In these instances, quick weight loss is desired.

Counseling for weight loss in athletes should include ways to adjust or modify diet and exercise. Nutritional supplements are unlikely to be effective. Pharmacological supplements may impair performance because those that act to increase energy expenditure, e.g., ephedrine and β_3 agonists, act on the sympathetic nervous system and therefore can increase tremor, cause nervousness, and exert effects on the cardiovascular system. Moreover, there may be differences between lean and obese individuals in thermogenesis so that leaner subjects may not show the same response to these drugs. Although anorexiant drugs enhance weight loss in obese subjects, the effects on individuals who are already relatively lean are not known. Furthermore, there is always a large inter-subject variability in response to drugs, and there are untoward side effects, ranging from mild gastrointestinal symptoms to life-threatening conditions such as pulmonary hypertension.

Athletes should be taught that "diet pills" are probably ineffective. Even if they were effective, the amount of weight loss would be small, and the weight would be regained when the diet pills were discontinued. Due to side effects, these pharmacological agents are more likely to impair performance than to improve it. A healthy diet with modifications to reduce energy intake is the best bet for reducing weight and maintaining optimal training and performance. It should be noted that for obese individuals, a relatively small weight loss, 5–10%, is associated with improvements in obesity-related co-morbidities (National Task Force on the Prevention and Treatment of Obesity, 1996). Thus, in the pharmacological treatment of obesity, the gains can outweigh the risks of the drug.

Wrestlers and bodybuilders commonly use diuretics for quick weight loss. These are effective in producing a 2–4% decrease in body weight in 24 h. Because these athletes consider diuretics safe, the potential for abuse is high. However, abuse of these drugs can be life threatening. There are several case reports of bodybuilders who developed severe muscle cramps and serious cardiac problems due to diuretic abuse. Diuretics cause a disturbance in electrolyte balance that leads to cardiac and skeletal muscle dysfunction. Athletes' lack of knowledge regarding the various kinds of diuretics and their specific interactions with certain foods and supplements make their use particularly dangerous.

Athletes undergoing resistance training who want to gain muscle mass will more than likely already be taking protein and amino acid supplements, creatine, and/or chromium. There is little evidence to support the efficacy of chromium as an anabolic agent. Creatine (about 20 g/d) consistently has been found to increase body weight by about 2–3 kg within a week. What is not known is whether this reflects an increase in skeletal muscle protein or an increase in water retention. Furthermore, creatine appears to be more effective in vegetarians and others who initially have lower body stores of creatine. Although the estimated daily need for creatine is about 2 g, and the average American diet contains only about 1 g, the body can produce creatine to compensate for the lack in the diet (Eichner, 1997). Perhaps the body's production of creatine cannot entirely compensate for the lack of dietary creatine in vegetarians.

Because 20 g/d of creatine increases body weight in a few days, after which a reduced dose is recommended (5 g/d; maintenance program), creatine is not considered to be harmful. However, there is concern that athletes may continue to take the 20 g/d dose, and consequences of this practice are not known. Twenty grams of creatine is about the amount contained in 5.5 kg of raw steak (Eichner, 1997).

Resistance-training athletes need more protein (1.4–1.8 g of protein $\cdot$ kg$^{-1}\cdot$d^{-1}) than what is recommended (0.8 g of protein$\cdot$kg$^{-1}\cdot$d^{-1}) by the Food and Nutrition Board (who set the recommended dietary allowances (RDA) of nutrients). However, most of these athletes eat sufficiently large volumes of food such that they are easily meeting their protein needs without additional supplements. There is little evidence to support the notion that protein supplements beyond this range will increase muscle mass. However, protein supplements are not considered dangerous, and they certainly present considerably less risk than do anabolic steroids. If athletes feel that protein supplements (or creatine supplements) are of benefit, then perhaps they should not be discouraged from taking them, especially if it prevents them from going on to try anabolic steroids.

Strength-training athletes who are determined to increase their protein intake to over 2.0 g of protein$\cdot$ kg$^{-1}\cdot$d^{-1} must be careful not to do this by ingesting additional red meat or whole eggs, which are high in fat. An inexpensive and good source of protein is dry milk powder (casein), which will provide all the necessary amino acids at less than half the cost of the "high-tech" protein supplements marketed to athletes. Although the high-tech supplements include a variety of additives to boost weight gain, they have never been tested to evaluate their efficacy, and it seems unlikely they would be more effective than diet alone or a supplement such as casein.

Several formulations of amino acid supplements have been purported to increase growth hormone and insulin, thereby resulting in muscle mass gain. Most studies have found that the amount of amino acids included in supplements marketed to athletes is not sufficient to cause a change in hormonal status or affect muscle mass. These supplements are costly and probably should be avoided because the consequences of using selected amino acids for a long period of time have not been determined. Large amounts of one amino acid may affect the body's absorption of other amino acids and result in gastrointestinal disturbances.

Anabolic-androgenic steroids have definitely been shown to increase muscle mass, whereas growth hormone increases body weight but possibly not muscle mass. The risks associated with using anabolic-androgenic steroids are serious, including liver damage, prostate enlargement, cardiomyopathy, personality change ("roid rage"), and, for adolescents, the premature closure of the epiphyses of growing bones. Inappropriate use of growth hormone (GH) can result in acromegaly, a thickening of bones leading to disfigurement. Also, GH produces enlarged internal organs, muscle and joint weakness, and cardiomyopathy. Clenbuterol, a β_2 agonist, increases muscle protein deposition in animals but has not yet been shown to increase muscle mass in humans. However, only a few studies of β_2 agonists are available using human subjects, and the doses used were probably less than those used by athletes. The side effects of using clenbuterol, which acts on the sympathetic nervous system, are increased tremor, heart palpitations, nervousness, headaches and myalgia.

Pharmacological agents to increase muscle mass are dangerous and can impair performance and health. It would certainly be a breach of ethics to prescribe or recommend these drugs for the purposes of improving athletic performance. Anabolic steroid use has filtered down to high school and even junior high school students, where the potential negative effects may have a greater impact. In 1990, Terney and McLain surveyed high school students about use of anabolic steroids and found that 5.5% of athletes and 2.4 % of non-athletes admitted to steroid use. They predicated that if the group were representative of the general population, then about 700,000 high school students around the country were using steroids. The problem has only worsened over the years (Thein et al., 1995; Wadler et al., 1994). Nutter (1997) reported that 5.3% of boys and 1.5% of girls in middle school (grades 6,7, and 8) reported anabolic steroid use. The mean age of the group assessed was 13.3 y, suggesting that the problem of anabolic steroid use extends to very young adolescents.

The late David Hough, MD, former Director of Sports Medicine at Michigan State University, offered a list of suggestions for athletes who are making choices about drug use and these are presented in Table 8-3. However, getting athletes to stop using these drugs is a serious challenge because they believe that others are using them and that they will not be able to compete successfully if they don't do likewise. What intervention can be used when winning is more important than the risk to health and well being? Coaches, trainers, and health professionals who deal with athletes must work together to develop ways to stop drug use.

The placebo effect for most supplements and pharmacological agents is very high. Because athletes believe these substances will enhance weight loss or gain, they may train harder or work more efficiently, which will likely result in improved performance. If nutritional supplements are not dangerous, and if their use prevents taking dangerous drugs, then perhaps ineffective but innocuous nutritional supplements should not be discouraged. However, we do not know if the use of harmless supplements will increase the likelihood of using more dangerous agents.

DIRECTIONS FOR FUTURE RESEARCH

Evidence on whether chromium and pyruvate are effective as weight loss agents is scant. Pyruvate is modestly effective in promoting weight loss and fat loss. However, because studies on the effectiveness of pyruvate (3-carbon compounds) were all done in the same laboratory, further studies are warranted to confirm and extend these findings. Study results for chromium are equivocal; a method for the accurate assessment of an individual's chromium status is needed to determine if chromium is an effective weight loss supplement for that individual. Other nutritional supplements that are marketed for weight loss, such as

TABLE 8-3. *Suggestions for the athlete making choices about drug use.* Data from Hough (1990).

1. Know the facts about drugs.
2. View your body as something to keep safe from harm and free from contamination.
3. Think about your plans for the future and your health.
4. Go for natural methods that allow you to look good and perform well.
5. Enjoy and appreciate your uniqueness; don't ever try to be somebody else.
6. When in doubt, check it out with somebody who really cares.
7. After considering all the possible consequences, have the courage to make a good decision based on healthy practices.

hydroxycitrate and carnitine, must be examined to determine their effectiveness.

Both thermogenic and anorexiant drugs have proven to be effective and relatively safe weight-loss agents in obese subjects. Further studies are underway to generate new drugs that can produce similar or greater weight loss without any side affects. The effect of these drugs coupled to an exercise program has received limited study. Although beneficial for obese subjects, use of these agents may be impractical for athletes because the side effects will likely impair performance. Although nicotine (smoking) can control weight in non-obese subjects, but its effect on thermogenesis and appetite appears to be different in males and females. The mechanism to explain the gender differences are not known.

Numerous nutritional weight-gain products exist, and athletes need to be able to discern advertising claims from reality. Chromium has not been proven to enhance muscle mass in most individuals, but research is needed to assess whether or not chromium may promote muscle accretion in those who are chromium deficient. Creatine causes a dramatic gain in body weight in less than a week. Research is needed to verify that this weight gain is caused by an increase in muscle protein, water accumulation, or another factor. Also, whether the status of the body's creatine stores will affect the response to creatine supplements needs to be examined.

Research is fairly clear on protein requirements of strength-training athletes to maintain nitrogen balance. However, whether or not very high protein intakes will promote further increases in muscle mass has not been determined. Protein supplements containing substances designed to boost muscle mass should be evaluated to determine their effectiveness. The effects of most nutritional supplements designed to increase muscle mass have been evaluated only in men, and their relative effectiveness in women should be documented.

Most studies of nutritional supplements for weight gain or weight loss have not controlled for diets of the subjects, and many have not controlled for subjects' physical activity. Also, sample sizes tend to be insufficient to detect small changes. Further well-controlled studies of dietary supplements are warranted.

One well-controlled study found that anabolic steroids do increase muscle mass in recreational strength-training individuals, and this study should be replicated for well-trained male and female athletes. Studies are fairly conclusive that growth hormone administration does not enhance muscle mass. Clenbuterol is the "new kid on the block" purported to increase muscle mass in dramatic ways. Although anecdotal evidence suggests that many athletes are using clenbuterol, there are no studies that have assessed the effects of clenbuterol on increasing muscle mass in athletes.

SUMMARY

"Over 30 scientific reports were published based on . . . . . . exhaustive studies . . . . all showing Chromium Picolinate flat out works. In fact, these scientific studies were so mega-conclusive, their reports were published in such respected publications like . . . . Cosmopolitan, McCalls, Allure, New Body, Women's Sport and Fitness . . . and USA Today." This quote appeared in a full page advertisement in the *Boston Globe*, March 26th, 1996. The ad, which is not unique, promised a 49-lb weight loss in only 29 d. Weight loss products offer little more than hope. The placebo effect can keep many of these products on the market for long enough to make sizable profits. Two studies investigated chromium effects on weight loss in overweight individuals, and the results were equivocal. In the one study to report that chromium was effective, only 1.26 kg of weight was lost in 10 wk. Despite advertisement claims to the contrary, there is little evidence that chromium is an effective weight loss agent.

Although a few studies have reported that pyruvate is an effective weight loss agent, the amount of weight loss attributed to the supplement was less than 1.7 kg in 21 d. Moreover, these studies used obese and overweight individuals as subjects. However, based on limited research, pyruvate is marketed as a weight loss product. It should be noted that dietary supplements are largely unregulated, so athletes should be wary of marketing claims, and health professionals, coaches, and athletic trainers should be cautious about recommending dietary supplements

Pharmaceuticals must undergo rigorous testing in well-controlled, large-scale clinical trials before they are approved for use. Thermogenic or anorexiant drugs have proven effective and relatively safe weight loss agents, but with some side effects, and in some cases these effects can be very dangerous. However, weight loss is relatively small and slow, and discontinuation of the drug results in return of the weight. Studies of these pharmacological agents have mostly been done with obese individuals so that the effects on those who are mildly overweight are not fully known. Although these drugs induce only a small weight loss in obese individuals, the weight loss is associated with health benefits; thus, their use justifies the risks. However, these agents are contraindicated for athletes because they may adversely affect performance due to side effects. Nicotine in the form of smoking does serve to control weight, but the mechanisms responsible are unclear; nicotine can likely impair performance because of the numerous adverse effects it has on the body. Diuretics, which induce quick weight reduction due to water loss, are commonly used by athletes who need to "cut weight" or "make weight" for competition. Although athletes consider diuretics safe, abuse can disrupt electrolyte balance and lead to cardiac and skeletal muscle disturbance.

Supplements such as chromium picolinate and creatine are considered natural alternatives to anabolic steroids to promote muscle mass gain. However, data have not substantiated these claims for chromium. Although there is a dramatic weight gain associated with creatine, it is not known if the weight gain is due to increases in muscle protein.

Weight-training athletes need to ingest more protein than the recommended dietary allowance (RDA) to maintain nitrogen balance, but these needs are generally met by the diet. The recommended amount of protein for strength-training athletes is 1.4–1.8 g of protein $\cdot$ kg$^{-1}\cdot$ d^{-1}. Although amino acid supplements are purported to increase the production of growth hormone and insulin to promote anabolism, most studies using amino acid doses recommended by the manufacturer have not found increases in blood concentrations of these hormones.

Anabolic steroids can increase muscle mass, even in those not participating in a resistance-training program. Growth hormone may be effective in increasing fat-free mass, but this is not necessarily caused by an increase in skeletal muscle mass. Recent attention has focused on the use of clenbuterol as means to increase muscle mass. Studies in animals have documented increased growth with clenbuterol, but there are no data on its effectiveness in humans. Although some pharmacological agents to increase muscle mass are effective, they are unsafe, unethical, illegal, and banned by several sports organizations.

Most nutritional or pharmacological agents have not been proven to provide quick, safe, and long lasting remedies for weight loss or muscle mass gain. Glossy advertisements for such products are enticing but often misleading or deceptive. The National Institutes of Health have recently established an Office of Dietary Supplements to address the rampant increase in dietary supplements. Despite media hype, popular belief, and wishful thinking, there are no miracle means to gain muscle mass and no magic cures for obesity. In 1973, Thomas Szasz wrote "Formerly, when religion was strong and science weak, men mistook magic for medicine; now, when science is strong and religion weak, men mistake medicine for magic."

ACKNOWLEDGEMENT

Thanks to Drs. Mike Sherman, Dennis McKay, and Xiaocai Shi for their excellent and expert reviews of this chapter. Their valuable contributions provided keen insight into these topics.

BIBLIOGRAPHY

Abenhaim, L., Y. Moride, F. Brenot, S. Rich, J. Benichou, X. Kurz, T. Higenbottam, C. Oakley, E. Wouters, M. Aubier, G. Simonneau, and B. Bégaud (1996). Appetite-suppressant drugs and the risk of primary pulmonary hypertension. *N.E.J.Med.* 335:609–616.

ADA Report (1997). Position of the American Dietetic Association: Weight management. *J. Am. Diet. Assoc.* 97:71–74.

Alén, M., K. Häkkinen, and P.V. Komi (1984). Changes in neuromuscular performance and muscle fiber characteristics of elite power athletes self-administering androgenic and anabolic steroids. *Acta Physiol. Scand.* 122:535–544.

Al-Zaki, T., J.Talbot-Stern (1996). A bodybuilder with diuretic abuse presenting with symptomatic hypotension and hyperkalemia. *Am. J. Emerg. Med.* 14:96–98.

American College of Sports Medicine (1987). Position stand on the use of anabolic-androgenic steroids in sports. *Med. Sci. Sports Exerc.* 19:534–539.

Anderson, R.A., and A.S. Kozlovsky (1985). Chromium intake, absorption and excretion of subjects consuming self-selected diets. *Am. J. Clin. Nutr.* 41:1177–1183.

Arch, J.R., and S. Wilson (1996). Prospects for beta 3-adrenoceptor agonist in the treatment of obesity and diabetes. *Int. J. Obes. Relat. Metab. Disord.* 20:191–19.

Armstrong, L.E., D.L. Costill, and W.J. Fink (1985). Influence of diuretic-induced dehydration on competitive running performance. *Med. Sci. Sports Exerc.* 17:456–461, 1981.

Ascoli, M., and D.L. Segaloff (1996). Adenohypophyseal hormones and hypothalamic releasing factors. In: Hardman, J.G., L.E. Limbird, P.B. Molinoff, R.W. Ruddon, A. G. Gilman (eds.) *Goodman and Gilman's The Pharmacological Basis of Therapeutics*, 9th ed. New York: McGraw-Hill, pp. 1363–1382.

Astrup, A., and S. Toubro (1993). Thermogenic, metabolic, and cardiovascular responses to ephedrine and caffeine in man. *Int. J Obesity* 17 (Suppl. 1), S41–S43.

Astrup, A., L. Breum, S. Toubro, P. Hein, and F. Quaade (1992a). The effect and safety of an ephedrine/caffeine compound compared to ephedrine, caffeine and placebo in obese subjects on an energy restricted diet. *Int. J. Obesity* 16:269–277.

Astrup, A., B. Buemann, N.J. Christensen, S. Toubro, G. Thorbek, O.J. Victor, and F. Quaade (1992b). The effect of ephedrine/caffeine mixture on energy expenditure and body composition in obese women. *Metabolism* 41:686–688.

Astrup, A., D. L.Hansen, and S. Toubro (1996). Ephedrine and caffeine in the treatment of obesity. *Int. J Obesity* 20:1–3.

Astrup, A., S. Toubro, S. Cannon, P. Hein, and J. Madsen (1991). Thermogenic synergism between ephedrine and caffeine in healthy volunteers: A double-blind, placebo-controlled study. *Metabolism* 40: 323–329.

Astrup, A., S. Toubro, N.J. Christensen, and F. Quaade (1992c) Pharmacology of thermogenic drugs. *Am. J. Clin. Nutr.* 55: 246S-248S.

Atkinson, R.L., and V.S. Hubbard (1994). Report on the NIH workshop on pharmacologic treatment of obesity. *Am. J. Clin. Nutr.* 60:153–156.

Audrain, J.E., R.C. Klesges, and L.M. Klesges (1995). Relationship between obesity and metabolic effect of smoking in women. *Health Psychol.* 14:116–123.

Bahrke, M.S., and C.E. Yesalis III (1994). Weight training: a potential confounding factor in examining the psychological and behavioral effects of anabolic-androgenic steroids. *Sports Med.* 18:309–318.

Bahrke, M.S., C.E. Yesalis III, and J.E. Wright (1996). Psychological and behavioural effects of endogenous testosterone and anabolic-androgenic steroids: an update. *Sports Med.* 22:367–390.

Balsom, P.D., B. Ekblom, B. Söderlund, B. Sjödin, and E. Hultman (1993a). Creatine supplementation and dynamic high-intensity intermittent exercise. *Scand. J. Med. Sci. Sports* 3:143–149.

Balsom, P.D., S.D.R. Harridge, K. Söderlund, B. Sjödin, and B. Ekblom (1993b). Creatine supplementation per se does not enhance endurance exercise performance. *Acta Physiol. Scand.* 149:521–523.

Balsom, P.D., K. Söderlund, and B. Ekblom (1994). Creatine in humans with special reference to creatine supplementation. *Sports Med.* 18:268–280.

Balsom, P.D.,K. Söderlund, B. Sjödin, and B. Ekblom (1995). Skeletal muscle metabolism during short duration high-intensity exercise: influence of creatine supplementation. *Acta Physiol. Scand.* 154:303–310.

Bhasin, S., T.W. Storer, N. Berman, C. Callegari, B. Clevenger, J. Phillips, T.J. Bunnell, R. Tricker, A. Shirazi, and R. Casaburi. (1996). The effects of supraphysiologic doses of testosterone on muscle size and strength in normal men. *N. Engl. J. Med.* 335:1–7.

Blundell, J.E., and A. Greenough (1994). Pharmacological aspects of appetite: implications for the treatment of obesity. *Biomed. Pharmacother.* 48:119–125.

Bray, G.A. (1996). Obesity. In: E.E. Ziegler and L.J. Fler, Jr. (eds). *Present Knowledge in Nutrition.* Washington, D.C.: Int. Life Sciences Institute, pp.19–32.

Breum, L., J.K. Pedersen, F. Ahlstrøm, and J. Frimodt-Møller. (1994) Comparison of an ephedrine/caffeine combination and dexfenfluramine in the treatment of obesity. A double-blind multi-centre trial in general practice. *Int. J. Obes.* 18:99–103.

Brownell, K.D. , and Rodin, J. (1994). The dieting maelstrom, *American Psychologist* 49: 781–791.

Bucci, L., J.F. Hickson, Jr., J.M. Pivarnik, I. Wolinsky, J.C. McMahon, and S.D.Turner (1990). Ornithine ingestion and growth hormone release in bodybuilders. *Nutr. Res.* 10:239–245.

Bucci, L., J.F. Hickson, Jr., I. Wolinsky, and J.M. Pivarnik. (1992). Ornithine supplementation and insulin release in bodybuilders. *Int. J. Sport Nutr.* 2:287–291.

Butterfield, G., W. Evans, P. Lemon, and K. Yarasheski. (Round Table) (1992). Protein needs of the active person. *Sports Science Exchange*.8:Summer.

Caldwell, J.E., E. Ahonen, and U. Nousiainen (1984). Differential effects of sauna -, diuretic-, and exercise-induced hypohydration. *J. Appl. Physiol.* 57: 1018–1023.

Caruso, J.F., J.F. Signorile, A.C. Perry, B. Leblanc, R. Williams, M. Clark, and M. M. Bamman (1995). The effects of albuterol and isokinetic exercise on the quadriceps muscle group. *Med. Sci. Sports Exerc.* 27:1471–1476.

Celejowa, I , and M. Homa (1970). Food intake, nitrogen and energy balance in Polish weight lifters during a training camp. *Nutr. Metab.* 12:259–274.

Chesley, A., J.D. MacDougall, M.A. Tarnopolsky, S.A. Atkinson, and K. Smith (1992). Changes in human muscle protein synthesis after resistance exercise. *J. Appl. Physiol.* 73:1383–1388.

Christ, D.M., G.T. Peake, P.A. Egan, and D.L.Waters (1988). Body composition response to exogenous GH during training in highly conditioned adults. *J. Appl. Physiol.* 65:579–584.

Clancy, S.P., P.M. Clarkson, M.E. DeCheke, K. Nosaka, P.S. Freedson, J.J. Cunningham, and B. Valentine (1994). Effects of chromium picolinate supplementation on body composition, strength, and urinary chromium loss in football players. *Int. J. Sport Nutr.* 4:142–153.

Claremont, A.D., D.L. Costill, W. Fink, and P. Van Handel (1976). Heat tolerance following diuretic induced dehydration. *Med. Sci. Sports Exerc.* 8: 239–243.

Clarkson, P.M., and S. Going (1996) Body composition and weight control, A perspective on females. In: O. Bar-Or, D.R. Lamb, and P.M. Clarkson (eds.) *Perspectives in Exercise Science and Sports Medicine Vol 9. Exercise and the Female:A Life Span Approach.* Carmel, IN: Cooper Publishing Group, pp. 147–214.

Connacher, A.A., Bennet, W.M., and R.T. Jung. (1992). Clinical studies with the β-adrenoceptor agonist BRL 26830A. *Am. J. Clin. Nutr.* 55: 258S-261S.

Cortez, M.Y., C.E. Torgan, J.T. Brozinick, R.H. Miller, and J.L. Ivy (1991). Effects of pyruvate and dihydroxyacetone consumption on the growth and metabolic state of obese Zucker rats. *Am. J. Clin. Nutr.* 53:847–853.

Criswell, D.S., S.K. Powers, and R.A. Herb (1996). Clenbuterol-induced fiber-type transition in the soleus of adult rats. *Eur. J. Appl. Physiol.* 74:391–396.

Daly, P.A., Krieger, D.R., Dulloo, A.G., Young, J.B., and Landsberg, L. (1993). Ephedrine, caffeine and aspirin: safety and efficacy for treatment of human obesity. *Int. J. Obes.* 17 (Suppl. 1):S73-S78.

Dawson, B., M. Cutler, A. Moody, S. Lawrence, C. Goodman, and N. Randall (1995). Effects of oral creatine loading on single and repeated maximal short sprints. *Aust. J. Sci. Med. Sport* 27:56–61.

Delanghe, J., J-P. De Slypere, M. De Buyzere, J. Robbrecht, R. Wieme, and A. Vermeulen (1989). Normal reference values for creatine, creatinine and carnitine are lower for vegetarians. *Clin. Chem.* 35:1802–1803.

Dodd, S.L., S.K. Powers, I.S.Vrabas, D. Criswell, S. Stetson, and R. Hussain (1996). Effects of clenbuterol on contractile and biochemical-properties of skeletal-muscle. *Med. Sci. Sports Exerc.* 28:669–676.

Deyssig, R., H. Frisch, W.F. Blum, and T. Waldhör (1993). Effect of growth hormone treatment on hormonal parameters, body composition and strength in athletes. *Acta Endocrinol.* 128:313–318.

Dulloo, A.G. (1993). Ephedrine, xanthines and prostaglandin-inhibitors: actions and interactions in the stimulation of thermogenesis. *Int. J. Obes.* 17 (Suppl. 1):S35-S40.

Dulloo, A.G., and D.S. Miller (1986). The thermic properties of ephedrine/methylxanthine mixtures: human studies. *Int. J. Obes.* 10:467–481.

Dulloo, A.G., J. Seydoux, and L. Girardier (1994). Paraxanthine (metabolite of caffeine) mimics caffeine's interaction with sympathetic control of thermogenesis. *Am. J. Physiol.* 267: E801–E804.

Earnest, C.P., P.G. Snell, R. Rodriguez, A.L. Almada, and T.L. Mitchell (1995). The effect of creatine monohydrate ingestion on anaerobic power indices, muscular strength, and body composition. *Acta Physiol. Scand.* 153: 207–209.

Eichner, E.R. (1997). Ergogenic aids: What athletes are using—and why. *Physician. Sportsmed.* 25(4): 70–83.

Elam, R.P. (1988). Morphological changes in adult males from resistance exercise and amino acid supplementation. *J. Sport Med. Phys. Fit.* 28:35–39.

Elam, R.P., D.H. Hardin, R.A.L.Sutton, and L. Hagen. (1989). Effects of arginine and ornithine on strength, lean body mass and urinary hydroxyproline in adult males. *J. Sports Med. Phys. Fit.* 29:52–56.

Evans, G.W. (1989). The effect of chromium picolinate on insulin controlled parameters in humans. *Int. J. Biosoc. Med. Res.* 11:163–180.

Fern, E.B., R.N. Bielinski, and Y. Schutz (1991). Effects of exaggerated amino acid and protein supply in man. *Experientia* 47:168–172.

Fitch, K.D. (1986). The use of anti-asthmatic drugs: do they affect sports performance? *Sports Med.* 3:136–150.

Flegal, K.M., R.P. Troiano, E.R. Pamuk, R.J. Kuczmarski, and S.M. Campbell (1995). The influence of smoking cessation on the prevalence of overweight in the United States. *N. Engl. J. Med.* 333:1165–1170.

Flisińska-Bojanowska, A. (1996). Effects of oral creatine administration on skeletal muscle protein and creatine levels. *Biol. Sport* 13:39–46.

Food and Nutrition Board, National Research Council (1989). *Recommended Dietary Allowances*, 10th Edition. Washington: National Academy Press, pp. 52–77.

Fogelholm, G.M., H.K. Näveri, K.T.K. Kiilavuori, and M.H.A. Härkönen (1993). Low-dose amino acid supplementation: no effects on serum human growth hormone and insulin in male weightlifters. *Int. J. Sports Nutr.* 3:290–297.

Fry, A.C., W.J. Kraemer, M.H. Stone, B.J. Warren, J.T. Kearney, C.M. Maresh, C.A. Weseman, and S.J. Fleck (1993). Endocrine and performance responses to high volume training and amino acid supplementation in elite junior weight lifters. *Int. J. Sport Nutr.* 3:306–322.

Geissler, C.A. (1993). Effects of weight loss, ephedrine and aspirin on energy expenditure in obese women. *Int. J. Obes.* 17 (Suppl. 1):S45–S48.

Goldberg J. Next target:Nicotine. *New York Times Magazine* 1996; August 4:22–27.

Gray, C.L., P.M. Cinciripini, and L.G. Cinciripini (1995). The relationship of gender, diet patterns, and body type to weigh change following smoking reduction: a multivariate approach. *J. Subst. Abuse* 7:405–423.

Green, A.L., E. Hultman, I.A. Macdonald, D.A. Sewell, and P.L. Greenhaff (1996). Carbohydrate ingestion augments skeletal muscle creatine accumulation during creatine supplementation in humans. *Am. J. Physiol.* 271:E821–E826.

Greenhaff, P.L., K. Bodin, K. Soderlund, and E. Hultman (1994). Effect of oral creatine supplementation on skeletal muscle phosphocreatine resynthesis. *Am. J. Physiol.* 266:E725–E730.

Greenway, F.L. (1992). Clinical studies with phenylpropanolamine: a metaanalysis.*Am. J. Clin. Nutr.* 55:203S-205S.

Griggs, R.C., W. Kingston, R.F. Jozefowicz, B.E. Herr, G. Forbes, and D. Halliday (1989). Effect of testosterone on muscle mass and muscle protein synthesis. *J. Appl. Physiol.* 66:498–503, 1989.

Guy-Grand, B. (1992). Clinical studies with d-fenfluramine. *Am. J. Clin. Nutr.* 55:173S-176S.

Guy-Grand, B., M. Apfelbaum, G. Crepaldi, A. Gries, P. Lafebvre, and P. Turner (1989). International trial of long-term dexfenfluramine in obesity. *Lancet* 2:1142–1145.

Hallmark, M.A., T.H. Reynolds, C.A. DeSouza, C.O. Dotson, R.A. Anderson, and M.A. Rogers (1996). Effects of chromium and resistive training on muscle strength and body composition. *Med. Sci. Sports Exerc.* 28:139–144.

Harris, R.C., K. Soderlund, and E. Hultman (1992). Elevation of creatine in resting and exercised muscle of normal subjects by creatine supplementation. *Clin. Sci.* 83:367–374.

Hasten, D.L., E.P. Rome, B.D. Franks, and M. Hegsted (1992). Effects of chromium picolinate on beginning weight training students. *Int. J. Sport Nutr.* 2:343–350.

Haupt, H.A., and G.D. Rovere (1984). Anabolic steroids: A review of the literature. *Am. J. Sports Med.* 12:469–484.

Hervey, G.R., A.V. Knibbs, L. Burkinshaw, D.B. Morgan, P.R.M. Jones, D.R. Chettle, and D. Vartsky (1981). Effects of methandienone on the performance and body composition of men undergoing athletic training. *Clin. Sci.* 60:457–461.

Hoffman, B.B., and R.J. Lefkowitz (1996). Catecholamines, sympathomimetic drugs , and adrenergic receptor antagonists. In: Hardman, J.G., L.E. Limbird, P.B. Molinoff, R.W. Ruddon, A. G. Gilman (eds.) *Goodman and Gilman's The Pharmacological Basis of Therapeutics*, 9th ed. New York: McGraw-Hill. pp. 199–248.

Hoffman, B.B., R.J. Lefkowitz, and P. Taylor (1996). Neurotransmission: The autonomic and somatic motor nervous systems. In: Hardman, J.G., L.E. Limbird, P.B. Molinoff, R.W. Ruddon, A. G. Gilman (eds.) *Goodman and Gilman's The Pharmacological Basis of Therapeutics*, 9th ed. New York: McGraw-Hill, pp.105–140.

Horswill, C.A. (1994). Physiology and nutrition for wrestling. In: D.R. Lamb, H.G. Knuttgen, and R. Murray (eds.) *Perspectives in Exercise Science and Sports Medicine. Vol 7. Physiology and Nutrition for Competitive Sport.* Carmel, IN: Cooper Pub. Group, pp. 131–180.

Horton, T.J., and C.A. Geissler (1991). Aspirin potentiates the effect ephedrine on the thermogenic response to a meal in obese but not lean women. *Int. J. Obes.* 15:359–366.

Hough, D.O. (1990). Anabolic steroids and ergogenic aids. *Am. Fam. Phys.* 41:1157–1164.

Hultman, E., K. Söderelund, J.A. Timmons, G. Cederblad, and P.L. Greenhaff (1996). Muscle creating loading in men. *J. Appl. Physiol.* 81:232–237.

Ingalls, C.P., W.S. Barnes, and S.B. Smith (1996). Interaction between clenbuterol and run training—Effects on exercise performance and MLC isoform content. *J. Appl. Physiol.* 80:795–801.

Isidori, A., A. Lo Monaco, and M. Cappa (1981). A study of growth hormone release in man after oral administration of amino acids. *Curr. Med. Res. Opin.* 7:475–481.

Jackson, E.K. (1996). Diuretics. In: Hardman, J.G., L.E. Limbird, P.B. Molinoff, R.W. Ruddon, A. G. Gilman (eds.) *Goodman and Gilman's The Pharmacological Basis of Therapeutics*, 9th ed. New York: Mc-Graw-Hill, pp. 685–713.

Jacobson, B.H. (1990). Effect of amino acids on growth hormone release. *Phys. Sportsmed.* 18:63–70.

Jensen, E.X., C. Fusch, P. Jaeger, E. Pelheim, and F.F. Horber (1995). Impact of chronic cigarette smoking on body composition and fuel metabolism. *J. Clin. Endocrinol. Metab.* 80:2181–2185.

Jorenby, D.E., D.K. Hatsukami, S.S. Smith, M.C. Fiore, S. Allen, J. Jensen, and T.B. Baker (1996). Characterization of tobacco withdrawal symptom: transdermal nicotine reduce hunger and weight gain. *Psychopharmacology* 128:130–138.

Kaats, G.R., K. Blum, J.A. Fisher, and J.A. Adelman (1996). Effects of chromium picolinate supplementation on body composition - A randomized, double-masked, placebo-controlled study. *Cur. Ther. Res.: Clin. Exper.* 57:747–756.

Kawachi, I., R.J. Troisi, A.G. Rotnitzky, E.H. Coakley, and G.A. Colditz (1996). Can physical activity minimize weight gain in women after smoking cessation? *Am. J. Pub. Health* 86:999–1004.

Kempen, K.P.G., W.H.M. Saris, J.M.G. Senden, P.P.C.A. Menheere, E.E. Blaak, and M.A. Van Baak (1994). Effects of energy restriction on acute adrenoceptor and metabolic responses to exercise in obese subjects. *Am. J. Physiol.* 267:E694–E701.

Kreider, R.B., V. Muriel, and E. Bertun (1993). Amino acid supplementation and exercise performance: analysis of the proposed ergogenic value. *Sports Med.* 16:190–209.

Kumpulainen, J.T. (1992). Chromium content of foods and diets. *Biol. Trace Elem. Res.* 32:9–18.

Lamb, D.R. (1984). Anabolic steroid in athletics: how well do they work and how dangerous are they? *Am. J. Sports Med.* 12:31–38.

Lambert, M. I., J. A. Hefer, R.P. Millar, and P.W. Macfarlane (1993). Failure of commercial oral amino acid supplements to increase serum growth hormone concentrations in male body-builders. *Int. J. Sports Med.* 3:298–305.

Landsberg, L., and J.B. Young (1993). Sympathoadrenal activity and obesity: physiological rationale for the use of adrenergic thermogenic drugs. *Int. J. Obes.* 17:S29–S34.

Laritcheva, K.A., N.I. Yalovaya, V.I. Shubin, and P.V. Smirnov (1978). Study of energy expenditure and protein needs of top weight lifters. In: J. Parizkova and V.A. Rogozkin (eds.) *Nutrition, Physical Fitness, and Health* Baltimore: University Park Press, pp. 155–163.

Lefavi, R.G., R.A. Anderson, R.E. Keith, G.D. Wilson, J.L. McMillan, and M.H. Stone (1992). Efficacy of chromium supplementation in athletes: emphasis on anabolism. *Int. J. Sport Nutr.* 2: 111–122.

Lemon, P.W.R. (1994). Are dietary protein needs affected by regular exercise? *Insider* 2 (3):October.

Lemon, P.W.R. (1995). Do athletes need more dietary protein and amino acids? *Int. J. Sport Nutr.* 5:S39–S61.

Lemon, P.W.R. (1992). Effect of exercise on protein requirements. In: C. Williams and J.T. Devlin (eds.) *Food, Nutrition, and Sports Performance*. London: E. and F. N. Spon, pp. 65–86.

Lemon, P.W.R. (1991). Protein and amino acid needs of the strength athlete. *Int. J. Sport Nutr.* 1:127–145.

Levitsky, D.A., and R. Troiano (1992). Metabolic consequences of fenfluramine for the control of body weight. *Am. J. Clin. Nutr.* 55:167S–172S.

Lipworth, B.J. (1996). Clinical pharmacology of the beta 3–adrenoceptors. *Br. J. Clin. Pharmacol.* 42:291–300.

Lombardo, J.A., R.C. Hickson, and D.R. Lamb. (1991). Anabolic/androgenic steroids and growth hormone. In: D.R. Lamb and M. H. Williams (eds.) *Perspectives in Exercise Science and Sports Medicine, Vol. 4, Ergogenics: Enhancement of Performance in Exercise and Sport*. Dubuque, IA: Wm. C. Brown Publishers, pp. 249–284.

Lönnqvist, F., A. Thörne, K. Nilsell, J. Hoffstedt, and P. Arner. (1995). A pathogenic role of visceral fat β_3–adrenoceptors in obesity. *J. Clin. Invest.* 95:1109–1116.

Loughton, S.J., and R.O. Ruhling (1977). Human strength and endurance responses to anabolic steroid and training. *J. Sports Med.* 17:285–296.

Lukaski, H.C., W.W. Bolonchuk, W.A. Siders, and D.B. Milne (1996). Chromium supplementation and resistance training:effects of body composition, strength, and trace element status of men. *Am. J. Clin. Nutr.* 63:954–965.

MacLachlan, M., A. A. Connacher, and R.T. Jung (1991). Psychological aspects of dietary weight loss and medication with the atypical beta agonist BRL 26830A in obese subjects. *Int. J. Obes.* 15:27–35.

Maltin, C.A., M.I. Delday, J.S. Watson, S.D. Heys, I.M. Nevison, I.K. Ritchie, and P.H. Gibson (1993). Clenbuterol, a β-adrenoceptor agonist, increases relative muscle strength in orthopaedic patients. *Clin. Sci.* 84:651–654.

Marable, N.L., J.F. Hickson, M.K. Korslund, W.G. Herbert, R.F. Desjardins, F.W. Thye (1979). Urinary nitrogen excretion as influence by a muscle-building exercise program and protein intake variation. *Nutr. Rep. Int.* 19: 795–805.

Martineau, L., M.A. Horan, N.J. Rothwell, and R.A. Little (1992). Salbutamol, a β_2-adrenoceptor agonist, increases skeletal muscle strength in young men. *Clin. Sci.* 83: 615–621.

McCarty, M.F. (1996). Chromium (III) picolinate (letter). *FASEB J.* 10:365–367.

Mertz, W. (1992). Chromium: History and nutritional importance. *Biol. Trace Elem. Res.* 32:3–8.

Miller, S. (1997). Quick fix: Do diet pills work? *Newsweek* April 21, 64.

Molnár, D. (1993). Effects of ephedrine and aminophylline on resting energy expenditure in obese adolescents. *Int. J. Obes.* 17 (Suppl.1) : S49–S52.

Morton, A.R., and K.D. Fitch (1992). Asthmatic drugs and competitive sport: an update. *Sports Med.* 14:228–242.

Mujika, I., J-C. Chartard, L. Lacoste, F. Barale, and A. Geyssant. (1996). Creatine supplementation does not improve sprint performance in competitive swimmers. *Med. Sci. Sports Exerc.* 28:1435–1441.

Munro, J.F., C. Scott, and J. Hodge (1992). Appraisal of the clinical value of serotoninergic drugs. *Am. J. Clin. Nutr.* 55:189S–192S.

Murphy, R.J.L., L. Beliveau, K.L. Seburn, and P.F. Gardiner (1996). Clenbuterol has a greater influence on untrained than on previously trained skeletal-muscle in rats. *Eur. J. Appl. Physiol.* 73:304–310.

Murray, R. (1995). Fluid needs in hot and cold environments. *Int. J. Sport Nutr.* 5 (suppl.), S62–73.

Napoli, R., and E.S. Horton (1996). Energy requirements. In: E.E.Ziegler and L.J. Filer, Jr. (eds.) *Present Knowledge in Nutrition.* 7th ed., Washington, DC:International Life Sciences Institute, pp. 1–6.

National Task Force on the Prevention and Treatment of Obesity (1996). Long-term pharmacotherapy in the management of obesity. *JAMA* 276:1907–1915.

Nielsen, B., R. Kubica, A. Bonnesen, I.B. Rasmussen, J. Stoklosa, and B. Wilk (1981). Physical work capacity after dehydration and hyperthermia. *Scand. J. Sports Sci.* 3:2–10.

Nielsen, F.H. (1996). Controversial chromium: does the superstar mineral of the mountebanks receive appropriate attention from clinicians and nutritionists? *Nutr. Today* 31:226–233.

Norregaard, J., S. Jorgensen, K.L. Mikkelsen, P. Tonnesen, E. Iversen, T. Sorensen, B. Soeberg B, and H.B. Jakobsen. (1996). The effect of ephedrine plus caffeine on smoking cessation and postcessation weight gain. *Clin. Pharmacol. Ther.* 60:679–686.

Norton, P., G. Falciglia, and D. Gist (1993). Physiological control of food intake by neural and chemical mechanisms. *J. Am. Diet. Assoc.* 93:450–457.

Nutter, J. (1997). Middle school students' attitudes and use of anabolic steroids. *J. Strength and Cond. Res.* 11:35–39.

O'Connor, H.T., R.M. Richman, K.S. Steinbeck, and I.D. Caterson (1995). Dexfenfluramine treatment of obesity: a double blind trial with post trial follow up. *Int. J. Obes.* 19:181–189.

Ööpik, V., S. Timpmann, and L. Medijainen (1995). The role and application of dietary creatine supplementation in increasing physical performance capacity. *Biol. Sport* 12:197–212.

Papadakis, M.A., D. Grady, D. Black, M.J. Tierney, G.A.W. Gooding, M. Schambelan, and C. Grunfeld (1996). Growth hormone replacement in healthy older men improve body composition but not functional ability. *Ann. Intern. Med.* 124:708–716.

Pasquali, R., and F. Casimirri (1993). Clinical aspects of ephedrine in the treatment of obesity. *Int. J. Obes.* 17:S65–S68.

Pasquali, R., F. Casimirri, N. Melchionda, G. Grossi, L. Bortoluzzi, A.M. Morselli Labate, C. Stefanini, and A. Raitano (1992). Effects of chronic administration of ephedrine during very-low-calorie diets on energy expenditure, protein metabolism and hormone levels in obese subjects. *Clin. Sci.* 82:85–92.

Pasquali, R., M.P. Cesari, N. Melchionda, C. Stefanini, A. Raitano, and G. Labo (1987). Does ephedrine promote weight loss and low-energy adapted women? *Int. J. Obes.* 11:163–168.

Perkins, K.A. (1997). Nicotine effects during physical activity. In: T. Reilly and M. Orme (eds.) *The Clinical Pharmacology of Sport and Exercise.* Amsterdam: Excerpta Medica, pp. 89–99.

Perkins, K.A., and J.E. Sexton (1995). Influence of aerobic fitness, activity level, and smoking history on the acute thermic effect of nicotine. *Physiol. Behav.* 57:1097–1102.

Perkins, K.A., L.H. Epstein, C. Forte, S.L. Mitchell, and J.E. Grobe (1995). Gender, dietary restraint, and smoking's influence on hunger and the reinforcing value of food. *Physiol. Behav.* 57:675–680.

Perkins, K.A., L.H. Epstein, J.E. Sexton, R. Solberg-Kassel, R.L. Stiller, and R.G. Jacobs (1992). Effects of nicotine on hunger and eating in male and female smokers. *Psychopharmacology* 106:53–59.

Perkins, K.A., L.H. Epstein, R.L. Stiller, M.H. Fernstrom, J.E. Sexton, R.G. Jacob, and R. Solberg (1991). Acute effects of nicotine on hunger and caloric intake in smokers and nonsmokers. *Psychopharmacology* 103:103–109.

Perkins, K.A., J.E. Sexton, and A. DiMarco (1996). Acute thermogenic effect of nicotine and alcohol in healthy male and female smokers. *Physiol. Behav.* 60:305–309.

Perkins, K.A., J.E. Sexton, A. DiMarco, and C. Fonte (1994). Acute effects of tobacco smoking on hunger and eating in male and female smokers. *Appetite* 22:149–158.

Pfohl, M., I. Blomberg, and R.-M. Schmülling (1996) Long-term changes of body weight and cardiovascular risk factors after weight reduction with group therapy and dexfenfluramine. *Int. J. Obes.* 18:391–395.

Prather, I.D., D.E. Brown, P. North, and J.R. Wilson (1995). Clenbuterol: a substitute for anabolic steroids? *Med. Sci. Sports Exerc.* 27:1118–1121.

Rásky, E., W.J. Stronegger, and W. Freidl (1996). The relationship between body weight and patterns of smoking in women and men. *Int. J. Epidemiol.* 25:1208–1212.

Redondo, D.R., E.A. Dowling, B.L. Graham, A.L. Almada, and M.H. Williams (1997). The effect of oral creatine monohydrate supplementation on running velocity. *Int. J. Sport Nutr.* 6:213–221.

Rudman, D., A.G. Feller, H.S. Nagraj, G.A. Gergans, P.Y. Lalitha, A.F. Goldberg, R.A., Schlenker, L. Cohn, I.W. Rudman, and D.E. Mattson (1990). Effects of human growth hormone in men over 60 years old. *N. Engl. J. Med.* 323:1–6.

Sanders-Bush, E., and S.E. Mayer (1996). 5–hydroxytryptamine (serotonin) receptor agonists and antagonists. In: Hardman, J.G., L.E. Limbird, P.B. Molinoff, R.W. Ruddon, A. G. Gilman (eds.) *Goodman and Gilman's The Pharmacological Basis of Therapeutics,* 9th ed. New York: McGraw-Hill, pp. 249–263.

Sawka, M. N., and K. B. Pandolf (1990). Effects of body water loss on physiological function and exercise performance. In: C.V. Gisolfi and D.R. Lamb (eds.) *Perspectives in Exercise Science and Sports Medicine, Vol. 3, Fluid homeostasis During Exercise.* Carmel,IN: Benchmark Press, Inc., pp. 1–31.

Schutz, Y., R. Munger, O. Dériaz, and E. Jéquier (1992). Effect of dexfenfluramine on energy expenditure in man. *Int. J. Obes.*16 (Suppl. 3):S61–S66.

Signorile, J.F., K. Banovac, D. Flipse, J.F. Caruso, and M. Gomez (1995). The effects of chronic administration of metaproterenol on muscle size and function. *Arch Phys. Med. Rehab.* 76:55–58.

Silverstone, T., and E. Goodall (1992). Centrally acting anoretic drugs: a clinical perspective. *Am. J. Clin. Nutr.* 55:211S-214S.

Söderlund, K., P.D. Bolsom, and B. Ekblom (1994). Creatine supplementation and high intensity exercise: influence on performance and muscle metabolism. *Clin. Sci.* 87 (Suppl.):120–121.

Spann, C., and M.E. Winter (1995). Effect of clenbuterol on athletic performance. *Ann. Pharmacother.* 29:75–77.

Spring, B. , J. Wurtman, R.Wurtman, A. El-Khoury, H. Godberg, J. McDermott, and R. Pingitore (1995). Efficacies of dexfenfluramine and fluoxetine in preventing weight gain after smoking cessation. *Am. J. Clin. Nutr.* 62:1181–1187.

Stahl, K.A., and T.F. Imperiale (1993). An overview of the efficacy and safety of fenfluramine and mazindol in the treatment of obesity. *ARCH Fam Med* 2:1033–1038.

Stearns, D.M., J.J. Belbruno, and K.E. Wetterhahn (1995). A prediction of chromium (III) accumulation in humans from chromium dietary supplements. *FASEB J.* 9:1650–1657.

Stearns, D.M., J.P. Wise,Sr., S. Patierno, and K.E. Wetterhahn (1995). Chromium (III) picolinate produces chromosome damage in Chinese hamster ovary cells. *FASEB J.* 9:1643–1649.

Steen, S.N. (1991). Nutrition considerations for the low-body weight athlete. In: J.R. Berning and S.N. Steen (eds.) *Sports Nutrition for the 90s: The Health Professional's Handbook.* Gaithersburg, MD: Aspen Publishers Inc., pp. 153–174.

Stinson, J.C., C.M. Murphy, J.F. Andrews, and G.H. Tomkin (1992). An assessment of the thermogenic effects of fluoxetine in obese subjects. *Int. J. Obes.* 16:391–395.

Stock, M.J. (1996). Potential for β-adrenoceptor agonists in the treatment of obesity. *Int. J Obesity* 20:4–5.

Stoecker, B.J. (1996). Chromium. In: E.E. Ziegler and L.J. Filer,Jr. (Eds.) *Present Knowledge in Nutrition* 7th ed., Washington, DC:International Life Sciences Institute, pp. 344–353.

Stroud, M.A., D. Holliman, D. Bell, A.L. Green, I.A. Macdonald, and P.L. Greenhaff. (1994). Effect of oral creatine supplementation on respiratory gas exchange and blood lactate accumulation during steady-state incremental treadmill exercise and recovery in man. *Clin.Sci.* 87:707–710.

Stunkard, A. (1982). Anorectic agents lower a body weight set point. *Life Sci.* 30:2043–2055.

Sturmi, J.E., and G.W. Rutecki (1995). When competitive bodybuilders collapse: A result of hyperkalemia? *Phys. Sportmed.* 23:49–53.

Suminski, R.R., R.J. Robertson, F.L. Goss, S. Arslanian, J. Kang, S. DaSilva, A.C. Utter, and K.F. Metz (1997). Acute effect of amino acid ingestion and resistance exercise on plasma growth hormone concentration in young men. *Int. J. Sport Nutr.* 7:48–60.

Szasz, T.S. (1973). *The Second Sin.* Garden City, NY:Doubleday Anchor, p. 128.

Taaffe, D.R., L. Pruitt, J. Reim, R.L. Hintz, G. Butterfield, A.R. Hoffman, and R. Marcus. (1994). Effect of recombinant human growth hormone on the muscle strength response to resistance exercise in elderly men. *J. Clin. Endocrinol. Metab.* 79:1361–1366.

Talcott, G.W., E.R. Fiedler, R.W. Pascale, R.C. Klesges, A.L. Peterson, and R.S. Johnson (1995). Is weight gain after smoking cessation inevitable? *J. Consult. Clin. Psychol.* 63:313–316.

Tarnopolsky, M.A., S.A. Atkinson, J.D. MacDougall, A. Chesley, S. Phillips, and H.P. Schwarcz (1992). Evaluation of protein requirements for trained strength athletes. *J. Appl. Physiol.* 73:1986–1995.

Tarnopolsky, M.A., J.D. MacDougall, and S.A. Atkinson (1988). Influence of protein intake and training status on nitrogen balance and lean body mass. *J. Appl. Physiol.* 64:187–193.

Taylor, P. (1996). Agents acting at the neuromuscular junction and autonomic ganglia. In: Hardman, J.G., L.E. Limbird, P.B. Molinoff, R.W. Ruddon, A. G. Gilman (eds.) *Goodman and Gilman's The Pharmacological Basis of Therapeutics,* 9th ed. New York: McGraw-Hill, pp. 177–197.

Terney, R., and L.G. McLain (1990). The use of anabolic steroids in high school students. *Am. J. Dis. Child.* 144:99–103.

Thein, L.A., J.M. Thein, and G.L. Landry (1995). Ergogenic aids. *Phys. Ther.* 75:426–439.

Toubro, S., A.V. Astrup, L. Breum, and F. Quaade (1993). Safety and efficacy of long-term treatment with ephedrine, caffeine and an ephedrine/caffeine mixture. *Int. J. Obes.* 17 (Suppl. 1): S69–S72.

Trent, L.K., and D. Thieding-Cancel (1995). Effects of chromium picolinate on body composition. *J. Sports Med. Phys. Fit.* 35:273–280.

WEIGHT LOSS AND GAIN **399**

Viru, A., M.Viru, R. Harris, V. Oopik, A. Nurmekivi, L. Medijainen, ans S. Timpmann (1993). Performance capacity in middle-distance runners after enrichment of diet by creatine and creatine action on protein synthesis rate. *Proceedings of the 2nd Maccabiah-Wingate International Congress on Sport and Coaching Sciences*, June 30–July 4, 1993, Wingate Institute, Netamnya, Israel, pp. 22–30.

Volek, J.S., and W.J. Kraemer. (1996). Creatine supplementation: Its effect on human muscular performance and body composition. *J. Nat. Strength Condit. Res.* 10:200–210.

Volek, J.S., W.J. Kraemer, J.A. Bush, T. Incledon, and M. Boetes (1997). Testosterone and cortisol in relation to dietary nutrients and resistance exercise. *J. Appl. Physiol.* 82:49–54.

Wade, N. (1972). Anabolic steroids: doctors denounce them, but athletes aren't listening [news]. *Science* 176:1399–1403.

Wadler, G.I. (1994). Drug use update. *Sports Med.* 78:439–455.

Wagner, JC. (1991). Enhancement of athletic performance with drugs. *Sports Med.* 12: 250–265.

Walberg-Rankin, J., C.E. Hawkins, D.S. Fild, and D.R. Sebolt (1994). The effect of oral arginine during energy restriction in male weight trainers. *J. Strength and Cond. Res.* 8:170–177, 1994.

Weintraub, M., and G. Bray. (1989). Drug treatment of obesity. *Med. Clin. N. Am.* 73:237–249.

Weintraub, M., P.R. Sundaresan, M. Madan, B. Schuster, A. Balder, L. Lasagna, and C. Cox (1992a). Long-term weight control study I (weeks 0–34): The enhancement of behavior modification, caloric restriction, and exercise by fenfluramine plus phentermine versus placebo. *Clin. Pharmacol. Ther.* 51: 586–594.

Weintraub, M., P.R. Sundaresan, B. Schuster, G. Ginsberg, M. Madan, A. Balder, E.C. Stein, and L. Byrne (1992b). Long-term weight control study II (weeks 34–104): An open-label study of continuous fenfluramine plus phentermine versus targeted intermittent medication as adjuncts to behavior modification, caloric restriction, and exercise. *Clin. Pharmacol. Ther.* 51: 595–601.

Weintraub, M., P.R. Sundaresan, B. Schuster, M. Moscucci, and E.C. Stein (1992c). Long-term weight control study III (weeks 104–156): An open-label study of dose adjustment of fenfluramine and phentermine. *Clin. Pharmacol. Ther.* 51: 602–607.

Weintraub, M., P.R. Sundaresan, B. Schuster, M. Averbuch, E.C. Stein, C. Cox, and L. Byrne (1992d). Long-term weight control study IV (weeks 156–190): The second double blind phase. *Clin. Pharmacol. Ther.* 51: 608–614.

Weintraub, M., P.R. Sundaresan, B. Schuster, M. Averbuch, E.C. Stein, and L. Byrne (1992e). Long-term weight control study V (weeks 190–210): Followup of participants after cessation of medication. *Clin. Pharmacol. Ther.* 51: 615–618.

Welle, S., C. Thornton, M. Statt, and B. McHenry (1996). Growth hormone increases muscle mass and strength but does not rejuvenate myofibrillar protein synthesis in healthy subjects over 60 years old. *J. Clin. Endocrinol.Metab.* 81: 3239–3243.

Wellman, P.J. (1992). Overview of adrenergic anorectic agents. *Am. J. Clin. Nutr.* 55:193S-198S.

Wilson, J.D. (1996). Androgens. In: Hardman, J.G., L.E. Limbird, P.B. Molinoff, R.W. Ruddon, A. G. Gilman (eds.) *Goodman and Gilman's The Pharmacological Basis of Therapeutics*, 9th ed. New York: McGraw-Hill, pp. 1441–1457.

Winslow, E., N. Bohannon, S.A. Brunton, and H.E. Mayhew (1996). Lifestyle modification: weight control, exercise, and smoking cessation. *Am. J. Med.* 101:25S-31S.

Wirth, V.J., and J. Gieck (1996). Growth hormone: Myths and misconceptions. *J. Sport Rehab.* 5:244–250.

Wise, S.D. (1992). Clinical studies with fluoxetine in obesity. *Am. J. Clin. Nutr.* 55:181S-184S.

Yarasheski, K.E., J.A. Campbell, K.Smith, M.J. Rennie, J. O.Holloszy, and D. M. Bier (1992). Effect of growth hormone and resistance exercise on muscle growth in young men. *Am. J. Physiol.* 262:E261–E267.

Yarasheski, K.E., J.J. Zachwieja, T.J. Angelopoulos, and D.M. Bier (1993). Short-term growth hormone treatment does not increase muscle protein synthesis in experienced weight lifters. *J. Appl. Physiol.* 74:3073–3076.

Yarasheski, K.E., J.J. Zachwieja, J.A. Campbell, and D.M. Bier (1995). Effect of growth hormone and resistance exercise on muscle growth and strength in older men. *Am. J. Physiol.* 268:E268–E276.

DISCUSSION

SHERMAN: Are there any regulations that exist related to the advertising or marketing of nutritional supplements for the purposes of either weight loss or weight gain, especially from the perspective of scientific support for efficacy?

CLARKSON: There is very little regulation. By and large, these supplements are not tested, and several studies that have tested actual supplements have found that what is in the supplement is not what's stated on the package. There needs to be regulation because these supplements can be dangerous. The NIH does have an office of dietary supplements, and I hope they will fund some studies of these supplements. We also need to educate the public concerning misuse of these supplements.

SHERMAN: You indicate that there is increased body mass following creatine supplementation. Would you comment on the effect of that change in body mass on changes in athletic performance?

CLARKSON: There have been several studies that showed that there is an improvement in brief exercises requiring short-term energy production, such as sprinting, or repetitive bouts of sprinting. If you scrutinize those data fairly carefully, not in every trial is there a benefit to creatine. It is fairly certain that there is no benefit in swimming performance. This conceivably could be due to an increased drag as body mass increases. It seems that creatine sometimes benefits repeated short-term exercise performance. This may be due to variability of performance measures and the variability in the individual response to creatine. If creatine stores are large initially, there may be a smaller response. We need better-controlled studies with large sample sizes.

SHERMAN: I believe pyruvate supplementation is now being marketed as a nutritional supplement for weight loss. I believe this is related to the observation of a lower RER after supplementation.

CLARKSON: Many weight-loss supplements are marketed based on one study with limited data. An interesting point about these weight-loss agents, or any ergogenic aid, is that they can get on the market fast —before studies can prove them ineffective. With supplements, there is always a dramatic placebo effect.

SHI: Chromium intake can increase insulin release, and insulin will stimulate fat utilization, which results in body weight loss. Insulin can also stimulate amino acid uptake, which causes weight gain. How can the human body differentiate the insulin stimulus for increasing body-fat utilization from that for increasing amino acid uptake?

CLARKSON: At first it was thought that chromium would increase lean body mass because of insulin's role in the uptake amino acids. When chromium was proven not to increase lean body mass, then it was thought that chromium would function to promote fat loss due to insulin's role in increasing fatty acid metabolism in the muscle cells.

MCKAY: If people are given an option, they are going to take pills rather than exercise or diet if they want to control their weight. What do you think the role of pharmacotherapy should be, in weight management?

CLARKSON: Fast weight loss is what people want. The role of pharmacology may be to give people a jump-start. If you ask someone who weighs 300 or 400 pounds to lose a pound a week, that is not going to be very exciting. Drugs may give people a quick start, but the program must also include some type of behavioral modification, including diet and exercise, so that people can be weaned off the drug and into a proper diet and exercise program. I would like to say, "Don't use the drugs at all," but I don't think that is practical. Anyone taking these drugs must be very, very clear on what the drugs can do and what the side effects are. There are 17,500 physicians who specialize in weight loss in this country and who prescribe these drugs. I don't think people are getting proper education on the effects of these drugs.

MCKAY: Most of us realize that behavioral modification and lifestyle changes are going to have to be incorporated with pharmacotherapy, and I agree that jump-starting these individuals through the use of pharmaceuticals may be very important. My second point is a basic principle of pharmacology, i.e., no drug has a single effect, and many of the effects are deleterious.

CLARKSON: Even though some drugs may not have side effects in small doses, athletes are taking them in megadoses, so the side effects may be even greater than normal.

MCKAY: Athletes, coaches and trainers may ignore many of the harmful side effects of the drugs and focus in on a single effect, such as weight loss or weight gain. I brought along with me a *Sports Illustrated* article from the April, 1997, issue. It includes a survey in which two scenarios were presented to 198 track sprinters, swimmers, power lifters, and other athletes, most of them U.S. Olympians or aspiring Olympians. Scenario 1: "You are offered a banned performance-enhancing substance with two guarantees—you will not be caught, and you will win. Would you take this substance?" One hundred and ninety-five athletes said "yes," and three said "no." Scenario 2: "You are offered a banned performance-enhancing substance that comes with two guarantees: you will not be caught, and you will win every competition in the next 5 y, but you will then die from the side effects of this substance. Would you take it?" More than half the athletes said "yes." My question is, how are we going to educate athletes, coaches and trainers about the use of drugs and weight management? They are going to look at advertisements in magazines and be tempted to use and abuse these agents.

CLARKSON: Chromium was very popular with athletes, and now it's not because scientific studies showed that it did not work. If we can prove without a doubt that a supplement doesn't work, that's the key. Our problem is that we don't have sufficient evidence in many cases. We should target coaches and trainers who must have some ethical responsibility to these young people to keep them healthy. If a drug works, athletes are not going to listen, but coaches and trainers may.

SPRIET: I believe that when assessing creatine studies we must realize the variability among people; not everyone responds. The best studies to examine performance are those that have also made creatine measurements in muscle. In studies that simply gave the supplement, did not make muscle measurements, and had negative performance outcomes, it may well be that half the subjects responded well while half did not. Also, the best evidence indicates that performance is more likely to be enhanced with creatine supplementation during repeated bouts of high-intensity exercise, implying that it is the ability to resynthesize phosphocreatine over a short period of time that affords the best possibility for showing a performance increase.

CLARKSON: I totally agree with you.

KENNEY: Is it true that there are few side effects of creatine supplementation other than muscle pulls and strains?

CLARKSON: Those effects are just anecdotal reports.

KENNEY: Also not documented, but rapidly emerging, is a high incidence of muscle cramping during high-intensity activity. Why do these athletes cramp when they are on the field when they take creatine? This cramping issue doesn't seem to be preventable by fluid electrolyte ingestion practices, at least not in the anecdotal evidence that I have seen. Do you have any insight into the mechanisms of increased muscle cramping with creatine use and what might be done to prevent it?

CLARKSON: I have been in contact with several companies who market creatine, and they say that people aren't drinking enough fluid with the creatine. However, I have spoken to at least 60 coaches or trainers throughout the country, and not one has noticed an increased incidence of cramping in their athletes.

KENNEY: They may not recognize it or believe it to be a serious side effect.

CLARKSON: That's possible.

SATTERWHITE: A drug used currently at the national and international level is beta-hydroxy-beta-methylbutyrate (HMB). What is known about that drug for preventing muscle breakdown during resistive training?

CLARKSON: I didn't find enough scientific information to include HMB in the chapter.

WALLBERG-RANKIN: We did a study feeding 0.2 g arginine/kg body weight. We did not see acute changes in growth hormone or blood arginine in response to this ingestion.

CLARKSON: Most of the earlier amino-acid studies infused the amino acids.

WALLBERG-RANKIN: Infusion is usually effective at increasing growth hormone, but feedings are often ineffective.

FIATARONE: I wonder about the β_2 agonists because there is a huge population of people who take these drugs for chronic obstructive pulmonary disease. None of them appear clinically to have benefits in terms of increased fat-free mass or decreased fat mass after years of exposure to these agents. Most of them now take selective β_2 agonists for pulmonary disease to try to limit side effects of the unselective agents.

CLARKSON: They use a smaller dose than what is used by athletes.

FIATARONE: A smaller dose, yes, but they are exposed to these agents for perhaps 30 y. By contrast, we see a lot of weight loss with Prozac taken by depressed people, when we don't want them to lose weight. I would think that if there were a marked effect of beta agonists on body composition, we would have seen it from hundreds of thousands of people who take these drugs clinically.

MAUGHAN: There does seem to be a benefit of the β_2 agonists when there is a loss of lean muscle tissue. In people who are immobilized after surgery, there seems to be good evidence that beta agonists can prevent that loss of lean tissue. Do athletes use beta agonists after injury?

CLARKSON: The single study that we have seen found benefits only to strength and found no difference in lean body mass or muscle mass. The predominate use of beta agonists is to increase muscle mass, not as rehabilitation.

EICHNER: Perhaps the best diet pill, and surely the safest, is the one called "placebo." As any physician can tell you, the placebo does wonders. You give a pill and tell the patient to expect weight loss, and they will lose weight. Even the color makes a difference. Give them a red pill, they say it revs them up; give them a blue pill, they say it makes them sleepy. You can even take patients with nausea, give them a medicine that normally causes nausea, tell them it will cure their nausea, and sure enough, it does. Seventy percent of people respond to placebo, which raises questions about the 30% who don't. So I suggest, not entirely in jest, that we prescribe placebo pills for inducing weight loss.

HOUTKOOPER: How effective are herbal products for weight loss?

CLARKSON: There are few well-controlled scientific studies in this area.

Index

Body fat distribution, 107–150; cardiovascular disease, risks of obesity, 108 110; measuring, 110; metabolic complications, 110–112

Body fat mass, adult standards, 86–87; aging changes effect, 248–251; assessment methods, 63–66; body composition screening practical implications, 83–85; children's standards, 87–91; fat balance maintenance/regulation, 14 15; FFM (fat-free mass), intensive care mortality factor, 62; loss justification in athletics, 208

Body potassium, fat assessment method, 63–66

Body water, fat assessment method, 63–66

Body weight, athletic goals, 223–224; brain peptides influence, 4–5; conceptual model for regulation, 3–4; regulation, 3–6; set-point regulation, 3–4

Bodybuilders, weight gain/loss practices, 204–207

Bone density, fracture resistance effect in children, 306–307

Bone mass, older adults aging effects, 250–251

Brain peptides, body weight influence, 4–5; leptin, 4–5; neuropeptide Y (NPY), 5

Bulimia nervosa, described, 158–159; prevalence among nonathletes, 166; warning signs, 179–180

CAD (coronary artery disease), childhood origins, 299–302; children's risk factor studies, 321–324; clotting/fibrinolysis indices in children, 306; fat patterning in children, 304–306; practical implications of childhood obesity intervention, 329–330

Calculations, energy expenditure, 9–12; macronutrient oxidation, 9–12

Cancer, obesity risks, 2

Carbohydrates, eating behaviors, 16–17; intake effect on macronutrient oxidation, 12; utilization during exercise, 23–27

Cardiovascular disease, body fat distribution, 108–110; obesity risk factors, 2

Cardiovascular fitness, defined, 297; physical training effect on children, 319–320

Cardiovascular health, defined, 298

CATCH study, school-based obesity intervention in children study, 328–329

Catecholaminergic agents, weight loss, 363–364

CHD (Coronary heard disease), 108

Childhood obesity, diet 315; physical activity, 311–314; practical implications of intervention, 329–330; resting energy expenditure, 310–311

Children, body composition studies, 320–321; body fat mass standards, 87–91; bone density effect on fracture resistance, 306–307; CAD/NIDDM metabolic syndrome, 299–302; cardiovascular fitness studies, 319–320; cardiovascular health versus cardiovascular fitness, 297–299; childhood obesity intervention practical implications, 329–330; clotting/fibrinolysis indices, 306; endothelial dysfunction, 303; etiology of childhood obesity, 310–316; fat patterning, 304–306; future research directions, 331–332; Georgia Prevention Institute

obesity/physical training study, 324; left ventricular geometry/function, 302–303; obesity-related CAD/NIDDM risk factor studies, 321–324; physical activity determinants, 309; physical training/exercise studies, 316–327; school-based intervention studies, 327–329

Cholesterol, levels in visceral obesity, 114–116

Chromium, dietary supplement for weight loss, 351–352; weight gain, 371–373

Creatine, weight gain, 373–376

Dancers, weight loss practices, 203

Dehydration, effects on physiology, 209; exercise performance effects, 218

Densitometry, versus DXA (dual-energy x-ray absorptiometry), 78; young adult body composition measurement method, 77

Dietary fats, intake effect on macronutrient oxidation, 13–14; utilization during exercise, 29–35

Dietary supplements, amino acids, 378–379; chromium, 351–352, 371–373; creatine, weight gain, 373–376; protein, 376–378; pyruvate, 354–356; weight gain, 373–379; weight loss, 351–356

Dietary treatment, visceral obesity, 127–130

Diets, childhood obesity, 315; children's energy expenditure studies, 317 319; endurance training effect on obese older adults, 266–269; macronutrient oxidation effects, 12–14; obesity risk factor, 2; resistance training effect on obese older adults, 269–270; versus exercise for weight loss, 41–42

Diuretics, weight loss, 369–371

DSED (Diagnostic Survey of the Eating Disorder), 162

DXA (dual-energy x-ray absorptiometry), body composition measure, 66–68; body composition estimation techniques, 66–71; laboratory body composition measurement methods, 75–79; versus densitometry

Dyslipidemic state, visceral obesity, 122–126

EAT (Eating Attitudes Test), eating disorder diagnostics, 162–163

Eating disorders, anorexia as exercise result in older adults, 273–275; anorexia athletica, 160–161; anorexia nervosa, 153, 157–158, 165; at risk sports, 152–153; athlete diagnostics, 163–164; athlete risk factors, 171–174; athletes versus nonathletes, 167–169; athletic prevalence studies, 166–170; body composition cultural trend pressures, 152–154; bulimia nervosa, 158–159, 166; by female/male athletes within a sport, 170; by sports comparisons, 169 170; clinical types, 156–159; development/prevalence of, 165–171; diagnostic methods, 162–165; DSED (Diagnostic Survey of the Eating Disorder), 162; EAT (Eating Attitudes Test), 162–163; EDI (Eating Disorder Inventory), 162–163; ethnic/racial group studies, 171; excessive exercise as cause, 154–156; excessive exercise factors in athlete, 173–17;

measurement calculations, 9–12; protein intake effects, 12–13
Macronutrient selection, exercise effect, 38–39
Males, age-adjusted percent body fat equations, 91; eating disorder diagnostic criteria, 161
Master athletes, body composition, 255–260
Meals, postexercise energy intake composition impact, 39–40
Metabolic complications, visceral adipose tissue, 110–112
Metabolic rate, weight loss effects, 213–215
Minerals, weight loss effects, 216–217
Mood, weight loss effects, 217–218
Multicompartment models, body composition estimations, 63–66; FFM (fat-free mass) assessment, 63–66; LBM (lean-body mass) assessment, 63–66; limitations, 67–68; measurement error minimization strategies, 66–68
Muscle mass, older adults aging effects, 250

National Health and Nutrition Examination Survey, obesity rates, 2
Neuropeptide Y (NPY), body weight regulation, 5
Nicotine, weight loss, 367–369
NIDDM (Non-insulin dependent diabetes mellitus), 108, 124; childhood origins, 299–302; children's risk factor studies, 321–324; fat patterning in children, 304–306; obesity risks, 2; practical implications of childhood obesity intervention, 329–330; skeletal muscle characteristics, 20
Nutrition, weight gain recommendations, 229–231; weight loss recommendations, 225–226; weight loss recover recommendations, 227–229
Nutritional supplements, amino acids, 378–379; chromium, 351–352, 371–373; creatine, weight gain, 373–376; protein, 376–378; pyruvate, 354–356; weight gain, 373–379; weight loss, 351–356

Obesity, body fat mass, 14–15; body weight regulation, 3–6; body weight regulation conceptual model, 3–4; cancer risks, 2; cardiovascular disease, 108; cardiovascular disease risks, 2; children's CAD/NIDDM risk factor studies, 321–324; controlled physical training for obese children, 324–326; diet/physical activity factors, 2; etiology of childhood obesity, 310–316; fat balance, 14–15; fat oxidation effects, 17–20; genetic versus environmental contributors, 6–7; macronutrient balance fluctuations, 8–14; macronutrient intake and oxidation integration, 15–17; National Health and Nutrition Examination Survey, 2; NIDDM (non-insulin dependent diabetes mellitus) risks, 2; osteoarthritis risks, 2; peripheral vascular disease risks, 2; physical inactivity relationship, 7–8; risks factors, 6–20; school based intervention studies, 327–329; screening for, 62; visceral adipose tissue, 111; weight stabilization at obese level, 15–16
Older adults, aerobic exercise body

weight/composition changes, 260–263; aging changes effect on weight/body composition, 245–251; anorexia resulting from exercise, 273–275; behavioral issues affecting body weight/exercise, 278; Behavioral Risk Factor Surveillance System Survey, 252; body fat mass aging effect, 248–251; diet/endurance training effect on obese subjects, 266 269; diet/resistance training effect on obese subjects, 269–270; energy intake exercise effects, 270–273; epidemiological studies of normal aging, 251–255; exercise intensity/frequency requirements, 277–278; exercise safety issues, 280; exercise/dietary modification weight control effect, 266– 270; fall risk, 62–63; FFM (fat-free mass) as mortality factor, 62; future research directions, 280–281; lean body mass aging effects, 252; master athlete body composition, 255–260; modality of exercise to choose, 275–276; muscle mass aging effects, 250; muscle mass aging effects, 250; new behavior initiation/adoption mechanisms, 279; obese subject exercise/diet choices, 276 277; physical activity barriers, 279–280; readiness to change assessment, 278 279; resistive exercise body weight/composition changes, 263–266; sarcopenia/osteoporosis contribution to mortality, 62
Osteoarthritis disease, obesity risks, 2
Osteoporosis (bone demineralization), older adult mortality factor, 62; female athlete eating disorder consequence, 176–178

Peripheral vascular disease, obesity risks, 2
Pharmacological agents, amphetamines, 356; anabolic-androgenic steroids, 382 384; androgenic receptors, 362–363; anoretic agents, 363–369; β_2 agonists, 379–382; catecholaminergic agents, 363–364; diuretics, 369–371; ephedrine, 357–358; ephedrine combinations, 361–362; ephedrine/caffeine, 358–359; ephedrine/caffeine/aspirin, 359–361; human growth hormone, 384–386; nicotine, 367–369; sertonergic agents, 364–367; thermogenic, 356–363; weight gain, 379 386
Physical activity, childhood obesity, 311–314; children's determinants, 309; exercise compensation, 41; future research directions, 45–46; obesity risk factor, 2; practical implications, 42–44
Physical inactivity, obesity relationship, 7–8
Physical training, cardiovascular fitness effect on children, 319–320; children's studies, 316–327; Georgia Prevention Institute obese children study, 324
Plasma cholesterol, levels in visceral obesity, 114–116
POMS (Profile of Mood States), weight loss practices, 217–218
Population specific equations, body composition, 74–75
Post-menopausal women, visceral obesity, 112–114, 116
Proteins, intake effect on macronutrient oxida-